THE GLOBAL HEALTHCARE MANAGER

THE **GLOBAL HEALTHCARE MANAGER**

Competencies, Concepts, and Skills

**Michael Counte, Bernardo Ramirez,
Daniel J. West Jr., William Aaronson, *Editors***

AUPHA

Health Administration Press, Chicago, Illinois

Association of University Programs in Health Administration, Washington, DC

23 22 21 20 19   5 4 3 2 1

Library of Congress Cataloging-in-Publication Data

Names: Counte, Michael A., editor.
Title: The global healthcare manager : competencies, concepts, and skills / Michael Counte, Bernardo Ramirez, Daniel J. West Jr., William Aaronson, editors.
Description: Chicago, Illinois : Health Administration Press (HAP) ; Washington, DC : Association of University Programs in Health Administration (AUPHA), [2019] | Includes bibliographical references and index.
Identifiers: LCCN 2018036759 (print) | LCCN 2018037874 (ebook) | ISBN 9781640550162 (eBook13) | ISBN 9781640550179 (Xml) | ISBN 9781640550186 (Epub) | ISBN 9781640550193 (Mobi) | ISBN 9781640550155 (print : alk. paper)
Subjects: LCSH: Health services administration. | World health.
Classification: LCC RA971 (ebook) | LCC RA971 .G562 2019 (print) | DDC 362.1--dc23
LC record available at https://lccn.loc.gov/2018036759

Acquisitions editor: Jennette McClain; Project manager: Michael Noren; Cover designer: James Slate; Layout: Cepheus Edmondson

Found an error or a typo? We want to know! Please email it to hapbooks@ache.org, mentioning the book's title and putting "Book Error" in the subject line.

For photocopying and copyright information, please contact Copyright Clearance Center at www.copyright.com or at (978) 750-8400.

Health Administration Press
A division of the Foundation of the American
  College of Healthcare Executives
300 S. Riverside Plaza, Suite 1900
Chicago, IL 60606-6698
(312) 424-2800

Association of University Programs
  in Health Administration
1730 M Street, NW
Suite 407
Washington, DC 20036
(202) 763-7283

BRIEF CONTENTS

DETAILED CONTENTS

Section III   Managing the Organization–Environment Interface

Section IV   Looking Ahead in Global Health Management

*Steven J. Szydlowski, DHA, Robert Babela, Benjamin K.
Poku, DrPH, Terra Anderson, Vladimir Krcmery, MD, PhD,
ScD, FRCP, Bruce J. Fried, PhD, Fevzi Akinci, PhD, Blair
Gifford, PhD, Steven G. Ullmann, PhD, Afsan Bhadelia,
PhD, and Felicia Knaul, PhD*

INTRODUCTION

The main focus of this textbook is on the growing global importance of the healthcare manager role and the corresponding need for managers to develop the necessary skills to improve healthcare organizations. The book's content is guided first by the notion that, to be an effective change agent in a complex and dynamic global health context, healthcare managers must possess and develop a specific body of knowledge and competencies. The book's second guiding principle is that the aim of effective global healthcare managers is to improve and maintain the health of individuals and populations.

Global Healthcare Management

This book does not focus on global health, international health, or world health systems; instead, all of these concepts provide the frame of reference for *global healthcare management*. A framework for global healthcare management is shown in exhibit I.1 and described in the paragraphs that follow. Employing this framework, the competent global healthcare manager can lead

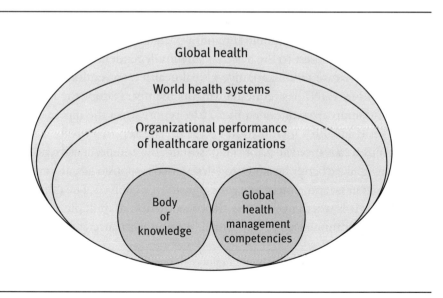

EXHIBIT I.1
Global Healthcare Management Framework

health provider teams and shape the performance of healthcare organizations in achieving individual and population health outcomes.

Global Health

Global health represents the broadest influence of our framework of analysis, and it circumscribes the context of our area of study. The term *global health* has a variety of definitions, many of which have derived from adaptations of public health and international health or evolved from earlier notions of hygiene and tropical medicine. Koplan and colleagues (2009), working with the Consortium of Universities for Global Health Executive Board, crafted and adopted the following comprehensive definition:

> Global health is an area for study, research and practice that places a priority on improving health and achieving equity in health for all people worldwide. Global health emphasizes transnational health issues, determinants and solutions; involves many disciplines within and beyond the health sciences and promotes interdisciplinary collaboration; and is a synthesis of population-based prevention with individual-level clinical care.

Other authors continue to discuss and define the elements of global health that remain essential and influence funding, education, leadership, governance, constituency behavior, international partnerships/cooperation, and policy. Health and sustainable development are inseparable. Meanwhile, interconnection and interdependence are fundamental to addressing the real challenges of global health that reside in what Frenk, Góméz-Dantes, and Moon (2014) call the "triple burden" of disease—the unfinished agenda related to communicable diseases; the growing worldwide importance of chronic diseases and longevity; and the health risks associated with globalization. As we shape the idea of a global society, we should shift our understanding of global health from the health of the poorest to the health of an interdependent global population.

As the nature of collaborative global health interventions evolves, the United Nations (UN) has requested that its members adopt the recommendations and strategies contained in a 2014 report from the director-general of the World Health Organization (WHO). The report calls for enhanced partnerships to advance the priorities of sustainable comprehensive healthcare systems; to achieve better health outcomes, shared responsibility, accountability, and inclusiveness; and to accelerate the transition to universal health coverage (UN 2014). It is worth noting that the coordination of multiple stakeholders presents significant challenges for global health governance.

World Health Systems

Most countries around the world have been experiencing a rapid evolution and transformation of their health systems. This trend was accelerated by the global health focus of the World Bank's 1993 World Development Report, titled *Investing in Health*. For the first time, the idea of "investing in health" moved beyond the health sector and into the realm of the ministries of finance, with significant attention to socioeconomic issues. Twenty years later, a *Lancet* Commission report set forth a framework for transforming global health within one generation, by the year 2035. The report highlighted four key premises (Jamison et al. 2013):

1. "There is an enormous payoff from investing in health."
2. "A 'grand convergence' in health is achievable within our lifetimes."
3. "Fiscal policies are a powerful and underused lever for curbing of non-communicable diseases and injuries."
4. "Progressive universalism, a pathway to universal health coverage, is an efficient way to achieve health and financial protection."

Starting in 2007, a series of UN-sponsored meetings began advancing the global health and foreign policy agenda. In December 2012, the UN member countries adopted a General Assembly resolution recognizing that governments have a responsibility to "scale up efforts to accelerate the transition towards universal access to affordable and quality health-care services" (UN 2012). Health systems around the word have already mobilized in pursuit of diverse strategies to achieve this goal within their very different and complex national settings.

Healthcare Organizational Performance

Every health system is dependent on first-contact hospitals that provide access to high-quality, appropriate care and use resources efficiently. Improving the performance of these first-contact hospitals is essential for strengthening any health system. A key objective of healthcare managers is to identify and suggest innovative, scalable solutions and conduct basic operations research using a practical, small-area demonstration strategy. Healthcare managers should use performance improvement techniques to measure output, improve processes, and develop managerial procedures.

Resource management involves the efficient and effective use of an organization's human, financial, and information resources. In healthcare settings, resources vary by country, region, geography, and locality, and many facilities and systems must operate under critical low-resource conditions. Effective healthcare managers possess appropriate skills for low-resource management and can obtain the best possible results under the circumstances. The combination of creativity, perseverance, and hard work can help overcome such issues as reduced access to medications, limited availability of equipment or supplies, and partial or restricted capability for advanced technological procedures.

Many organizations and authors have classified countries, or regions within countries, based on the level of socioeconomic and other types of resources available. This approach has led to such classifications as *least developed countries*, *low-income countries*, and *lower middle-income countries*, which many times reflect the priorities or interests of a particular development program. The challenge remains to apply management strategies that truly promote global health development. As Filerman (2013) suggests, some classification systems and nomenclatures can stand in the way of a unifying approach for global health development that addresses quality of life and health status across all populations without boundaries.

A number of frameworks have been set forth for the improvement of organizational performance in healthcare. For example, the WHO's framework, titled *Everybody's Business: Strengthening Health Systems to Improve Health Outcomes*, proposes six "building blocks" (WHO 2007):

1. Good *health services delivery* performance
2. A *health workforce* that achieves the best possible health outcomes
3. Reliable and timely *health information*
4. Equitable and cost-effective access to *medical products, vaccines, and technologies*
5. A *health financing system* that ensures needed services with financial protection and incentives for efficient use of services
6. Effective *leadership and governance* that ensures the involvement of the constituency in all aspects of health services

The Role of the Global Healthcare Manager

The role of the global healthcare manager has changed dramatically as areas of management have developed, as healthcare organizations have evolved and transformed, and as health reforms have been implemented around the world. The growth and diffusion of managerial concepts, theories, and technologies present unique challenges, and the challenges faced by healthcare managers vary depending on organizational level, type of facility or organization, country or region, resource level, and other factors. To meet these challenges, healthcare managers must possess appropriate knowledge and competencies.

Body of Knowledge and Competencies

Members of the Association of University Programs in Health Administration (AUPHA) Global Healthcare Management Faculty Forum, under the leadership of Dr. Daniel Dominguez and with the collaboration of the editors of this textbook, developed a body of knowledge (BOK) for global healthcare management, and that BOK has been adapted for this book. As the authors of the various chapters developed their learning objectives and competencies (which are presented at the start of each chapter), we modified the BOK into the final version provided in the appendix.

The BOK facilitates the development of a variety of competencies, including cognitive abilities, behavioral skills, attitudes, and characteristics, that support effective and appropriate professional interactions across a variety of cultural contexts. Within the profession of healthcare administration, such competencies would include (1) current and relevant knowledge of global health issues; (2) attitudes and behaviors required for multicultural understanding and effective transcultural communication; (3) the conceptual and analytical skills required for identifying and effectively applying global managerial best practices; and (4) attitudes, behaviors, and skills necessary for developing international partnerships, networks, and other collaborative and professional relationships for research, global learning abroad, teaching/coaching, and service learning.

Readers of this book can use the BOK in the appendix to further develop their competencies across any training or educational curricula. The first column shows the key domains or topics, and the second column describes the areas of knowledge. Consistent with the principles of the Bloom taxonomy, the BOK focuses on the two basic levels—knowledge and comprehension—for undergraduate students, and it emphasizes the four top levels—application, analysis, synthesis, and evaluation—for graduate students. Finally, the third column in the appendix indicates some subdisciplines and areas of application that fit within each of the domains or topics.

The Goal and Organization of This Textbook

The goal of this textbook is to provide students and practitioners with an integrative framework of knowledge and policy that addresses the growing diffusion of diverse managerial concepts, theories, and technologies. The book analyzes key concepts from the perspectives of clinicians and administrators of various nations, recognizing opportunities for public and private differences. The focus of the book is not directed toward global health or macro-level policy concerns; instead, such concerns serve only as a contextual framework for the effective leadership and decision-making processes of healthcare managers in their organizations.

The authors of this book developed the chapter contents to assist students in developing leadership and managerial competencies to become effective healthcare managers. The competencies and learning objectives are listed at the start of each chapter. The learning objectives focus on concepts that the students are expected to master, and the attainment of competencies requires application and practice. The level of competency attained will grow through achievement of the learning objectives, as well as through work experience and opportunities provided through discussion questions, vignettes, cases, and other exercises.

The text takes into consideration several major cross-cutting themes affecting the globalization of healthcare management, stimulating the reader to think about the intersection and interrelation of the chapters' content. The book also provides opportunities for application and reflection through case studies, vignettes, and practical recommendations, as well as such tools as checklists and guidelines.

Cross-Cutting Themes

Major cross-cutting themes throughout the book include the following:

1. *Sociocultural factors.* The book recognizes the unique qualities and characteristics of every country and its cultures. To work effectively, managers need to understand that organizations are social systems composed of individuals and groups. Culture helps shape values, behaviors, attitudes, and the nature of work.

2. *Clinician–manager relationships and leadership.* Positive outcomes in healthcare require the formation of clinical/management teams, with professionals and health workers from a variety of disciplines working together to address complex problems. Effective teams are typically supported by leaders who respect the team members and help develop, carry out, and evaluate processes that enhance quality of care, performance, and patient safety.

3. *Performance improvement and value-based management.* This theme focuses on mechanisms that improve health outcomes, support provider and patient satisfaction, and lower the cost of healthcare. These mechanisms include, but are not limited to, management and reimbursement models such as risk sharing and pay-for-performance, as well as innovative mobile/virtual technologies that focus on wellness and value.

4. *Resource management.* This theme considers how resources are distributed among organizations in the same country, within diverse types of healthcare systems (e.g., public, private, charitable), and within the same type of healthcare system but in different geographical/cultural/social/economic subregions. It particularly recognizes the management challenges associated with low availability of resources.

5. *Decision making, data analytics, and evidence-based management.* With advances in information technology, more effective collection and analysis of data become critically important for management decisions. Many countries have adopted electronic health record systems that allow for the collection of substantial amounts of data. Through data analytics, managers can become better informed about quality of care, the costs and benefits of various clinical procedures, and measures of organizational efficiency and effectiveness. The available evidence and

analytical insights can facilitate the evaluation of managerial practices and support decision making to achieve organizational improvement.

Sections and Chapters of the Book

This book is organized into four sections, with the chapters of each section contributing to a common theme. Section I, "Essential Health Services Management Concepts and Practices," focuses on organizational structure, financing and financial management, human resources, and information technology. Section II, "Leadership, Organizational Design, and Change," addresses leadership principles, governance, strategic planning, marketing, ethics, and organizational change. Section III, "Managing the Organization–Environment Interface," focuses on the impact of the external environment on organizational performance. The chapters of this section discuss health policy, demographic shifts, and the growing importance of population health management and long-term care. Section IV, "Looking Ahead in Global Health Management," concludes the text with a look at future trends in global health.

Detailed summaries of the individual chapters are provided in the paragraphs that follow.

Section I—Essential Health Services Management Concepts and Practices
Chapter 1—Functions, Structure, and Physical Resources of Healthcare Organizations

The central idea of this chapter is that function defines structure. Healthcare organizations vary—not only from country to country but also within each country—as they address access, quality, and cost issues influenced by social, economic, and political factors. The principles described in this chapter can be applied to ambulatory, acute, chronic, and home care organizations with varying levels of resources and local organizational response capacity.

The first part of the chapter examines the key functions of healthcare organizations, with an emphasis on the need for a continuum of patient-centered care. The chapter reviews the main components of a healthcare organization and the ways those components interact to produce and measure outcomes and drive performance improvement. It then explores and contrasts ways of designing and structuring organizations to effectively and efficiently carry out the key functions. Finally, the chapter proposes a scheme for the analysis and design of physical resources and functions to support the successful operation of a healthcare organization. This chapter provides important context for the rest of the chapters in section I, as well as for the quality and process design discussions later in the book.

Chapter 2—Healthcare Systems, Financing, and Payments

The purpose of this chapter is to provide a general overview of global healthcare expenditures, to discuss the macroeconomic drivers of variation among countries, and to provide insight into the primary models that countries have used to finance and deliver healthcare. The chapter starts by defining *healthcare financing* and exploring its functions, from revenue collection to pooling to purchasing and setting the benefits package. It also provides an introduction to the mechanics of health insurance and a discussion of the natural incentives associated with the way clinical providers are paid. The chapter provides relevant groundwork for the more detailed financial, quality, and managerial content contained in later chapters.

Chapter 3—Financial Management of Healthcare Organizations

This chapter focuses on micro-level considerations unique to the types of financial decisions faced by healthcare managers in complex national and multinational environments. It begins with a discussion of the primary long-term financial planning process and the major financial decision-making tools used by healthcare managers. It then describes the long-term financial risks and implications that organizations must address when operating within existing markets, when expanding their scale or scope of operations within existing markets, or when entering new markets. The chapter also discusses the primary short-term financial planning methods and the short-term financial risks and implications that organizations face when financing day-to-day healthcare delivery in national and multinational settings.

Chapter 4—Human Resource Management in a Global Context

Within a global context, the healthcare sector is essentially a human enterprise, and the connections that exist between people engaging in health work has been of the utmost importance. This chapter, therefore, focuses on human resources (HR) principles and effective HR management practices. Best practices (based on evidence-based management), sociocultural perspectives, and the impact of culture are incorporated in the discussion, as are lessons from the global health workforce. Additional HR lessons deal with self-management and emotional intelligence in the context of being an effective manager and leader of others.

Chapter 5—Information Technology for Healthcare

This chapter seeks to provide a basic understanding of information technology in healthcare. It offers an introduction to electronic health records (EHRs), discussing the exchange of data between records and the ways EHR data can be used in clinical support systems to improve patient care. The chapter also addresses privacy, security, and the protection of patient information. The chapter concludes with a discussion of the steps involved in assessing, selecting, and implementing EHR systems.

Section II — Leadership, Organizational Design, and Change
Chapter 6 — Principles of Effective Leadership

Efforts to improve healthcare outcomes and quality require competent and effective leaders. Global healthcare leaders must possess the knowledge, skills, and competencies to develop and modify systems of care, build effective inter-professional teams, and drive continuous change and improvement. This chapter examines leadership qualities, traits, and characteristics; the leader's responsibilities and professional identity; and contemporary leadership issues—all while allowing for country-specific and regional variation. Applied examples help underscore the importance of managing resources wisely, ensuring sustainable projects, and meeting the needs of vulnerable populations. Discussion questions, case studies, and vignettes provide opportunities for the application and integration of key concepts and ideas.

Chapter 7 — Strategic Management and Marketing

This chapter introduces the basic process of strategic planning, and it connects that process with the strategic marketing efforts needed to help the organization meet its goals and objectives. Examples and short cases from various countries and from different sectors of the healthcare arena promote systems thinking from diverse perspectives. After completing this chapter, readers will be able to draft a strategic plan with the ability to communicate with desired audiences through targeted channels of communication.

Chapter 8 — Process Design and Continuous Quality Improvement for Operational Change in Global Health

A variety of operations management principles, models, tools, techniques, and quality improvement (QI) methods are widely prevalent across global health settings, and this chapter provides an overview of several that are most relevant for global health students and managers. The tools described in this chapter, once mastered and applied, can help ensure process improvements that truly add value to clients, constituents, stakeholders, communities, and the health sector as a whole. A key point highlighted by the chapter is that health management professionals and policymakers must understand the level of operational change desired and choose QI instruments that are most appropriate for that change and for their organizations or systems.

Chapter 9 — Managerial Ethics in Global Health

This chapter addresses managerial ethics in the global health context. It discusses the importance of ethics in managerial decisions, with attention to the additional sensitivity that is required in situations where two or more cultures come together. The chapter provides examples of the difficult ethical issues that may arise in global health contexts.

Chapter 10—Boards and Good Governance

An organization's governing body, often called the board of directors or board of trustees, is a group of community, business, and health sector leaders who make decisions about the organization's purpose, plans, and overall direction. One of the aims of this chapter is to show how health system leaders in low-resource countries can explore the power of the board to foster conditions in which the people who deliver and manage health services are more likely to succeed. The chapter lists 5 key practices and 11 essential elements of good infrastructure for effective board work.

Section III—Managing the Organization–Environment Interface
Chapter 11—Health Policy Design

This chapter aims to help readers develop the knowledge base necessary to understand, effectively influence, and adapt to global (national) health policies. It focuses on key concepts of policy design that are employed throughout the world and are of particular importance for health managers and organizational leaders.

Chapter 12—Global Demographics and the Management of Long-Term Services and Supports

Global healthcare delivery systems in the twenty-first century face numerous demographic challenges, many of which are associated with the aging of the population and the growing number of individuals with chronic and disabling conditions. The ways countries address these issues will depend heavily on their traditions and cultures, their healthcare systems' plans and policies, and their access to resources and technology. This chapter provides an overview of the demographic, historical, and cultural forces affecting the demand for long-term care, and it discusses management issues such as the need for trained staff in the long-term care field and the use of technology in care management. In addition, the chapter highlights five countries at different stages of aging—Japan, Sweden, China, Turkey, and the United States—and examines their unique experiences and solutions.

Chapter 13—Managing the Health of Populations

This chapter helps readers develop the knowledge and skills necessary to understand, plan for, and manage the health of a constituent population. It focuses on key concepts in population health management strategies that are employed around the world and are of particular importance to health managers.

Section IV—Looking Ahead in Global Health Management
Chapter 14—Future Trends in Global Health

This chapter describes current and future global health trends that are affecting healthcare managers and health system design. Areas of focus include health policy, technology, public health, human rights, workforce planning, changes in health sectors, catastrophic events, and trends in consumer behavior. The chapter takes a forward-looking approach to critical issues that have an impact on global health status.

Epilogue

The epilogue concludes the book with an overview and summary of the key elements of global healthcare management, with an emphasis on the interrelations between global health, global health systems, and the performance and leadership of healthcare managers. It synthesizes the book's content into a set of building blocks to support future healthcare managers and foster effective healthcare management across the globe.

Instructor Resources

This book's Instructor Resources include an instructor's manual, Power-Point slides, and a test bank.

For the most up-to-date information about this book and its Instructor Resources, go to ache.org/HAP and browse for the book's title or author names.

This book's Instructor Resources are available to instructors who adopt this book for use in their course. For access information, please email hapbooks@ache.org.

References

Filerman, G. L. 2013. "The Role of Health Services Administration Education in Global Health Development: A New Perspective." *Journal of Health Administration Education* 30 (4): 241–50.

Frenk, J., O. Góméz-Dantes, and S. Moon. 2014. "From Sovereignty to Solidarity: A Renewed Concept of Global Health for an Era of Complex Interdependence." *Lancet.* Published January 4. www.thelancet.com/pdfs/journals/lancet/PIIS0140-6736(13)62561-1.pdf.

Jamison, D. T., L. H. Summers, G. Alleyne, K. J. Arrow, S. Berkley, A. Binagwaho, F. Bustreo, D. Evans, R. G. A. Feachem, J. Frenk, G. Ghosh, S. J. Goldie, Y. Guo, S. Gupta, R. Horton, M. E. Kruk, A. Mahmoud, L. K. Mohohlo, M. Ncube, A. Pablos-Mendez, K. S. Reddy, H. Saxenian, A. Soucat, K. H. Ultveit-Moe, and G. Yamey. 2013. "Global Health 2035: A World Converging Within a Generation." *Lancet*. Published December 3. www.globalhealth2035.org/sites/default/files/report/global-health-2035.pdf.

Koplan, J. P., T. C. Bond, M. H. Merson, K. S. Reddy, M. H. Rodriguez, N. K. Sewankambo, and J. N. Wasserheit. 2009. "Towards a Common Definition of Global Health." *Lancet*. Published June 2. www.thelancet.com/journals/lancet/article/PIIS0140-6736(09)60332-9/.

United Nations (UN). 2014. "Report of the Director-General of the World Health Organization on Partnerships for Global Health." Published September 26. https://documents-dds-ny.un.org/doc/UNDOC/GEN/N14/549/23/PDF/N1454923.pdf?OpenElement.

———. 2012. "Global Health and Foreign Policy." General Assembly Resolution A/67/L.36. Published December 6. www.un.org/ga/search/view_doc.asp?symbol=A/67/L.36.

World Health Organization (WHO). 2007. *Everybody's Business: Strengthening Health Systems to Improve Health Outcomes: WHO's Framework for Action*. Accessed March 23, 2018. www.who.int/healthsystems/strategy/everybodys_business.pdf.

I

ESSENTIAL HEALTH SERVICES MANAGEMENT CONCEPTS AND PRACTICES

FUNCTIONS, STRUCTURE, AND PHYSICAL RESOURCES OF HEALTHCARE ORGANIZATIONS

Bernardo Ramirez, MD, Antonio Hurtado, MD,
Gary L. Filerman, PhD, and Cherie L. Ramirez, PhD

Chapter Focus

The key idea of this chapter is that form follows function, and function defines structure. Healthcare organizations vary—not only from country to country, but also within each country—as they address issues of access, quality, and cost that are influenced by social, economic, and political factors. The principles described in this chapter can be applied to ambulatory, acute, chronic, and home care organizations with varying levels of resources and local organizational response capacity. The first section of this chapter examines the key functions of healthcare organizations, with an emphasis on the need for a continuum of patient-centered care. Later sections review the main components of healthcare organizations and the ways they interact to achieve desired outcomes and performance improvement. The chapter explores ways of designing, structuring, and analyzing organizations to effectively and efficiently manage physical resources and carry out key functions.

Learning Objectives

Upon completion of this chapter, you should be able to

- distinguish the key functions of healthcare organizations and relate them to the priorities of access, cost, and quality;
- develop mechanisms to assess the performance of healthcare organizations;
- design a structure for an organization that takes into consideration the resources available in a given community to achieve the best possible health outcomes;

- plan and prioritize the physical resources needed to effectively accomplish the organization's key functions, taking into account the available resources in that particular system; and
- integrate physical, human, and technological resources to provide appropriate clinical, support, managerial, and supply chain services in a healthcare organization, taking into consideration all legal, accreditation, and regulatory mandates.

Competencies

- Demonstrate an understanding of system structure, funding mechanisms, and the way healthcare services are organized.
- Balance the interrelationships among access, quality, safety, cost, resource allocation, accountability, care setting, community need, and professional roles.
- Assess the performance of the organization as a part of the health system.
- Use monitoring systems to ensure that corporate and administrative functions meet all legal, ethical, and quality/safety standards.
- Effectively apply knowledge of organizational systems, theories, and behaviors.
- Demonstrate knowledge of governmental, regulatory, professional, and accreditation agencies.
- Interpret public policy, and assess legislative and advocacy processes within the organization.
- Effectively manage the supply chain to achieve timeliness and efficiency of inputs, materials, warehousing, and distribution, so that supplies reach the end user in a cost-effective manner.
- Adhere to procurement regulations in terms of contract management and tendering.
- Effectively manage the interdependency and logistics of supply chain services within the organization.

Key Terms

- Facility design
- Healthcare system
- Health technology assessment (HTA)
- Prearchitectural medical functional program
- Regionalization
- Sustainability

Key Concepts

- Facility design
- Facility management
- Low-resource management
- Medical equipment

- Operations management
- Organizational design
- Performance improvement
- Physical resources management

Introduction

We can define the most important functions of healthcare organizations using a systemic analysis inspired by Avedis Donabedian's (1988) original conception of structure, process, and outcomes. Exhibit 1.1 shows how, as the population and the healthcare organization interact, the system aligns the available or required resources to produce the key notions of utilization, access, productivity, efficiency, and effectiveness, which interact to shape the organization's performance. Performance, meanwhile, depends on the competent actions of healthcare managers and other human resources in the organization.

Since the mid-1900s, the functions, responsibilities, and competencies of healthcare managers have developed in different ways around the world. In the United States and Canada, the role primarily developed as a postgraduate specialty supported by the W. K. Kellogg Foundation under the umbrella of

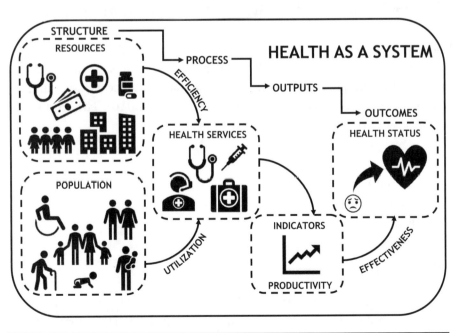

EXHIBIT 1.1
Elements of Health Systems Analyzed with a Systemic Approach

Sources: Data from Bradbury and Ramirez-Minvielle (1995); Donabedian (1966).

the Association of University Programs in Health Administration (AUPHA). A handful of university programs were established in 1948. As demand grew and the healthcare field expanded, new graduate and undergraduate university programs developed in a number of schools related to health or management disciplines (Counte, Ramirez, and Aaronson 2011).

Around the world, a number of countries—and a number of locations inside countries—have developed a strong alignment of professional healthcare managers across healthcare organizations; other locations, however, have almost no notion of healthcare management as a profession. In some countries, clinicians are promoted to serve in managerial roles at healthcare organizations without first having had the opportunity to acquire management competencies (West et al. 2012). The International Hospital Federation (IHF) has created a special interest group in health management to promote the professionalization of the discipline and the use of a leadership competency framework to improve the impact of managers at all levels of organizations and health systems (IHF 2015).

healthcare system
The arrangement of people, institutions, and resources that deliver healthcare services to meet the needs of a target population. The system's framework aligns resources to support the key performance domains of access, utilization, efficiency, quality, sustainability, and learning.

The main functions of **healthcare systems** and organizations in the continuum of care are financing, provision of health services, stewardship, and resource development (Frenk, Góméz-Dantes, and Moon 2014). Of these functions, provision of health services and resource development are key, and they are the ones further explored in this chapter. Provision of health services starts with sound planning and effective/efficient organization. Financing is addressed in chapters 2 and 3, and stewardship is discussed in chapters 6 and 11.

The Performance of Health Systems: Six Core Domains

Healthcare organizational performance around the world was the focus of an extensive study sponsored by the World Bank, in which investigators conducted a thorough literature review and developed a guide to concepts, determinants, measurement, and intervention design (Bradley et al. 2010). The World Bank report examined six core performance domains:

1. Access
2. Utilization
3. Efficiency
4. Quality
5. Sustainability
6. Learning

The first four domains are related to the "iron triangle" of healthcare, a concept that was introduced by Kissick (1994) and later provided the basis for the "triple aim" initiative developed by the Institute for Healthcare Improvement (IHI). Kissick's iron triangle consists of access, quality, and cost containment, whereas the IHI's "triple aim" adds the dynamics of population health (IHI 2012).

Access incorporates several dimensions—physical access, financial access, linguistic access, and information access—that are supplemented by service availability and the provision of nondiscriminatory services. Equitable treatment should be provided regardless of gender, race, ethnicity, religion, age, or any other physical or socioeconomic condition. Utilization includes dimensions of patient or procedure volume relative to capacity or population health characteristics. Efficiency is determined by cost- or staff-to-service ratios and by patient or procedure volume. Quality includes clinical and management quality, as well as patient experience.

The last two domains—**sustainability** and learning—are key to ensuring constant, self-propelled growth in an ever-changing, complex environment such as healthcare. *Sustainability* in healthcare can be defined as "the capacity of health services to function with efficiency, including the financial, environment and social interaction that guaranties an effective service now and in the future, with a minimum of external intervention and without limiting the capacity of future generations to fulfill their needs" (Ramirez, Oetjen, and Malvey 2011, 134). Sustainability can be considered from two distinct perspectives or dimensions. The first perspective focuses on the sustainability of processes that create a basic functional network throughout the organization, allowing for flexibility and quality improvement—both of which are necessary for the dynamic change environment of healthcare. The second perspective deals with organizational sustainability, and it includes five multidimensional pillars:

sustainability The capacity for a healthcare organization to function efficiently and in a manner that supports effective service both presently and in the future.

1. The *environmental pillar* represents the initial point of focus for sustainability, and it includes—but is not limited to—the use of clean and renewable energy and the conservation of the natural environment. This pillar incorporates recycling techniques to preserve the quality of the atmosphere, to reuse solid and liquid waste, and to safely dispose of contaminants.
2. The *sociocultural pillar* strengthens community support and promotes the identification of key cultural, ethnic, and other values among the community of staff, patients, and users. It incorporates population health and social marketing strategies.
3. The *institutional capacity development pillar* promotes the strategic management of the organization. It aims to strengthen competencies at all levels and instill an empowering knowledge management culture, facilitating coordinated efforts of governance, leadership, and personnel integration and participation.

4. The *financial pillar* ensures the delivery of healthcare programs and activities that are cost effective and efficient in the use of resources. It is indispensable for achieving the organization's goals and objectives.
5. The *political pillar* involves staff, patient, and community advocacy to advance the interests of the organization.

Finally, the learning domain empowers the organization to adapt to change and to explore and adopt innovations. It incorporates efforts to use data audit and feedback processes, to distribute relevant information and provide patient education through partnerships with the constituency, and to implement training and continuing education initiatives for the healthcare workforce.

The Challenge of Organizing Health Services Resources to Achieve Optimum Performance

The provision of universal access to optimal prevention, care, cure, and rehabilitation can be considered an ultimate goal of healthcare. Most governments, either directly or indirectly, subscribe to this goal; the challenge is—given the limitations of resources and entrenched infrastructure—achieving the greatest possible return on the investment toward reaching it. All countries, regardless of their level of wealth or industrialization, are limited in their ability to achieve this goal, often because of political philosophies expressed as public policy. Even those nations in the most favorable positions often lack the will or capacity to translate their knowledge of what is possible into practice for the benefit of all people.

Over many years of technological development and interaction among professional, political, and economic forces, three enduring organizational foci have emerged for achieving the optimum health status for a population. They are (1) hospitals, (2) primary care provision, and (3) regionalization.

Hospitals
In every country, hospitals are the most visible symbol of healthcare development and care for the sick. They represent public assurance that there is a place for people to go for care when needed. Hospitals are also important economic engines, generating employment and anchoring the economies of communities. They consume a large portion of the health sector resources in many countries.

The hospital is arguably the most complex contemporary organization to manage. Hospitals, particularly in developing countries, struggle internally with inadequate management and governance; limited sources of income; insufficient human resources; poorly planned, financed, and maintained physical plants; and rudimentary quality controls. At the same time, they are often buffeted by such external forces as regulations, competition, inadequate payment systems, and conflicting service demands.

Experts from a number of countries, the World Health Organization (WHO), and the international development agencies of industrialized nations came together in an extraordinary meeting to address the challenges facing hospitals today and going forward (German Federal Ministry for Economic Cooperation and Development [BMZ] / German Corporation for International Cooperation [GTZ] and WHO 2010). The meeting was based on the premise that the role of hospitals should change within the upcoming decade, and it sought to clarify the critical issues concerning hospital reform. It also sought to formulate a plan to address those issues. There was no official follow-up to the meeting, but the consensus sent a powerful message to the policy community. The key issues identified by the meeting are as follows (BMZ/GTZ and WHO 2010):

- Clarifying the role and function of hospitals in the health system
- Political dimensions and expectations of hospitals
- Hospital isolation in the face of blurring demarcations
- Linkages between hospitals and other levels of the health system
- Cost and benefit of technological progress
- Data to measure hospital performance in relation to population outcomes
- Universal coverage and accessibility
- Hospital financing within overall health spending
- Hospital governance and autonomy
- The legal framework within which hospitals operate
- Human resources
- Involvement of private hospital actors
- Hospitals in a global health marketplace
- Hospitals and the wider economy

There is no better summary of the challenges facing hospital and health system administrators and planners.

Primary Care Provision

The development of primary care has emerged as the central strategy to achieve universal access, comprehensive care, and cost containment, not only in developing countries but also in industrialized countries. The goal for low-resource societies is to provide essential services that are realistically within their reach, with community participation. WHO (1978) has promoted primary care development since the Alma-Ata Declaration of 1978. The declaration was formulated by public health leaders who were largely committed to the position that healthcare is a right and that the state has the responsibility to provide it.

Alma-Ata created an enduring tension between two "ideal" models—a hospital-centric ideal model of health system development, with overtones of private practice and specialization, and an ideal model based on publicly supported community-based primary care providers, with the hospital in a supporting role. The conflict between the two ideal models was summarized by Frenk, Ruelas, and Donabedian (1989, 1):

> In most developing countries the concern is that . . . [hospitals] already absorb such a high proportion of resources that they seriously threaten any effort to achieve full coverage of the population. Furthermore, it is widely believed that a health care system centered around hospitals is intrinsically incompatible with the geographic, economic, and cultural attributes of many populations. In addition, the mix of services offered by hospitals . . . is believed to poorly match the prevailing epidemiologic profile and the population needs for preventive and continuous care.

Gillam (2008, 537) assessed the practical impact of the Alma-Ata Declaration on governments' policies and actions, noting that "early efforts at expanding primary care in the late 1970's and early 1980's were overtaken in many parts of the developing world by economic crisis, sharp reductions in public spending, political instability, and emerging disease. The social and political goals of Alma Ata provoked early ideological opposition and were never fully embraced in market oriented, capitalistic countries. Hospitals retained their disproportionate share of local health economies."

In setting out a model of a preferred future, the WHO (2008, 55) states: "Primary-care teams cannot ensure comprehensive responsibility for their populations without support from specialized services, organizations and institutions that are based outside the community served . . . [and] typically concentrated in a 'first referral level district hospital.'" Assuming that, in many countries, most of the existent service deliverers are controlled by the system designers, the model calls for coordination of all resources to be vested in the primary health team, presumably mandated by law in most cases. Under that premise, "The primary-care team becomes the mediator between the community and the other levels"(WHO 2008, 55).

It is important to emphasize that primary care systems are ultimately dependent on hospitals. To be comprehensive, a system must have a hospital available to treat complicated, often life-threatening cases. The system also must be able to receive trauma cases from rural employment and transportation situations that far exceed the competencies and resources of primary care. Patients who are unable to access community and primary care services have been known to travel great distances to reach the nearest hospital in case of emergency.

Regionalization

Regionalization is the third enduring organizational focus, but a specific definition of the term is evasive. The term has as many definitions as it has plans and applications. Roemer (1965) stated that regionalization cannot be defined on the basis of experience but that agreement can be reached with regard to its objectives. The following general objectives have emerged, with a degree of agreement across applications, as central to the regionalization process:

- The efficient utilization of limited health resources
- The efficient utilization of expensive health resources
- The provision of adequate, appropriate, and accessible health services to a population
- The improvement and maintenance of standards of health services provision

    The application of the concept of regionalization to healthcare provision can be traced back more than a hundred years. The event that had the broadest global impact was the United Kingdom's 1920 "Interim Report on the Future of Medical and Allied Services," commonly known as the Dawson report, after Sir Bertrand Dawson, a physician to the British royal family. The report proposed a comprehensive national organization of health services that was organized around base hospitals and integrated most services in defined regions of the country (Consultative Council on Medical and Allied Services, Great Britain 1920). The United Kingdom implemented the report's basic principles in the country's National Health Service over the course of 28 years. The Dawson report has influenced health systems in a variety of countries, particularly in Europe.

    Dawson proposed dividing the country into regions that would (eventually) meet most of the preventive and curative health needs of the population. Specialized, scarce, and expensive services for a wider area (or country) would be available on referral but not duplicated at the regional level. The services of hospitals would be defined according to a classification system, thereby ensuring access to basic services while avoiding competition and underuse. The influence of Dawson's emphasis on the integration of preventive and curative resources to achieve a more effective investment balance cannot be overstated.

    Hospital-centered regionalization has become a widely discussed approach to health system organization in a number of countries, particularly in Europe but also elsewhere. For instance, the Chilean National Health Service reorganization program, which started in the 1960s, created hospital areas with the understanding that a hospital would have full responsibility for the health of the population within its service area. With all health activities linked to the hospital, clinical physicians would have to be directly involved in

regionalization
A broad organizational concept with a variety of applications; its key aims include efficient use of limited and expensive health resources, the provision of accessible health services to a defined population, and the development of standards for health services provision.

the field programs, potentially leading to the effective integration of preventive and curative medicine. At the time of the program's implementation, private hospitals were not included; the director of the area was to be the director of the largest (frequently, the only) hospital in the area.

The rationalization of health-provision resources to serve a defined population—be it a country, region, district, or community—is a very appealing idea. In theory, it is most likely to succeed in a central command-and-control political system, wherein one owner has control over all the components. However, that theory assumes that the full range of essential services exists or is accessible in each region. Application becomes more complicated—and potentially unrealistic—when applied to pluralistic environments with diverse financing schemes, multiple ownerships, local governments, advocacy organizations, and competing demands. Also, of course, additional complications follow from the differing political philosophies about the role of the state.

One key organizational issue focuses on how to integrate new knowledge into the capital planning process. Another issue deals with reducing the duplication of diagnostic services that can be provided electronically to many hospitals. An additional question is how to create incentives in the capital management process that will modify internal organization and **facility design** to support such changes (Edwards, Wyatt, and McKee 2004).

facility design
The design of the space in which a business's activities take place. The planning and layout of that space have a significant impact on the flow of work, materials, and information through the system.

Kenya's pluralistic environment provides an example of how the role of the private sector can be constrained by the lack of access to capital. A substantial portion of care is provided by private for-profit and faith-based hospitals that have difficulty obtaining loans. As a result, funds are not available to start new hospitals, or to improve or replace existing facilities (Barnes et al. 2010). In Benin, banks generally loan only to large, well-established hospitals that are managed or owned by well-known doctors, and smaller enterprises are rarely considered. Capital funding limitations can also result from poor management skills, difficulties with property titles, and lack of collateral (Strengthening Health Outcomes Through the Private Sector [SHOPS] Project 2013).

Addressing these issues will require an understanding of global experience and an emphasis on the development of leadership and management competencies. The professionalization of healthcare managers will be indispensable in advancing the effective and efficient use of organizations' resources.

Organizational Planning and Design

Organizational planning and design enable managers to align the healthcare organization's functions and resources with its mission, vision, values, goals, and objectives. The planning process incorporates a variety of tools to facilitate work relations and interactions, efficient resource allocation, and effective decision making.

The challenges facing healthcare managers can be either internal or external to the organization. One of the most important internal challenges involves the increasing technical complexity of the services being provided, which stems from continually changing medical technologies and the diversity and professional autonomy of the health professionals who interact in the delivery of services. Other internal and external challenges are associated with healthcare managers' need to balance the components of the iron triangle. Balancing access and equity with efficient, cost-effective services and quality outcomes requires robust organizational design and planning, as well as flexibility to confront the dynamic conditions of the healthcare environment.

Organizational designs take as many forms as needed to address the uniqueness of a dynamic organization. The designs are usually reflected in an organizational chart that describes the relations, authority, responsibilities, and interactions of the different units and individuals. Other documents and tools—such as organizational manuals, job descriptions, policies, regulations, and legal or administrative documents—also describe the various functions, resources, and responsibilities in more detail. A number of these tools are described throughout this book. Some tools commonly used in the planning process are flowcharts, affinity diagrams, Gantt charts, and balanced scorecards. In large and complex organizations, and across countries and healthcare systems, increasingly comprehensive information systems and the application of informatics are now indispensable.

Several questions need to be answered before an appropriate organizational design can be determined. For example, how can we design an organization that responds to the pace of change and complexity of the external environment? How can we create a simple enough organization that presents clear responsibilities for all areas of the organization while responding to complex interrelations and problems that need to be solved? How can we incorporate clinicians and managers in the decision-making process? How do we create strong supporting guidelines throughout the organization while at the same time allowing some level of autonomy and empowerment for the providers and units (Baker, Narine, and Leatt 1994)?

An organizational chart can be presented in a variety of ways, and there is no clear "best" organizational design. Most organizations will use combinations of design types, most of which derive from three basic formats—functional design, divisional design, and matrix design. Functional design is the most traditional of the formats, and it is well suited to organizations that offer well-defined services or products, respond to slower environmental changes, and have clearly defined stakeholders. Divisional design works better in larger organizations with multiple product or service lines that can be grouped into larger divisions. Finally, matrix design is most appropriate for organizations that must respond to rapid changes in technology or highly dynamic or competitive environments. A variation of the matrix design is the program design, which combines substantive areas and strong, well-differentiated programs with complex and unique requirements for performance. These design formats have been used in all types of healthcare organizations, and each includes elements that can effectively contribute to organizational success. It is relatively common for organizations to adopt hybrid models or change their organizational designs to respond to specific circumstances.

Management of Physical Resources

How do organizational processes determine the physical design and structure of healthcare organizations? This discussion will focus on two main elements. The first element involves the planning processes of healthcare units, of which a critical component is the development of a **prearchitectural medical functional program** that defines the services to be offered and the resources required. The second element involves the supplies and utilities needed by healthcare units (e.g., electric power, water, fuels, medicinal gases, telephones, internet), which can be provided by either public services or private companies. The processing and distribution of these supplies take place in the "house of machines," which serves as the nuclear resource for the units' function and connects the operation of all systems (e.g., electric, hydrosanitary, air conditioning, telecommunications, information technology). These activities enliven the elements and allow the optimal operation of functional units or facilities, administrative services, and support services as an integrated, efficient, and effective operation.

prearchitectural medical functional program
A planning document that serves as a road map for the design of a facility; it identifies functional program areas and defines such aspects as users, operational scenarios, design criteria, and square footage needed.

Clinical units, administrative units, and the resources of general support services that were defined in the corresponding prearchitectural medical program are distributed among the hospital buildings. Each functional unit has its own structure with respect to physical, human, material, and technological resources. The units carry out processes that transform the resources into services, the results of which are generally evaluated with indicators of quantitative and qualitative performance. Each unit receives general support services, including maintenance of architectural finishes, furniture, facilities, and equipment; cleaning and disinfection; disposal of waste; and the supply of inputs required for operation. These elements and their interrelations are illustrated in exhibit 1.2.

The construction and operation of healthcare units are strongly regulated by laws, rules, and norms of compulsory observance, typically to ensure quality, preservation of the environment, and health and safety in the workplace. The operation of the units generates liquid, solid, and gaseous waste, the management of which must be in accordance with legal provisions intended to control the pollution of air, land, and water mantles and to avoid risks to the health of patients, users, service providers, vendors, and visitors to the units. Because of safety concerns, particular interest exists with regard to proper management of

EXHIBIT 1.2
Management of Physical Resources in Healthcare Units

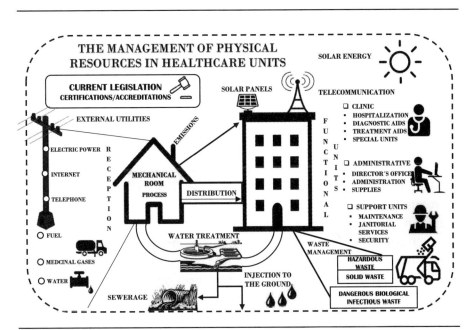

THE MANAGEMENT OF PHYSICAL RESOURCES IN HEALTHCARE UNITS

equipment and substances that emit radiation and biological products capable of generating infections.

Current trends support the efficient use of energy and the use of renewable energy to promote a less costly and more environmentally friendly operation. Such trends can be seen in the use of solar panels for the heating of water and photovoltaic cells for the generation of electric power, as well as intelligent systems that control lighting and air conditioning.

Water management seeks to ensure water availability, storage, and potability, to maintain both a continuous supply and a critical reserve in case water availability is suspended, which may happen during natural disasters. Potable water is critical both for ingestion and for use in processes of care that require efficient washing of hands, surfaces, and equipment. Wastewater treatment plants can be used to recycle water and reduce consumption, leveraging water to recharge the subsoil, to water gardened areas, and to use in health services.

Solid waste management is of the utmost importance. Classifications for solid waste management include organic and inorganic waste, potentially contaminated waste, and waste that requires special management because of strict regulations regarding its collection, storage, transportation, and disposal.

Health units' internal and external communication requires a complex telecommunication infrastructure, internet connectivity, and systems that allow the efficient management of voice messages and data. Such systems are particularly important for the electronic registration of various transactions and interactions necessary for the operation of the unit.

The Planning Process

During the planning process for the construction of healthcare units, a number of elements are taken into consideration: location and geographical area of influence; the target population, with its demographic and epidemiologic profile; the types of services to be offered; and market analysis with respect to offer and demand of services both public and private.

Based on the preliminary information, a prearchitectural medical functional program is developed. This program defines the services that will be offered and any required physical spaces in accordance with the applicable regulations. A key challenge is to articulate the requirements to create functional units equipped with all the necessary resources to ensure their correct operation. At the same time, additional challenges involve making sure that the interrelations between the clinical units and the support services establish a pattern of consistent functionality and maximize efficiency to users, staff, and suppliers of goods and services. The dimensions and orientation of the land to be used for the construction will affect the number and configuration of the levels to be built, as well as the distribution of services to be provided.

The functional medical program provides the basis for the development of the architectural project, which in turn will produce functional units with appropriate furniture and equipment. Given the highly specialized and constantly evolving nature of hospital services and medical technology, this plan needs to be developed by a group of experts in hospital design, with participation of both architects and the operators of health units.

The architectural project must comply with the established framework of laws, regulations, and standards. It should keep in mind the following considerations:

- Installed capacity that responds to the needs of the target population, as well as the provision of personal clinical services
- Sufficiency of resources to achieve the goals and objectives (productivity) outlined in the business plan
- Functionality (efficiency and effectiveness) in compliance with current regulations, to ensure regular and emergency access to clinical healthcare services with comfort and security for staff, third-party suppliers, patients, and their families

Once the clinical and support units (e.g., outpatient care, emergency care, hospitalization wards, diagnostic support units, general and administrative services) and their specific capacities (e.g., numbers of offices, cubicles, operating rooms, warehouses, waiting rooms) have been defined, the final considerations for the functional plan involve determining the medical and instrumental equipment required for the operation of the various units. Decisions made at this point will depend on the financial resources available and the level of complexity expected for a particular medical facility.

Once the prearchitectural functional program has been developed and adjusted, the executive project defines all systems, facilities, and equipment that will require supplies and utilities such as water, drainage, electric power, hydrosanitary services, air conditioning, medical gases, fuel, and telecommunications. These needs are reflected in a program with a phase-in plan that considers the stages required for construction, facilities, equipment, preoperation, and commissioning of the units in question.

The next step involves carrying out the executive project, which requires the development of the operating systems necessary for the installation and provision of the projected utilities and supplies. Project leaders should consider environmental and safety implications and ensure full compliance with regulations and standards for construction and facilities. They should also take into account the requirements that may need to be met in the future to achieve certification from accreditation agencies, such as The Joint Commission in the United States.

Execution of the project requires a project management program that elaborates required tasks, equipment and other resources, and the responsible parties. The project management program takes into consideration the span of time required for various activities and tasks, sets targets for their conclusion, and facilitates coordination between components. A variety of project management software programs are available to assist with this step. Depending on the unit's magnitude and complexity, the management of the project or supervision of work can also be contracted to a third-party company that has experience with similar units.

Of particular importance is the definition of the management model to be used to operate the healthcare unit. Selection of this model considers the strategic framework (i.e., mission, vision, values, goals, and objectives); the organizational model; the desired measures of effectiveness; the distribution of resources and workforce; internal operation manuals; work regulations; rules, both internal and external; and market and/or operational plans and programs. Specific calculations need to be made for the supply and consumption of various materials, including items needed for office operations; food and medical supplies; emergency and regular maintenance materials; and tools and equipment.

Health need assessments and the steps outlined in this section can determine the amount of investment required, as well as the cost of the operation, for a unit. This information, in turn, can inform the development of a business plan to identify the feasibility and sustainability of the proposed facility or unit.

Functional Unit Requirements

The requirements for the operation of a health unit should be assessed using the management model, with attention to organizational design, the staff or personnel necessary to meet the established work shifts, job positions and descriptions, organizational procedures and manuals, rules and regulations, and necessary inputs. Planning for the design, operation, and use of resources is influenced by such factors as the type of services provided, the medical and technological delivery capacities, the availability of resources, and the country's level of development (taking into account health expenditure as a percentage of the gross domestic product). It is also influenced by the part of the health sector in which the unit is going to operate. The public and social security sectors have well-defined models and prototypes, and most countries have specific rules for the private sector.

The functional units of the clinical area correspond to the provision of direct services to patients and include outpatient care, auxiliary diagnostic, auxiliary treatment, hospitalization, and specialized care units. The architectural design should consider the locations and resources required for the operation of each functional unit—incorporating both clinical services and support services—to ensure optimal access, flow, and comfort for users, providers, and suppliers. Flows should be accurately defined for the movement of users and staff, as well as for food, clean and dirty clothes, solid and potentially contaminated waste, mobile equipment, and operating supplies. The aim is to establish an infrastructure that facilitates efficient processes and stimulates productivity and satisfaction for users and staff.

Clinical services generally include the categories of outpatient services; support services, such as laboratory diagnosis and imaging; support treatment services, such as surgical and obstetric units; and hospitalization and adult special care units, such as intensive care units and burn centers. Clinical services support is given largely through nursing, which is the main pillar for patient care and an indispensable aspect for hospitalization, outpatient care, and clinical support areas. Support services—which are discussed in greater detail in the next section—include food and dietary services, cleaning and disinfection, gardening, security, waste management, and maintenance of buildings, installations, and equipment. Management services—which include senior management and middle management and supervision—are grouped by such functions as direction, quality management, management of resources (human, material, technological, and financial), public relations, and marketing.

All functional units and support services must have a management model that is documented in a procedures manual, with components dedicated to structure, processes, and expected outcomes. It should also have programs relating to quality, protection of the environment, and health and safety at work, as well as an annual operating budget and program that defines the goals, objectives, strategies, and measurable results. Each unit and service can be turned into a cost center that allows more detailed and accountable operations.

Exhibit 1.3 provides a guide for analyzing the main elements of structure, process, and outputs/outcomes that interact in the operation of a functional unit. The accompanying vignette uses an example from Brazil to illustrate some operational issues.

EXHIBIT 1.3
Functional Unit
Process

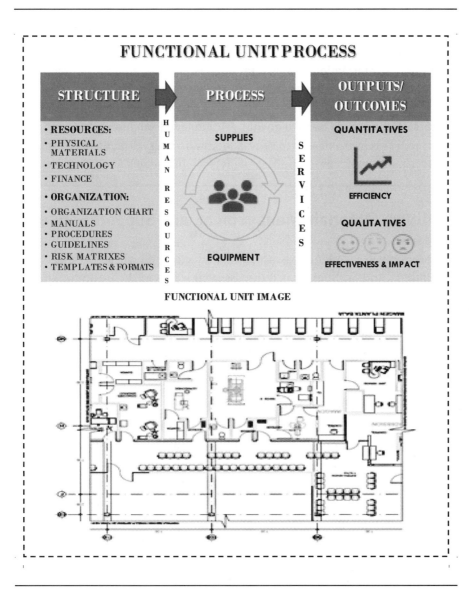

FUNCTIONAL UNIT PROCESS

FUNCTIONAL UNIT IMAGE

Vignette: Operations Management in Brazilian Hospitals

by Ana Maria Malik

Research on private nonprofit hospitals with between 30 and 800 beds revealed that bed management in the state of São Paulo, Brazil, is practically nonexistent (Raffa 2017). Although *management* is slowly becoming a

(continued)

buzzword, efficiency is not a real concern, and bed occupancy generally is not planned. Barriers to bed management initiatives include (1) problems with health information systems; (2) doctors being treated as though they "own" the beds, meaning that their approval (either formally or informally) is needed for use of the beds; and (3) a lack of discharge planning for inpatients, leading many beds to go idle. Additional information in the original Portuguese is available at http://gvsaude.fgv.br/sites/gvsaude.fgv.br/files/tese_claudia_raffa_21_03.pdf.

Facilities, Materials Management, and Support Services

This section will examine key issues for the effective and efficient management of buildings and facilities. It will discuss such topics as the planning, design, construction, and remodeling of facilities; housekeeping and environmental services; safety and security; issues with medical and nonmedical equipment; health technology assessment (acquisition, management, and audits); food services; purchasing, receiving, storing, distributing, processing, and controlling supplies; and the future of materials management.

Facilities Conservation and Maintenance

Management of the physical infrastructure focuses on the conservation, maintenance, and operation of buildings, facilities, and equipment. The department responsible for this area represents a key structural element both for the functioning of the unit's services and for the development of the processes that transform inputs into services. Its main objective is to ensure the good condition of the property and the maintenance of the facility and equipment, allowing for a correct and continuous operation with high levels of energy efficiency and security. The department achieves this objective through the work of trained personnel who apply both routine and preventive programs, as well as corrective actions when needed.

Effective management requires building plans that are organized by system and by architectural area, as well as an inventory of installed equipment with technical specifications, warranties, service providers, and maintenance programs. The facility must also have a stock of spare parts and supplies to use for replacement, as well as tools and equipment needed for corrective actions. Electronic devices can facilitate the registration of equipment.

The hospital operator should design and implement the necessary means to ensure the timely, permanent, efficient, effective, safe, and reliable operation of all infrastructure, facilities, general and special equipment, administrative and fixed furniture, and public services. Operations should comply with a rigorous "program of daily routines" that includes preventive, corrective, and reagent procedures, responding to the various particularities of each functional unit. Activities must be based on strict procedures yet also designed with flexibility to allow for technological updating, continued innovation, and responses to changes in demand that may occur over the course of the contractual term.

Public Areas Services, Maintenance, and Energy Efficiency

Key objectives of this area are to maintain optimal conditions of the facilities with regard to appearance, conservation, and functionality and to ensure the continuity and operation of all facilities, fluids, energy, systems, and equipment. Such efforts require an adequate annual program of preventive maintenance in compliance with the requirements of the present description, performance indicators, and applicable and existing legislation.

The operator should be responsible for the preventive and corrective maintenance of administrative and fixed furniture and building equipment, as well as all the facilities of the hospital or organization. Key priorities include ensuring the provision of services for the public; meeting the needs of normal, continuous, and permanent use of all areas and services of the organization; ensuring a high level of safety; and providing efficient solutions that contribute to the preservation of the environment.

Medical Gases Management and Distribution

The aim of this service is to ensure the permanent supply, conditions of use, and operation of various types of medicinal gases. Such gases are needed to assist patients and to support the operation of systems and equipment. The operator must ensure the proper management of medicinal gases through the most modern infrastructure and technology, meeting the needs of the hospital and maintaining conditions of safety and efficiency in accordance with the scale of the project. The operator must ensure the quantity, quality, continuity, and reliability of gas services with absolute respect for applicable laws. This area also must comply with the buildings', installations', and equipment requirements for accreditation and certification, as specified in the appropriate manuals, and any other terms and conditions established in contracts and their annexes. Service should also ensure the correct management of processes and subprocesses detailed in the approved operation manual.

Medical Equipment Maintenance and Supply / Health Technology Assessment

The central objective of this service is to carry out all management procedures concerning the operation, maintenance, and replacement of medical equipment and instruments. A related objective is to design and implement training and ongoing technical assistance for the correct use and operation of all of the required equipment, with specially qualified personnel for each item and task, to ensure operational excellence in all functional units. The operator should be

---

Vignette: Health Technology Assessment in Brazilian Hospitals

by Ana Maria Malik

Research has revealed ongoing challenges with health technology assessment in Brazilian hospitals (Francisco 2017). A regulatory agency, ANVISA, was created in 2000, and a national council, CONITEC, originated in 2006 and was institutionalized in 2011. In addition, a national network for HTA, known as REBRATS, was created in 2008, and it consists of 80 health facilities, 27 of which are hospitals. A research study sampled those hospitals by region and interviewed participants of the HTA units; the interviewees largely acknowledged that their actions had not been effective. An earlier study, developed in 2011 and published in 2015, had produced similar findings: The units did not have their own budgets, their staff used time that was left over from other hospital activities, and they had no evidence that their efforts saved money or improved outcomes. In short, the hospitals did not really know what to do with their HTA units. Additional information in the original Portuguese is available at http://gvsaude.fgv.br/sites/gvsaude.fgv.br/files/dissertacao_-_fernando_de_rezende_francisco.pdf.

---

health technology assessment (HTA) The systematic evaluation of health technology and its properties, effects, and impacts; a multidisciplinary process for evaluating social, economic, organizational, and ethical issues related to health technology.

committed to the provision of safe, effective, and timely service, with absolute respect for the laws in force and compliance with established processes and subprocesses. Within this category of services, **health technology assessment (HTA)** represents a multidisciplinary process for evaluating social, economic, organizational, and ethical issues related to health technology. Several international resources and organizations related to the HTA function are listed at the end of this chapter. The accompanying vignette provides further illustration of key issues related to technology assessment.

Housekeeping, Janitorial, and Environmental Services

The chief objective of this area is to implement a cleaning service and manage common waste in all facilities and spaces of the hospital or organization. Adherence to established standards and safe practices allows optimum medical and nonmedical operation in terms of hygiene and aesthetics, while also reducing the risk of nosocomial infections and disease transmissions. Such efforts foster a sense of well-being among patients and personnel and project a positive image of the organization. The operator should be fully committed to the provision of a safe, effective, and timely service for common waste management and cleaning, with attention to applicable laws and the sustainability of the processes and products used.

Safety and Security

This service area focuses on safeguarding all functional areas of the hospital or facility and ensuring security, order, and personal integrity for patients, employees, visitors, and others. Established standards should foster and contribute to a culture of security, civil protection, self-protection, and order, in which both users and assets are preserved and safe from risk. The organization should project an image of safety through compliance with contractual requirements and applicable laws.

Materials Management and Warehouses

This service deals with the acquisition, receipt, storage, custody, inventory control, and distribution of the supplies, materials, tools, and equipment needed for the operation of the hospital or facility. This service should provide for logistics and the daily functioning of the institution in conditions of safety and high quality. The operator should be responsible for managing all the inputs required for the correct performance of functional units, especially those where medical tasks are performed. The operator is also responsible for maintaining an up-to-date inventory of property, furniture, and equipment, all in optimal conditions of order, cleanliness, and safety, for each of the areas of warehouse (e.g., medical materials warehouse, equipment and furniture warehouse, discontinued items warehouse).

Pharmacy Services

The main function of pharmacy services is to procure, prepare, distribute, store, and control drugs and other curative materials. Drug and medication management is critical in the overall operation of healthcare organizations, particularly with the disproportionate increases in drug costs and the abundance of new medications available in local, country, and world markets. The management of these critical resources is subject to a wide variety of regulations and market conditions, which are mostly specific to particular countries. The operation of the medication system is affected by such factors as the way physicians prescribe and use drugs and medications; the way pharmacists prepare, dispense, and distribute drugs and medications; the administration of medications by nurses and other health professionals; the administrative processing, control, and reimbursement mechanisms established by the health organization and its departments; and applicable regulations.

Food and Nutrition Services

Nutrition is an indispensable element of good clinical outcomes in healthcare organizations. This resource-intensive area involves more than just the hygienic and efficient procurement, processing, and distribution of high-quality meals to patients and staff. It involves specialized requirements for human resources, food and supplies, equipment, furniture, and large spaces throughout the facility.

Such spaces include, but are not limited to, kitchens, offices, cafeterias, dining rooms, elevators, warehouses, and storage areas. Food and nutrition services also require thoughtful and creative controls and budgeting. Many organizations use outside catering groups to provide some or all of these services. Some aspects of food services can be revenue generating.

Summary

This chapter has discussed the essential functions and structural components of healthcare organizations, with attention to the key challenges that healthcare managers face when aligning the structure and physical resources with the organization's mission, goals, and objectives. Different types of healthcare organizations and the varied health systems around the world present continuous and dynamic challenges for managers, who must thoughtfully reshape, realign, and redesign their management of resources to achieve value-based outcomes.

Discussion Questions

1. Using the diagram in exhibit 1.1, analyze how the various elements function and interact in a particular healthcare organization with which you are familiar. Then do similar analyses of the regional healthcare system to which that organization belongs and the national healthcare system to which the region belongs.

2. Review the *Leadership Competencies for Healthcare Services Managers* framework developed by the International Hospital Federation (available at www.ihf-fih.org/resources/pdf/Leadership_Competencies_for_Healthcare_Services_Managers.pdf). Work with your immediate peers to determine which competencies you have developed and which you need to work on to improve your individual and group performance. If you wish to expand on this exercise, take the competency questionnaire at http://healthmanagementcompetency.org/en/base.

3. How do the five pillars of sustainability apply to your organization? Are there certain actions you can take to develop one or more of those pillars? If so, make a plan of action, and set some measurable objectives for the task.

4. What is your idea of primary healthcare? Can you design a strategy to adapt primary healthcare to one of the services or programs in your organization? If possible, work with a team of peers on this exercise.

5. Describe the type of organization used in a particular department or service area of a hospital or healthcare organization with which you

are familiar. Review the current organizational chart, consider the department's relations with other departments, and propose ways to improve.

6. Review exhibit 1.2. Compare and contrast the elements in the diagram with those of a healthcare unit with which you are familiar. Think of two areas where improvements could be made, and design a plan to address them.

7. What is the process for designing or redesigning a healthcare facility? Think of a new service or program that would require physical resources and facilities, and apply the process to that case.

8. What are the key elements to management of medical equipment and supplies? Think of a specific piece of medical equipment, and identify the key elements for ensuring a good and efficient maintenance process.

9. What is health technology assessment? Look up some HTA agencies in your country, and examine the resources they have available.

10. Interview one or two key individuals in the food and nutrition service of a hospital or healthcare organization. Ask them to identify two of the most important issues or problems they face in their service or department. Develop a plan of action to address one of those issues.

Additional Resources

Health Planning
- World Health Organization, "Sub-national and District Management: Planning and Budgeting for Services": www.who.int/management/district/planning_budgeting/en/

Performance Improvement
- World Health Organization, "Strengthening Management Capacity": www.who.int/management/strengthen/en/
- World Health Organization, "The Health Manager's Website": www.who.int/management/en/
- World Health Organization, "Management for Health Services Delivery" (examples of diverse country experiences, with documents and reports): www.who.int/management/country/en/

Health Technology Assessment
- Health Technology Assessment International (HTAi), a global scientific and professional society: www.htai.org/htai/about-htai/

- International Network of Agencies for Health Technology Assessment (INAHTA), a network of agencies in various countries: www.inahta.org
- HTA Glossary, with definitions of various HTA terms: http://htaglossary. net/HomePage
- World Health Organization, "Health Technology Assessment: International HTA Networks": www.who.int/health-technology-assessment/ networks/en/

Health Facilities Design and Management
- World Health Organization, "Management of Health Facilities": www. who.int/management/facility/en/

Facilities and Materials Management
- World Health Organization, "Management of Resources and Support Systems: Drugs and Supplies": www.who.int/management/resources/ drugs/en/
- World Health Organization, "Management of Resources and Support Systems: Equipment, Vehicles and Building": www.who.int/ management/resources/equipment/en/

References

Baker, R., L. Narine, and P. Leatt. 1994. "Organizational Design for Health Care." In *The AUPHA Manual of Health Services Management*, edited by R. J. Taylor and S. B. Taylor, 103–17. Gaithersburg, MD: Aspen.

Barnes, J., B. O'Hanlon, F. Feeley III, K. McKeon, N. Gitonga, and C. Decker. 2010. "Private Health Sector Assessment in Kenya." World Bank working paper no. 193. Accessed September 15, 2017. http://documents.worldbank.org/ curated/en/434701468048274776/pdf/552020PUB0Heal10Box349442 B01PUBLIC1.pdf.

Bradbury, R. C., and B. Ramirez-Minvielle. 1995. "Continuous Quality Improvement in Latin American Health Systems." *Journal of Health Administration Education* 13 (1): 165–78.

Bradley, E. H., S. Pallas, C. Bashyal, P. Berman, and L. Curry. 2010. "Developing Strategies for Improving Health Care Delivery: Guide to Concepts, Determinants, Measurement, and Intervention Design." World Bank Health, Nutrition, and Population (HNP) discussion paper. Published June. http://site resources.worldbank.org/HEALTHNUTRITIONANDPOPULATION/ Resources/281627-1095698140167/DevelopingStrategiesforImproving HealthCareDelivery.pdf.

Consultative Council on Medical and Allied Services, Great Britain. 1920. "Interim Report on the Future Provision of Medical and Allied Services." Accessed March 29, 2018. www.nhshistory.net/Dawson%20report.html.

Counte, M., B. Ramirez, and W. Aaronson. 2011. "Global Health Management Education: Essential Competencies and Major Curricular Challenges." *Journal of Health Administration Education* 28 (2): 227–36.

Donabedian, A. 1988. "The Quality of Care: How Can It Be Assessed?" *JAMA* 260 (12): 1743–48.

———. 1966. "Evaluating the Quality of Medical Care." *Milbank Quarterly* 44 (3 Pt. 2): 166–203.

Edwards, N., S. Wyatt, and M. McKee. 2004. *Configuring the Hospital in the 21st Century.* European Observatory on Health Systems and Policy policy brief no. 5. Accessed September 15, 2017. http://apps.who.int/iris/bitstream/10665/107597/1/E84697.pdf.

Francisco, F. R. 2017. "Aplicação de avaliação de tecnologias em saúde (ATS) na tomada de decisão em hospitais." Fundação Getúlio Vargas. Accessed April 10, 2018. http://gvsaude.fgv.br/sites/gvsaude.fgv.br/files/dissertacao_-_fernando_de_rezende_francisco.pdf.

Frenk, J., O. Góméz-Dantes, and S. Moon. 2014. "From Sovereignty to Solidarity: A Renewed Concept of Global Health for an Era of Complex Interdependence." *Lancet.* Published January 4. www.thelancet.com/pdfs/journals/lancet/PIIS0140-6736(13)62561-1.pdf.

Frenk, J., R. Ruelas, and A. Donabedian. 1989. "Hospital Management Staffing and Training Issues." Working paper. Washington, DC: World Bank.

German Federal Ministry for Economic Cooperation and Development (BMZ) / German Corporation for International Cooperation (GTZ), and the World Health Organization (WHO). 2010. Report on meeting about the role of hospitals in today's health systems, October 12–13, Geneva, Switzerland. Unpublished summary.

Gillam, S. 2008. "Is the Declaration of Alma Ata Still Relevant to Primary Health Care?" *BMJ* 336 (7643): 536–38.

Institute for Healthcare Improvement (IHI). 2012. "IHI Triple Aim Initiative." Accessed August 5, 2017. www.ihi.org/Engage/Initiatives/TripleAim/Pages/default.aspx.

International Hospital Federation (IHF). 2015. *Leadership Competencies for Healthcare Services Managers.* Accessed August 3, 2017. www.ihf-fih.org/resources/pdf/Leadership_Competencies_for_Healthcare_Services_Managers.pdf.

Kissick, W. L. 1994. *Medicine's Dilemmas.* New Haven, CT: Yale University Press.

Raffa, C. 2017. "Análise das variáveis do ambiente interno para o gerenciamento de leitos em organizações hospitalares privadas." Fundação Getúlio Vargas. Accessed April 9, 2018. http://gvsaude.fgv.br/sites/gvsaude.fgv.br/files/tese_claudia_raffa_21_03.pdf.

Ramirez, B., R. M. Oetjen, and D. Malvey. 2011. "Sustainability and the Health Care Manager." *Health Care Manager* 30 (2): 133–38.

Roemer, M. I. 1965. *Medical Care in Relation to Public Health.* Geneva, Switzerland: World Health Organization.

Strengthening Health Outcomes Through the Private Sector (SHOPS) Project. 2013. "Benin Private Health Sector Assessment." United States Agency for International Development (USAID) brief. USAID / Abt Associates. Published September. http://abtassociates.com/AbtAssociates/files/50/5009aaae-6662-434a-aad1-7a5934f0eb9b.pdf.

West, D. J. Jr., G. Filerman, B. Ramirez, and J. Steinkogler. 2012. *CAHME Phase II: International Healthcare Management Education.* Commission on Accreditation of Healthcare Management Education. Accessed July 26, 2017. www.cahme.org/CAHME/CAHME_Resources/CAHME_Resources%20Reports/CAHME/Resources/CAHME_Reports.aspx?hkey=ac299497-81ef-4a5d-8cf8-0be7a45882c1.

World Health Organization (WHO). 2008. "Primary Care: Putting People First." In *The World Health Report.* Accessed March 29, 2018. www.who.int/whr/2008/08_chap3_en.pdf.

———. 1978. "Declaration of Alma-Ata. International Conference on Primary Health Care, Alma-Ata, USSR, 6-12." Accessed March 29, 2018. www.who.int/social_determinants/tools/multimedia/alma_ata/en/.

HEALTHCARE SYSTEMS, FINANCING, AND PAYMENTS

Jason S. Turner, PhD, Kevin D. Broom, PhD, Maysoun Dimachkie Masri, ScD, Francisco Yepes, MD, DrPH, and Ariel Cortés, MD, PhD

Chapter Focus

This chapter aims to provide a general overview of global healthcare expenditures, discuss the three macroeconomic drivers of variation among countries, and provide insight into the four primary models that countries have employed to finance and deliver healthcare. The chapter also gives a brief introduction into the mechanics of health insurance, and it concludes with a discussion of the natural incentives associated with the ways clinical providers are paid. The chapter provides important context for understanding the more detailed financial, quality, and managerial content that follows in later chapters.

Learning Objectives

Upon completion of this chapter, you should be able to

- explain basic concepts in health economics and health financing;
- differentiate the health system financing functions of revenue collection, pooling, and purchasing;
- identify the primary factors that drive variations in national healthcare expenditures;
- describe the macroeconomic tools used to constrain costs and allocate services;
- analyze the relationship between the four major organizational methods of healthcare and the factors of production;
- explain the mechanics of insurance and the way premiums are set;
- evaluate the role of healthcare payments in determining healthcare utilization and total expenditures; and
- articulate domestic financing and payment mechanisms.

Competencies

- Demonstrate an understanding of system structure, funding mechanisms, and the way healthcare services are organized.
- Balance the interrelationships among access, quality, safety, cost, resource allocation, accountability, care setting, community need, and professional roles.
- Effectively use risk management principles and programs, such as risk assessment and analysis and risk mitigation.

Key Terms

- Breakeven point
- Contingent loss
- Expected medical cost
- Fee-for-service (FFS)
- Fiscal space
- Health status risk
- Health system financing
- High-deductible health plan (HDHP)
- Keynesian economics
- Laissez-faire economics
- Loading factors
- Medical care risk
- National health insurance
- Pay for performance (P4P)
- Pooling
- Prospective payment system (PPS)
- Risk aversion
- Social insurance
- Underwriting methodology
- Universal coverage
- Utility

Key Concepts

- Healthcare delivery models
- Healthcare financing
- Health expenditures
- Health insurance
- Health interventions
- Marginal utility
- Price sensitivities
- Profit incentive
- Provider payment methods
- Risk management
- Supply and demand

Introduction

The world's countries, on average, allocate almost 10 percent of their gross domestic product (GDP) to healthcare goods and services (World Bank 2018).

However, the costs and financing of healthcare vary significantly from country to country. Whereas the countries of the European Union rank fairly close to the global average, the countries of Latin America, the Middle East, and South Asia dedicate a smaller portion of their GDP to healthcare—7.2 percent, 5.3 percent, and 4.4 percent, respectively, in 2014. The countries of North America, on the other hand, spend a higher-than-average percentage—16.5 percent of GDP in 2014. The ways that nations and societies organize their healthcare goods and services are equally varied. Approaches range from unregulated free-market systems that rely heavily on citizens' disposable income to centrally planned, government-based systems that are supported by general tax revenue. Although many nations lean to one side of the spectrum or the other, most

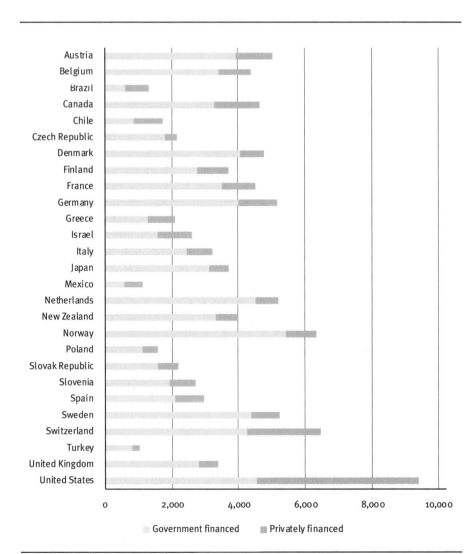

EXHIBIT 2.1
National Expenditures per Capita (purchasing power parity)

Source: Data from World Bank (2017).

employ a mosaic of approaches borrowing from both extremes. The wide range of per-capita expenditures and funding approaches is illustrated in exhibit 2.1.

This chapter will introduce the basic functions of healthcare financing, and it will support those concepts with practical applications. It will discuss national health expenditures and common delivery approaches, as well as some of the mechanisms employed in those approaches to constrain costs. The chapter will examine, from a macroeconomic perspective, the ways countries fund and dispense healthcare goods and services. It will explore various healthcare financing models; provide a general overview of insurance mechanisms; discuss the purchasing of healthcare services; and consider how the various provider payment methods relate to cost containment.

Health System Financing

health system financing
The process of collecting, allocating, and distributing revenues to cover health services for a designated population.

In short, **health system financing** is the process of collecting, allocating, and distributing revenues to cover health services for a designated population. The World Health Organization (WHO) defines *health financing*, in greater detail, as the "function of a health system concerned with the mobilization, accumulation and allocation of money to cover the health needs of the people, individually and collectively, in the health system" (WHO 2008). WHO states that "the purpose of health financing is to make funding available, as well as to set the right financial incentives for providers, to ensure that all individuals have access to effective public health and personal health care" (WHO 2000, 95).

Every country experiences demographic changes and epidemiological transitions that influence the population's healthcare needs and the demand for specific healthcare services. As a result, each country has a unique context, with different healthcare financing challenges arising at different times. As a result, health financing policy cannot simply be imported from one country to another. Nonetheless, systems in every country perform similar key functions with regard to healthcare financing. All healthcare systems raise revenues for the health system (revenue collection), often from a variety of sources. All systems accumulate these revenues on behalf of a designated population (pooling), and they all transfer these resources to service providers (purchasing) (Kutzin et al. 2017).

Revenue Collection
Countries need to raise adequate revenues for the provision of healthcare, and they must ensure that the flow of funds is stable and predictable. A number of organizations have attempted to estimate the amount of healthcare spending considered necessary for an adequate system. The WHO's (2010) *World Health Report*, for instance, has recommended that public spending on health

not be lower than 4 to 5 percent of GDP. Further updates have suggested that governments of low-income countries should spend at least $86 per capita (in 2012 US dollars) to deliver essential health interventions (Jowett et al. 2016). However, even if a government wants to increase public spending on health, the lack of **fiscal space** may limit the extent to which such actions are possible. *Fiscal space* can be defined as "the availability of budgetary room that allows a government to provide resources for a desired purpose without any prejudice to the sustainability of a government's financial position" (Heller 2005). Increasingly, countries are facing difficult resource constraints in providing healthcare services to their populations.

fiscal space
The flexibility of a government in determining where to spend revenue.

Revenues for the healthcare sector can be collected through a number of possible sources, each of which distributes the financial burden differently and affects who will have access to healthcare. Direct taxation is based on the earnings of households or businesses, and the taxes are paid directly to the government or through a public agency that collects the funds. Examples include income taxes and corporation taxes. Indirect taxation takes the form of excise or consumption taxes on specific goods or services that may or may not be intended to influence health behavior. Indirect taxes can be used to target health-related behavioral choices, whether by improving access to healthy dietary options, creating incentives for behaviors associated with improved health outcomes, or discouraging less healthy options. Examples of consumption taxes include taxes on cigarettes, alcoholic beverages, unhealthy foods, and sugary nonalcoholic beverages (Shibuya et al. 2003; WHO 2016).

Additional sources of healthcare funding may include revenues from state-owned industries, such as oil and gas industries, and external grants and loans provided by the World Bank. When private revenue sources are used for healthcare, they typically take the form of out-of-pocket payments made by the patient at the time of service and individual prepayment of voluntary health insurance.

Pooling

Fund **pooling** involves the accumulation of health revenues on behalf of a defined population for eventual transfer to providers (McIntyre and Kutzin 2016). When funds are pooled, through either voluntary participation or various taxation mechanisms, and expenses are predicted for a defined population, individuals are exchanging uncertain health-related expenses that will occur at some point in the future for budgetable and predictable expenses. The pooling function is a risk-mitigation tool that exchanges an uncertain contingent loss (i.e., the possibility of falling ill and needing care) for predetermined fees (e.g., taxes, insurance premiums). Pooling allows health systems to redistribute resources among people with a diverse set of health risks—some of which are high cost and require intense utilization and others that require minimal to

pooling
The accumulation of health revenues on behalf of a defined population for eventual transfer to providers; pooling mitigates risks by grouping individuals together to share current or future medical expenses.

no interventions. Three main factors should be considered when analyzing pooling arrangements:

1. *The size of the pool.* Does the system have one large pool to cover the whole population, or does it have separate smaller pools? For example, one pool might cover the health needs of civil servants, another might include only salaried private-sector workers, and yet another might cover the poor.
2. *The risk mix.* What is the underlying health of the people whose healthcare costs are covered? Does the pool include individuals with preexisting conditions? Does it include young and healthy individuals, or is it primarily older people or those with chronic conditions? Does the pool include people with a diverse set of health risks?
3. *Participation.* Is participation in the pool voluntary or compulsory?

Purchasing

Purchasing involves the allocation of funds to providers that deliver healthcare goods and services (McIntyre and Kutzin 2016). It can be characterized as either passive or strategic. Passive purchasing transfers funds to providers without using information about either performance or need. Strategic purchasing, on the other hand, uses incentives and administrative mechanisms to allocate funds in a way that promotes quality improvement and efficiency of healthcare services. A strategic healthcare system purchaser makes choices based on (1) the population needs for various healthcare services, (2) the availability of effective medical interventions, (3) the relative cost-effectiveness of interventions, (4) the utilization of services, and (5) the quality and efficiency of services delivered by providers. The various provider payment methods—ranging from salary to fee-for-service to capitation to global budgets—will be discussed later in the chapter.

Case Study: Healthcare Financing in the United Arab Emirates

The United Arab Emirates (UAE) is made up of seven emirates: Abu Dhabi, Ajman, Dubai, Fujairah, Ras al-Khaimah, Sharjah, and Umm al-Qaiwain. Healthcare in the UAE is regulated at both the federal and emirate levels. The Ministry of Health and Prevention regulates the health sector at the federal level, sets national health policies, and regulates the northern emirates. The Dubai Health Authority (DHA) and the Health Authority of Abu Dhabi (HAAD) regulate the healthcare sector in Dubai and Abu Dhabi, respectively.

The UAE government is seeking to improve its healthcare infrastructure and expand its healthcare sector to reach higher international standards.

Access the healthcare financing data sets provided by WHO and/or the World Bank for the UAE in the years from 2000 to 2014. Tabulate and graphically present the following core indicators:

- Total health expenditure (THE) per capita (in international and US dollars)
- THE as a percentage of GDP
- General government health expenditure as a proportion of total general government expenditure (GGHE/GGE)
- The ratio of household out-of-pocket (OOP) payments for health to THE

Case Study Discussion Questions

1. Given the UAE's economic situation, is the percentage of the national budget that goes toward health reasonable? Compare the UAE to two other countries in the Middle East and North Africa (MENA) region. Also compare it to a high-income country (HIC) of your choice. Do your findings for the UAE reflect a strong government commitment to health? Review and summarize the strategic plan for HAAD and DHA. Discuss.
2. What does the assessment of OOP catastrophic expenditure show in terms of health finance mechanisms? Focusing on this issue, compare the UAE to two other countries within the MENA region and to a HIC of your choice. Discuss.
3. Build a health outcomes country profile (including life expectancy, maternal mortality, infant mortality, and communicable and noncommunicable diseases) for the UAE.
4. Based on your analysis, offer one healthcare financing policy recommendation.

National Healthcare Expenditures

The provision of healthcare requires time, education, training, specialized machinery, and a host of other finite resources. However, at the most basic level, total healthcare expenditures are a function of three factors: (1) the population receiving health-related services, (2) the number of services rendered per individual in the population, and (3) the underlying costs of the services being provided. For the purposes of this chapter, these factors will be referred to as *population*, *intensity*, and *price*. When the population, intensity of utilization, and price per service increase, so do national expenditures.

To allow for cross-national comparisons and to control for the significant population differences that exist among nations, expenses are often expressed per capita. However, even when population variances are accounted for, substantial differences in expenditure persist, as shown in exhibit 2.1. This remaining variation is driven by differences in price per service and in the intensity of services being consumed per individual. For example, individuals in Taiwan may receive more prescription drugs to treat hypertension than people in Italy do, and those prescriptions may be more expensive in one country than in another.

Variation in price and utilization intensity is anchored to the unique sociocultural values of nations and their related approaches to organizing and paying for healthcare. Governments often intervene in markets in an attempt to optimize outcomes and arrive at levels of price and intensity that reflect national desires. Such actions are consistent with **Keynesian economics**—a school of economics, named after John Maynard Keynes, that maintains that active government involvement to influence demand (primarily) can lead to optimal economic performance. A Keynesian approach might adjust the supply of healthcare providers and facilities, limit the pricing power of providers, or implement some mixture of those approaches. Alternatively, governments may pursue an approach more consistent with **laissez-faire economics**, in which markets are allowed to reach equilibrium in an environment with limited government intervention.

National Interventions

The differing approaches to government intervention can be illustrated by comparing France and the United States. Much of the French system, especially its more costly acute care aspects, is centrally planned, with controls on both supply and price. The United States, meanwhile, uses a more laissez-faire approach.

Within France, the Ministry of Social Affairs, Health, and Women's Rights is responsible for developing a national strategy to provide care and promote the health of French citizens. The strategy intentionally manages the number and location of public hospitals, public health programs, and publicly financed health centers (Rodwin 2003; Rodwin and Sandier 1993). Moreover, controls on capital expenditures and construction were introduced in 1970, and they set standards in place for the acquisition of new medical technologies (Rodwin and Sandier 1993). Even if demand exists for additional services, government-mandated supply constraints put a cap on the number and intensity of services that can be rendered. At the same time, the central government works with regional authorities to set budgets for hospitals, ambulatory care, mental health, and services to older adults and people with disabilities, along with general pricing controls. More than 78 percent of France's healthcare expenditures are funded through the French government, with the remaining 22 percent funded through private markets.

Keynesian economics
A school of economics, named after John Maynard Keynes, that maintains that active government involvement to influence demand (primarily) can lead to optimal economic performance.

laissez-faire economics
A school of economics that maintains that government involvement in the economy creates market frictions and interference that detract from optimal economic performance.

Exhibit 2.2 uses a classical supply-and-demand curve to help illustrate the effect of interventions like those implemented in France. As France limits the supply of healthcare providers, the quantity of services consumed shifts from quantity point G toward quantity point H, and the price of goods increases from price point B toward price point C. The restricted supply leads to a distinct possibility of unmet demand. Individuals would then be willing to pay more to have their healthcare needs or demands met, and prices would naturally drift higher. However, by simultaneously limiting the price of healthcare services through the use of a fixed and centrally planned budget, a second constraint is introduced. Prices are kept from drifting upward, because total expenses (price of goods × quantity of goods) are determined beforehand. The resulting downward government pressure on price and the government-imposed restriction of supply allow France to allocate its resources in a manner and at a cost acceptable to its constituents, at point E (price point B and quantity point H).

The United States, like Singapore and South Korea, has opted for a less planned system, relying more heavily on a laissez-faire, private market approach. More than 51 percent of all US healthcare expenditures are financed by individuals or employers within the United States (World Bank 2017). The US government does not regularly employ supply constraints, although such constraints may be used by private health insurers and some clinical training programs. Outside of some state-sponsored certificates of need, healthcare providers and facilities are generally able to practice where they wish. Moreover, with the exception of some distinct subpopulations, healthcare providers are able to charge what consumers and private insurers are willing to pay. Under this approach, the price and quantity of services are at the intersection of the demand and supply curves, at point F (quantity point G and price point B).

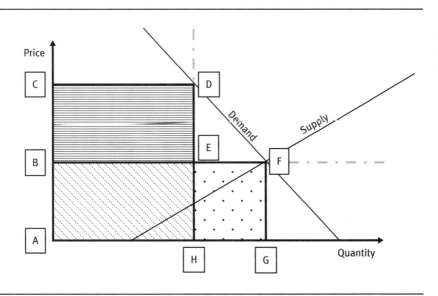

EXHIBIT 2.2
Impact of
Supply and
Demand
Constraints

Regardless of a nation's dependence on or intervention in markets, national health expenditures per capita remain a function of average cost per service and the average number of services per individual.[1] In exhibit 2.2, the rectangle formed by points ABFG represents the area where no supply or pricing constraints have been introduced. Rectangle ACDH represents the area in which the supply of healthcare is limited and no constraint is placed on pricing. Restrictions on supply may include, for example, constraints on the number of imaging machines, caps on the number of specialists, or checks on the number and placement of long-term and acute care facilities. In such instances, fewer services are rendered, but the cost per service is significantly higher, because individuals have unmet demand and are willing to pay more. The potential reduction in national health expenditures is therefore muted, and an increase in total expenditures may even occur.

To counter the higher costs per service that may accompany supply-side restrictions, governments and private insurers may adopt mechanisms to reduce consumer demand simultaneously. Such mechanisms, applied to exhibit 2.2, can effectively reduce the ACDH rectangle (supply-side limitations only) to the area of the ABEH rectangle (supply-side and demand-side limitations). Many demand-side mechanisms aimed at reducing expenditures rely on individual price sensitivities; they use pricing tools (e.g., copayments, deductibles, increased price sharing) to drive down the quantity of healthcare services rendered and, consequently, total healthcare expenditures. From a classical economics perspective, as individuals are asked to bear more financial responsibility, their willingness to consume decreases, and they generally seek fewer healthcare services. Although exceptions certainly exist in instances involving urgent or lifesaving care, the tendency for price increases to drive down consumption remains true in aggregate.

Another way to limit the quantity of services rendered is to limit people's eligibility to receive healthcare goods and services. When fewer individuals are available to consume healthcare, the aggregate number of services provided decreases. Similarly, changing what healthcare services are covered under a plan can also lower medical expenses. If a benefit scheme becomes more restrictive, individuals will not be able to consume the number of healthcare services they would have consumed without the restrictions. In both scenarios (limits on eligibility and restrictions on the services covered), total medical expenses are reduced at the cost of unmet demand. Individuals may be left without coverage or, if they are insured, without coverage for a particular intervention.

Predicting Healthcare Costs

contingent loss
A financial loss that occurs if an adverse health event occurs.

Regardless of the differences in the ways healthcare delivery systems are organized, the mechanisms for predicting general health expenditures remain remarkably similar (Lynch 1992). Governments or insurance firms, collectively referred to as *payers*, exchange an individual's **contingent losses** (in the event that the individual falls ill or needs or seeks care) for a fee. That fee may be a direct premium paid for by the consumer (as in the case of private insurance), or it may be paid for indirectly through tax revenues (as is the case with universal or social insurance coverage).

In a well-functioning system, payers first estimate the contingent losses or expenses for the covered population. The estimate incorporates the size of the eligible population, the intensity of utilization per person, and the cost of services to be provided. To determine total health expenditures, payers must project the probability that members of a predetermined target population will need or seek care. This probability represents the **health status risk** (also called the *population health risk*). The health status risk is then paired with the **medical care risk**—the estimated cost of providing care in the event that an individual seeks an intervention. Multiplying the probability of needing healthcare (health status risk) with the interventional costs (medical care risk) gives rise to the **expected medical cost** for an individual.

The expected medical costs can then be applied across the entire insured population to arrive at a global estimate of healthcare costs.[2] The process of calculating the expected medical costs is commonly known as the **underwriting methodology**. It relies on large data sets and actuarial tables to determine the average health status and medical care risk for a target population. The calculation and use of predicted medical expenses typically depend on national, social, and cultural norms. The methodology may reflect the idea of solidarity among individuals, with mutual aid between the sick and well, or it may stress individual responsibility and autonomy.

After medical expenses are projected, the **loading factors**—the overhead costs incurred while administering to the insured population—are considered. These administrative expenses cover such areas as auditing, clinician and facility oversight, utilization management, and, in the cases of private, investor-owned firms, profit. If the projected medical and administrative costs are unacceptably high, overhead expenses can be cut, or demand- and supply-side tools may be employed. The aggregate costs (medical plus overhead expenses) drive a total fee that must be paid out of pocket, through a supplementary insurance premium, through an employer/employee tax, or from government tax revenue.

Healthcare Delivery Models

Ultimately, governmental financing of healthcare aims to balance the benefits associated with the provision of health services with the negative impacts often associated with taxation. By funding a portion or the entirety of healthcare expenses, nations provide access to goods and services that increase life spans and improve workforce productivity through higher functionality and reduced absenteeism. More generally, they are providing access to healthcare that contributes

health status risk
The probability that a member of a target population will need or seek care; also called *population health risk*.

medical care risk
The cost of providing care in the event that an individual seeks an intervention.

expected medical cost
A measure calculated by multiplying the health status risk for an individual by the medical care risk.

underwriting methodology
The process of pooling individuals together and calculating the expected medical costs; it requires prediction of both health status risk and medical care risk for the population.

loading factors
The overhead costs incurred while administering to the insured population.

positively to both the productivity and the psychosocial fabric of the country. At the same time, however, the provision of those services requires a financing mechanism that introduces market frictions, imperfections, and transaction costs that distort the supply and demand of healthcare (Rice 1997; Romer and Romer 2007). Excise, employment, income, or consumption taxes that are too large can potentially have a number of negative consequences. Although debate on the issue continues (Blanchard and Perotti 1999), high effective tax rates have the potential to hinder capital investment, discourage innovation, and serve as a drag on employment markets (Eaton and Rosen 1980; Pissarides 1998).

Another concern is that healthcare can potentially crowd out other important areas related to national well-being, such as education, infrastructure, and social assistance programs. Among Organisation for Economic Co-operation and Development (OECD) member countries, total government spending as a percentage of GDP varies from a low of 33.46 percent in Switzerland to a high of 56.96 percent in Finland (see exhibit 2.3). Of those government expenditures, health-related goods and services account for an average of 16.21 percent. By individual country, that percentage ranges from 6.45 percent in Slovakia to more than 27.44 percent in the United States.

National health expenses are heavily influenced by the way healthcare is paid for and delivered. Although no two countries organize their healthcare in the same way, nations generally subscribe to one of four primary models: (1) universal coverage, (2) social insurance, (3) national insurance, or (4) private pay. Any model selected can be supplemented with elements of the remaining models, and more nuanced classification schemes can be pursued (Cortés 2017; Joumand, André, and Nicq 2010). For example, Sweden uses a universal model to deliver 95 percent of all care; the remaining 5 percent is distributed using a private pay insurance model to cover some elective services (Thomson et al. 2012).

Universal Coverage

universal coverage
A healthcare delivery model that is financed through general tax revenue and covers all citizens; also called the Beveridge model.

Universal coverage is paid for through general tax revenue and covers all citizens (Doron 1994). It is sometimes called the Beveridge model, in honor of William Beveridge, who instituted England's national program in 1948. Within the universal coverage model, central and regional governments are tasked with estimating health status and medical care risk for their entire population while simultaneously keeping costs in check. Most universal systems have little to no cost sharing, so they must employ supply-side tools to more heavily influence the healthcare infrastructure and overall expenses. This aim is primarily achieved through government management and ownership of facilities and healthcare equipment or through direct provider employment (Reid 2010; Simonet 2010). For example, Spain has a universal coverage model that is financed by the taxes of the entire population, has an extensive network of health centers, and does not usually have a copayment for health services (except for pharmaceutical copayments). The

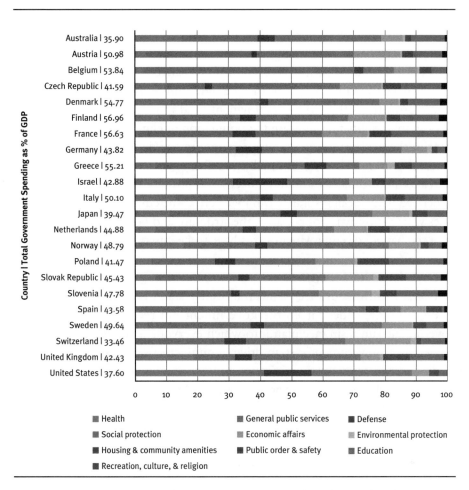

EXHIBIT 2.3
Government
Spending by
Category (2014)

Source: Data from the Organisation for Economic Co-operation and Development (2018).

United Kingdom, Italy, New Zealand, and Greece are also among the countries with universal coverage; not surprisingly, exhibit 2.1 shows that government expenditures account for the majority of their total healthcare expenditures.

Social Insurance Systems

Social insurance systems, or tax-based systems, were heavily influenced by Prussian Chancelor Otto von Bismarck, who instituted a social welfare program in the nineteenth century to cover accidents, disability, and retirement for the Prussian working population (Lee and Mir 2014; Wallace 2013). As a result, they are sometimes known as Bismarck systems. Unlike universal coverage, where the factors of production are predominantly owned by the government, the healthcare infrastructure within social insurance systems can be owned by either the government or private industry. Much of Latin America, Germany, and Japan have pursued the social insurance model, and such nations generally fund their programs through employment-related taxes. The associated tax

social insurance
A healthcare delivery model in which a benefits package is funded through employment-related taxes; the healthcare infrastructure in such systems can be owned by either the government or private industry.

revenue is then earmarked and set aside for future health expenses. These funds are kept separate from other tax revenues to avoid being subject to legislative impulses and to prevent comingling. In many countries, these funds are managed by independent entities separate from the government.

Social insurance programs may be significantly affected by general economic downturns that affect employment (and the associated tax revenue), demographic shifts that increase the population of eligible citizens, or reductions in the proportion of workers paying into the designated health funds. Whereas universal coverage is usually paid from general tax revenues that can be reallocated to meet a country's needs and priorities, the designated funds associated with social insurance can make cross-subsidizing more difficult. In cases where subsidy is not possible, the structure and benefits of the program have to change, or employment taxes have to be raised.

National Health Insurance

national health insurance
A healthcare delivery model in which providers are independent from the government but receive payment from a government-run insurance plan into which everyone is required to pay.

National health insurance blends the Bismarck and Beveridge models. Providers are independent from the government but receive payment from a government-run insurance plan into which everyone is required to pay. The single-payer, government system drives a number of benefits. Overhead and loading factors are kept to a minimum, because there is no marketing or profit incentive for the payer. Moreover, as a result of the single-payer system, governments are able to exert significant pricing controls to constrain costs. They can also curtail utilization by limiting the benefits covered by insurance. Tommy Douglas successfully championed national health insurance within Canada in 1962 (Reid 2010). The model was later pursued by South Korea and Taiwan.

Private Insurance or Out-of-Pocket Systems

Private insurance programs are financed through individual or employer contributions, and they are built upon the same foundation of health and medical care risk prediction. Programs in private insurance markets must be able to entice individuals to participate. Governments—those of Australia or Singapore, for instance—may use tax credits or other financial incentives to encourage people's participation in private markets, but private insurers do not have the force of government to compel participation. To induce membership, these private programs must promise to make average participants better off than they would be if they did not participate in the insurance market. From a classical economics perspective, competition for membership and revenue drives costs down, and market forces match the provider infrastructure to consumer preferences. The factors of production are held privately with little or no government influence.

Even in countries where universal coverage or social insurance is offered by a government, supplemental private markets almost always exist to provide access to goods or services that might not be covered by the existing national plan or that require significant wait time. The prevalence of supplemental, private insurance is highly dependent on the benefits and wait times of the Beveridge, Bismarck, and national health insurance models.

High-deductible health plans (HDHPs) are a variant of private insurance and out-of-pocket systems, and they have become increasingly popular as a way of allocating health goods and services. HDHPs cover "catastrophic," or very high-cost, medical services, are often paired with health savings accounts, and have high deductibles or copayments. The product's premise is to offer a low-cost premium and to expose the healthcare consumer to the financial consequences of their consumption behavior. Evidence suggests that consumers in HDHPs may not be effective price shoppers and may avoid preventive services and needed ambulatory care. Such plans may have a differential impact on people with low socioeconomic status or those with chronic conditions (Waters et al. 2011; Zhang et al. 2017).

high-deductible health plan (HDHP)
A variant of private insurance and out-of-pocket systems that covers "catastrophic" services, is often paired with a health savings account, and has high deductibles or copayments.

Vignette: Latin American Health Systems

Health systems in Latin America offer various mixes of the healthcare delivery models discussed in this section.

Colombia has a two-tier system that covers 96.6 percent of the population (OECD 2015). One tier provides access to both for-profit and not-for-profit insurance products, primarily uses private providers, and covers 49.2 percent of the population. The second tier covers 45.3 percent of the population, is government subsidized, uses both for-profit and not-for-profit insurance products, and uses public providers. Both tiers must offer the same package of services. Chile has a dual system covering 70 percent of the population, with a public insurance product financed by a mix of employment and general taxes. The public insurance product uses both private and public providers. The other 30 percent of the population is covered by private, for-profit insurers, partially financed by employment-related taxes, additional premiums, and out-of-pocket payments.

Brazil's Unified Health System (UHS), financed by general taxes, covers 100 percent of the population, as well as foreign nationals. It provides access to public providers and facilities. In reality, however, 25 percent of the population opts to pay private insurers to guarantee access, reduce wait times, and use services not covered by the UHS.

The Costa Rican system is financed by a mix of employment and general tax revenues, and it provides access to (primarily) public providers through a public social insurance organization. It covers approximately 85 percent of the population.

The Mechanics of Insurance

Private insurance exists in nearly every nation, either as the primary method for distributing healthcare or as a supplemental system. For private or supplemental insurance to succeed, the people seeking coverage must have **risk aversion**—meaning that the insured population has declining marginal utility. An alternative way of thinking about this population is that the people's **utility** is affected more severely by a loss than by a gain of the same magnitude. Although most individuals have behaviors and preferences that are indifferent to risk or even risk seeking, most individuals have some measure of risk aversion when it comes to health.

In a stylized and simplistic example of how private insurance markets function, imagine two states of health mapped onto a declining marginal utility curve (see exhibit 2.4). The vertical axis represents the measure of an individual's satisfaction or economic utility, and the horizontal axis represents income or wealth. As income increases, so does utility, but it does so at a declining rate. The relationship is nonlinear. More income creates more utility, but the impact of the additional income declines as the population or individual makes more money.

In the example in exhibit 2.4, imagine that individuals have a 50 percent chance of being healthy and having no medical expenses and a 50 percent chance of being sick. If individuals are healthy, they have the full $40,000 in discretionary funds. If sick, they incur $20,000 in healthcare expenses or lost wages. Because medical expenses reduce discretionary

risk aversion
A tendency to reduce uncertainty; in healthcare, this uncertainty is primarily associated with adverse medical events and the associated financial costs.

utility
The representation of the satisfaction experienced by consumers of goods and services; the higher the satisfaction, the greater the associated utility.

EXHIBIT 2.4
Declining Marginal Utility Curve

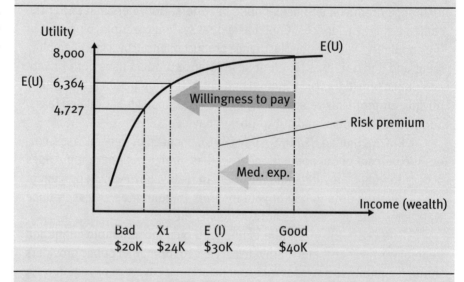

income to $20,000, individuals who are healthy and have more discretionary income have a higher utility (8,000 units) than those who are sick and have less income (4,727 units).

Unfortunately, individuals cannot determine in which state of health they will find themselves. However, through the use of underwriting techniques, insurance firms can estimate average medical expenses by calculating the probability of a person falling ill (health status risk) and the costs associated with seeking care (medical care risk). In our example, we have established that the probability of illness is 50 percent (or 0.5) and the cost associated with seeking care is $20,000. By multiplying the 0.5 probability by the $20,000 in medical goods and services, we arrive at expected medical costs of $10,000.

Expected medical costs = (0.5 probability of health × $0
in medical expenses) + (0.5 probability of sickness × $20,000
in medical expenses) = $10,000

If this scenario is replicated multiple times, over multiple years, or applied to a population with similar risk factors, individuals should expect to incur $10,000 in medical expenses, which would leave them with an expected income of $30,000.

To understand how individuals are enticed to participate in voluntary insurance programs based on the promise of a higher average utility, we need to calculate the expected utility in addition to the expected medical costs or income. The expected utility is calculated in the same manner as the expected income. In the healthy state, individuals have $40,000 in disposable income and 8,000 utility units. In the sick state, they have $20,000 in income and 4,727 utility units. Given the two states of the world, with a 50 percent chance of health and higher utility and a 50 percent chance of sickness and lower utility, an expected utility can be computed.

Expected utility = (0.5 probability of sickness × 4,727 utility units)
+ (0.5 probability of full health × 8,000 utility units) = 6,364

This number represents the average, expected level of satisfaction that will occur for the individual or the population in the absence of any insurance.

Voluntary insurance works precisely because of the concave nature of the utility curve and the fact that the expected income and the income associated with the expected utility are not the same. In our example, in the absence of insurance, individuals will, on average, experience a level of utility or satisfaction near 6,364. To achieve that level of utility, individuals would need $24,000 in disposable income. A well-functioning insurance

(continued)

market guarantees individuals higher utility by charging a premium that leaves them with more than $24,000 in disposable income. The resulting utility after paying for insurance is higher than where the individual would expect to be in the absence of coverage. The insurance guarantees that the individual will never experience the full $20,000 income loss associated with falling ill. The difference between the income in the good state and the income associated with expected utility is referred to as the *consumers' willingness to pay*. If insurers charge too much—such that less than $24,000 is left in disposable income—consumers will opt to go without insurance. The premium drops the expected utility below where the consumer would be, on average, without the insurance.

For insurance firms to remain viable, they must charge enough to pay the expected medical costs while also generating enough money to cover the administrative costs associated with claims administration, contracting, marketing, and so on (i.e., loading factors). As long as the insurance firms charge a premium that covers medical expenses and loading factors while also leaving individuals with more than $24,000 in disposable income, individuals will opt to purchase insurance, and the insurance firm will meet its medical expense and administrative obligations.

Provider Payment Mechanisms

Not surprisingly, the ways that healthcare providers are paid also influence practice patterns, the consumption of goods, and, ultimately, national health expenditures. Because clinicians receive specialized training and certifications that the general citizenry does not receive, information asymmetry exists between patients and providers. As a result, clinicians have the ability to induce demand and consumption that may or may not be needed or beneficial. Patients must rely not only on the superior training of those providing care but also on the belief that clinicians will act in their best interests. Ample evidence suggests that providers change their practice behavior in response to changes in how they are paid (Barnum, Kutzin, and Saxenian 1995; Colla et al. 2012; Yip and Eggleston 2001). Sometimes, these changes are conscious responses, and sometimes they result from unconscious variability in the practice of medicine. Governments and private insurers have taken note of provider responses and attempted to align payment incentives with desired clinical behavior.

Although providers may be paid in a variety of ways, these ways are largely variants of two main payment models: (1) a fee-for-service model and (2) a prospective payment system or fixed payment model.

EXHIBIT 2.5
Fee-for-Service
Profit Incentive

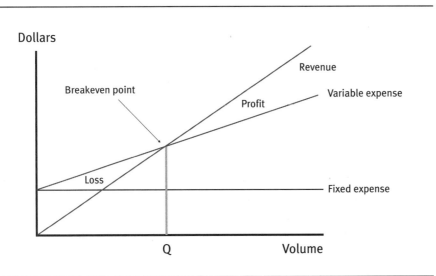

Fee-for-Service Payment Models

Under a **fee-for-service (FFS)** model, providers are paid on a per-occurrence basis, and the profit incentive functions as shown in exhibit 2.5. Fixed expenses remain flat, and variable expenses increase as more services are rendered. At the same time, revenue also depends on the volume of services. If no services are provided, providers do not generate any revenue. At low volumes, revenue is being generated, but it does not offset the fixed and variable expenses. When total revenues equal total expenses, providers are said to have reached the **breakeven point**. In the FFS environment, providers want to deliver as much care as possible to get as far past the breakeven point as is allowable. Every service provided after the breakeven point has been reached leads to additional profit.

Because the natural provider response under an FFS model is to supply as many services as possible, a number of governments have opted to pay frontline primary care physicians using this framework. From a resource allocation perspective, primary care physicians are the first party responsible for managing patient health, and they are substantially less expensive than specialists and hospitals. By encouraging high volume at the primary care level, an FFS framework has the ability to reduce the projected medical expense by actively managing everything from chronic disease to preventive services in such a way that more advanced and expensive medicine is altogether avoided. In other words, an FFS payment scheme incentivizes primary care physicians to keep patients out of facilities. Singapore, Switzerland, Germany, and Australia are among the countries that have moved primary care payment to an almost exclusive FFS basis.

fee-for-service (FFS)
A payment model in which providers are paid on a per-occurrence basis.

breakeven point
The point at which total revenues equal total expenses.

Prospective Payment System Models

Whereas the FFS model incentivizes providers to deliver as many services as possible, **prospective payment system (PPS)** or fixed payment models provide an incentive to limit volume. The profit incentive for such models is shown in exhibit 2.6. Under a PPS model, providers are paid a predetermined, flat fee to render predetermined services to a predetermined population for a predetermined period. In this environment, revenue per individual or facility is flat within the predetermined time frame. As clinicians or facilities provide more services, their fixed costs remain flat, and their variable costs increase. Because the revenue is flat and the total expenses are growing, expenses will at some point equal the revenue. This point represents the breakeven point. Once the breakeven point has been reached, any additional services rendered result in financial loss. Thus, providers can maintain financial viability or achieve profits by constraining the volume of services rendered.

Global budgets, capitation, case rates, diagnosis-related groups, and composite rates are all modified fixed payment models. Recognizing that facilities and specialists tend to be significant cost drivers, nations such as Australia, New Zealand, and France have moved toward the use of global budget and case-based payment models to keep facilities and high-cost providers from delivering more services than necessary. The danger in these environments is not overproduction of healthcare services but rather underproduction.

Pay-for-Performance and Value-Based Contracting

A number of governments have begun pairing fixed payment models with performance and quality incentives (Aryankhesal, Sheldon, and Manion 2013; Bowser et al. 2013). These **pay-for-performance (P4P)** models, sometimes

EXHIBIT 2.6
Prospective Payment System Profit Incentive

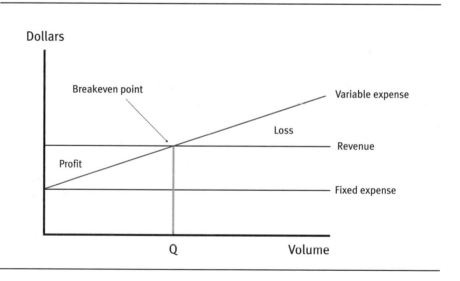

called *value-based contracting or purchasing arrangements*, reward or penalize providers depending on their adherence to predetermined standards. This approach can mitigate the potential underprovision of care associated with fixed payment models while also encouraging providers to meet quality standards. Providers may receive P4P adjustments in the form of an increase or decrease to the case rate or global budget, or, in some circumstances, as a one-time deposit (Damberg et al. 2009). Regardless of the form, the P4P incentives aim to drive improvements in quality and to offset the additional costs incurred by providers in adhering to clinical best practices. Successful P4P programs have tended to be narrow and targeted, and they have documented improvements in composite measures of quality; overall, however, research findings about the impact of P4P programs on health outcomes appear mixed (Wilson 2013).

Population health initiatives have been explored as another methodology for reducing total health expenditures. Initiatives such as community smoking-cessation programs and the heavy taxation of soft drinks aim to keep individuals healthy and reduce the likelihood of falling ill and seeking care. Many population health interventions have yet to be globally adopted, and research concerning their effectiveness is limited.

Summary

Contextual understanding of how healthcare is organized and funded within a particular country is a critical aspect of global healthcare management. Successful healthcare organizations appreciate the unique sociocultural factors that influence the adoption of various structures and processes, ranging from Keynesian interventions to approaches rooted in laissez-faire economics. Moreover, successful healthcare enterprises have the ability to position themselves to take advantage of private and social insurance opportunities, understand clinical payment methodologies and incentives, and can effectively predict not only healthcare-related risk but international business risk as well. In the next chapter, the focus will transition from the macroeconomic level to the organizational level. Specifically, it will address how a global operation identifies and manages risk, finds capital, and ensures effective asset management within foreign cultural, institutional, and economic environments.

Notes

1. National health expenditures = Quantity of services (Total population × Average number of services per person) × Average cost per service.

2. Depending on the forum, the expected medical costs for a population may also be called the *pure premium* or the *actuarially fair premium.*

Discussion Questions

1. Health financing systems distribute resources through revenue raising, pooling, and purchasing arrangements. Describe these healthcare financing functions, and give two examples of each for a healthcare system of your choice.
2. Knowledge of the characteristics of the various sources of revenue can help us understand the healthcare financing situation in a particular country. Direct taxes are one source of revenue collected for health services. List and explain the other sources, and give specific country examples.
3. What are the three macroeconomic drivers of national health expenditures?
4. What are the primary healthcare delivery methods that countries have employed, and how do they attempt to influence the factors of production?
   a. Which use demand-side tools?
   b. Which use supply-side tools?
5. What role does a nation's sociocultural foundation play in determining the delivery model and supply-and-demand mechanism used to influence health expenditures?
6. When are individuals likely to participate in voluntary insurance markets? Why?
7. Why do well-functioning insurance markets require the insured population to be risk averse?
8. How do payments to clinicians influence health expenditures?
   a. What is the natural provider response in a fee-for-service environment?
   b. What is the natural provider response in a capitated, fixed payment, or diagnosis-related group environment?
   c. How have payers attempted to mitigate that impact?

References

Aryankhesal, A., T. A. Sheldon, and R. Manion. 2013. "Role of Pay-for-Performance in a Hospital Performance Measurement System: A Multiple Case Study in Iran." *Health Policy and Planning* 28 (2): 206–14.

Barnum, H., J. Kutzin, and H. Saxenian. 1995. "Incentives and Provider Payment Methods." *International Journal of Health Planning and Management* 10 (1): 23–45.

Blanchard, O., and R. Perotti. 1999. "An Empirical Characterization of the Dynamic Effects of Changes in Government Spending and Taxes on Output." National Bureau of Economic Research. Published July. www.nber.org/papers/w7269.

Bowser, D. M., R. Figueroa, L. Natiq, and A. Okunogbe. 2013. "A Preliminary Assessment of Financial Stability, Efficiency, Health Systems and Health Outcomes Using Performance-Based Contracts in Belize." *Global Public Health* 8 (9): 1063–74.

Colla, C. H., N. E. Morden, J. S. Skinner, J. R. Hoverman, and E. Meara. 2012. "Impact of Payment Reform on Chemotherapy at the End of Life." *Journal of Oncology Practice* 8 (3S): e6s–e13s.

Cortés, A. E. 2017. "Grupos relacionados por el diagnóstico: Evaluación de la factibilidad de implementación en hospitales en Colombia." Universidad Rey Juan Carlos, Madrid, Spain.

Damberg, C. L., K. Raube, S. S. Teleki, and E. Dela Cruz. 2009. "Taking Stock of Pay-for-Performance: A Candid Assessment from the Front Lines." *Health Affairs* 28 (2): 517–25.

Doron, A. 1994. "The Effectiveness of the Beveridge Model at Different Stages of Socio-economic Development: The Israeli Experience." In *Beveridge and Social Security: An International Retrospective*, edited by J. Hills, J. Ditch, and H. Glennerster, 189–202. Oxford, UK: Clarendon Press.

Eaton, J., and H. S. Rosen. 1980. "Taxation, Human Capital, and Uncertainty." *American Economic Review* 70 (4): 705–15.

Heller, M. P. S. 2005. "Understanding Fiscal Space." International Monetary Fund. Published March. www.imf.org/external/pubs/ft/pdp/2005/pdp04.pdf.

Joumand, L., C. André, and C. Nicq. 2010. "Health Creation System, Efficiency and Institutions." Working document no. 769. Organisation for Economic Co-operation and Development, Department of Economics, Paris, France.

Jowett, M., M. P. Brunal, G. Flores, and J. Cylus. 2016. *Spending Targets for Health: No Magic Number.* World Health Organization. Accessed April 11, 2018. http://apps.who.int/iris/bitstream/handle/10665/250048/WHO-HIS-HGF-HFWorkingPaper-16.1-eng.pdf.

Kutzin, J., S. Witter, M. Jowett, and D. Bayarsaikhan. 2017. *Developing a National Health Financing Strategy: A Reference Guide.* World Health Organization. Accessed April 11, 2018. www.who.int/health_financing/documents/health-financing-strategy/en/.

Lee, D. S., and H. R. Mir. 2014. "Global Systems of Health Care and Trauma." *Journal of Orthopaedic Trauma* 28: S8–S10.

Lynch, M. E. 1992. *Health Insurance Terminology: A Glossary.* Washington, DC: Health Insurance Association of America.

McIntyre, D., and J. Kutzin. 2016. "Health Financing Country Diagnostic: A Foundation for National Strategy Development." World Health Organization. Accessed April 11, 2018. http://apps.who.int/iris/bitstream/handle/10665/204283/9789241510110_eng.pdf.

Organisation for Economic Co-operation and Development (OECD). 2018. "Central Government Spending." Accessed February 18. https://data.oecd.org/gga/central-government-spending.htm.

———. 2015. *OECD Reviews of Health Systems: Columbia 2016*. Paris, France: OECD Publishing.

Pissarides, C. A. 1998. "The Impact of Employment Tax Cuts on Unemployment and Wages; The Role of Unemployment Benefits and Tax Structure." *European Economic Review* 42 (1): 155–83.

Reid, T. R. 2010. *The Healing of America: A Global Quest for Better, Cheaper, and Fairer Health Care*. New York: Penguin.

Rice, T. 1997. "Can Markets Give Us the Health System We Want?" *Journal of Health Politics, Policy and Law* 22 (2): 383–426.

Rodwin, V. G. 2003. "The Health Care System Under French National Health Insurance: Lessons for Health Reform in the United States." *American Journal of Public Health* 93 (1): 31–37.

Rodwin, V. G., and S. Sandier. 1993. "Health Care Under French National Health Insurance." *Health Affairs* 12 (3): 111–31.

Romer, C. D., and D. H. Romer. 2007. "The Macroeconomic Effects of Tax Changes: Estimates Based on a New Measure of Fiscal Shocks." National Bureau of Economic Research working paper. Published July. www.nber.org/papers/w13264.

Shibuya, K., C. Ciecierski, E. Guindon, D. W. Bettcher, D. B. Evans, and J. C. Murray. 2003. "WHO Framework Convention on Tobacco Control: Development of an Evidence Based Global Public Health Treaty." *BMJ* 327 (7407): 154–57.

Simonet, D. 2010. "Healthcare Reforms and Cost Reduction Strategies in Europe: The Cases of Germany, UK, Switzerland, Italy and France." *International Journal of Health Care Quality Assurance* 23 (5): 470–88.

Thomson, S., R. Osborn, D. Squires, and M. Jun (eds.). 2012. *International Profiles of Health Care Systems, 2012: Australia, Canada, Denmark, England, France, Germany, Italy, Japan, the Netherlands, New Zealand, Norway, Sweden, Switzerland, and the United States*. Commonwealth Fund. Published November. www.commonwealthfund.org/~/media/Files/Publications/Fund%20Report/2012/Nov/1645_Squires_intl_profiles_hlt_care_systems_2012.pdf.

Wallace, L. S. 2013. "A View of Health Care Around the World." *Annals of Family Medicine* 11 (1): 84.

Waters, T. M., C. F. Chang, W. T. Cecil, P. Kasteridis, and D. Mirvis. 2011. "Impact of High-Deductible Health Plans on Health Care Utilization and Costs." *Health Services Research* 46 (1): 155–72.

Wilson, K. J. 2013. "Pay-for-Performance in Health Care: What Can We Learn from International Experience?" *Quality Management in Health Care* 22 (1): 2–15.

World Bank. 2018. "Health Expenditure, Total (% of GDP)." Accessed April 11. http://data.worldbank.org/indicator/SH.XPD.TOTL.ZS.

———. 2017. "World Development Indicators: Health Systems." Accessed April 11, 2018. http://wdi.worldbank.org/table/2.12.

World Health Organization (WHO). 2016. "Fiscal Policies for Diet and Prevention of Noncommunicable Diseases: Technical Meeting Report, 5–6 May 2015, Geneva, Switzerland." Accessed April 11, 2018. http://apps.who.int/iris/bitstream/handle/10665/250131/9789241511247-eng.pdf.

———. 2010. *The World Health Report—Health Systems Financing: The Path to Universal Coverage.* Accessed April 11, 2018. http://apps.who.int/iris/bitstream/handle/10665/44371/9789241564021_eng.pdf.

———. 2008. "Health Systems Financing." Published June. www.who.int/healthinfo/statistics/toolkit_hss/EN_PDF_Toolkit_HSS_Financing.pdf.

———. 2000. *The World Health Report 2000—Health Systems: Improving Performance.* Accessed April 11, 2018. www.who.int/whr/2000/en/.

Yip, W., and K. Eggleston. 2001. "Provider Payment Reform in China: The Case of Hospital Reimbursement in Hainan Province." *Health Economics* 10 (4): 325–39.

Zhang, X., A. Haviland, A. Mehrotra, P. Huckfeldt, Z. Wagner, and N. Sood. 2017. "Does Enrollment in High-Deductible Health Plans Encourage Price Shopping?" *Health Services Research.* Published October 23. https://onlinelibrary.wiley.com/doi/pdf/10.1111/1475-6773.12784.

FINANCIAL MANAGEMENT OF HEALTHCARE ORGANIZATIONS

Kevin D. Broom, PhD, Jason S. Turner, PhD, David Wyant, PhD, Francisco Yepes, MD, DrPH, and Ariel Cortés, MD, PhD

Chapter Focus

In this chapter, we focus on micro-level considerations unique to the types of financial decisions that managers face when health organizations operate within complex national and multinational environments. We first discuss the primary long-term financial planning process and the major financial decision-making tools used by healthcare managers. We next examine the long-term financial risks and implications that organizations must adequately address when operating within existing markets, when expanding their scale or scope of operations within existing markets, and when entering new markets. Later in the chapter, we discuss the primary short-term financial planning skills used by healthcare managers. Finally, we address a number of the short-term financial risks and concerns that organizations face when financing the day-to-day healthcare delivery in national or multinational settings.

Learning Objectives

Upon completion of this chapter, you should be able to

- identify and prioritize the primary concepts and tools used by health managers for both long- and short-term financial decision making;
- analyze major sources of financial risk to global operations when transitioning from national to multinational settings;
- assess the major sources of investment capital for healthcare organizations, both within national settings and across multinational settings; and
- modify long- and short-term financial management processes for foreign cultural, institutional, and economic environments.

Competencies

- Analyze problems, promote solutions, and encourage decision making in support of short- and long-term financial goals.
- Evaluate whether proposed actions align with and financially support the organizational business/strategic plan.
- Effectively understand and implement risk management principles and programs, such as risk assessment and analysis and risk mitigation.
- Use principles of project, operating, and capital budgeting in support of strategic decision making.
- Effectively use accounting principles and financial management tools, such as financial plans and measures of performance.
- Plan, organize, and monitor organizational resources to ensure optimal health outcomes and effective quality and cost controls.

Key Terms

- Balanced scorecard
- Capital access
- Capital budgeting
- Capital market depth
- Capital project analysis
- Capital rationing
- Capital structure
- Capitation
- Cash concentration system
- Cash management
- Commercial paper
- Derivative
- Discounted payback period
- Factoring receivables
- Forward contract
- Global budget
- Hedging
- Internal rate of return (IRR)
- Joint venture
- Licensing/franchising
- Management by exception
- Medical tourism
- Net present value (NPV)
- Payback period
- Public–private partnership
- Retained earnings
- Revenue cycle
- Strategic management process
- Transfer pricing
- Transparency
- Value-based payment (VBP)
- Variance analysis
- Working capital management

Key Concepts

- Budget development
- Budget execution
- Capital projects
- Cash flows
- Debt and equity
- Exchange rates
- Financial management

- Healthcare payment models
- Market depth
- Market entry
- Multinational operations
- Risk management
- Strategic management

Introduction

The preceding chapter addressed a variety of macro-level considerations for the global environments in which healthcare organizations operate, such as how a nation or society allocates healthcare goods and services, whether through a capitalist, free market approach or a centrally planned, government-based system. In this chapter, we build upon that material by focusing on micro-level considerations unique to the financial decisions of healthcare managers when their organizations operate in complex, often multinational, environments. We first discuss key financial management concepts and skills, and then we address the long- and short-term financial considerations that organizations must adequately address when entering new markets, when expanding the scale or scope of operations within existing markets, and when financing the provision of healthcare in multinational settings. Rather than using this chapter to conduct a "deep dive" into the mechanics of these topics (which is beyond the scope of this textbook), we discuss them conceptually and point to sources that provide much greater detail regarding the specific tools used to make decisions. Thus, we frame the critical content that should be developed within more-focused courses addressing financial management for healthcare managers. In discussing these topics, we also address the various contexts that may apply, from purely market-based settings to purely government-run settings.

Critical Financial Management Concepts

Regardless of the type of healthcare organization, the competitive environment in which it exists, or the country (or countries) in which it operates, all healthcare managers are expected to make wise decisions that positively affect the long-term financial health of the organization. Managers must exhibit the critical knowledge, skills, and abilities necessary to make those decisions in support of the strategic direction set by high-level executive leaders. Moreover, they must be valued participants in the planning and execution processes designed by functional-area experts (e.g., financial officers, comptrollers, treasurers) who are driven to achieve that strategic direction.

The budgeting process represents one of the most critical ways in which managers can support the direction of the organization, and it is often the first major dilemma a manager faces upon starting a job. Early and mid-careerists normally fall into a position of responsibility where they must serve as stewards of financial resources entrusted to them for the purposes of accomplishing a specified mission. Managers must understand the sources of those financial resources and the relationships between workload, costs, and financial solvency. They also must understand their role in both the budget development process and the budget execution process. Although these two processes normally occur concurrently—typically, planning of future-year budgets occurs while the current-year budget is being executed—we will discuss them in stages.

The Revenue Cycle

revenue cycle
The time frame between the delivery of care and the receipt of payment.

The major sources of funding—collectively referred to as *revenue*—for healthcare delivery are payments made through some sort of market-based system or through a government entity. The payments can come before care is delivered, or they may occur after care is delivered. The time frame between the delivery of care and the receipt of payment is called the **revenue cycle**. In market-based settings, this cycle can be very short (payment in cash at the time of care delivery) or very long (invoicing well after care delivery).

The revenue cycle includes the set of activities necessary for a provider to get paid. Generally, these activities include documenting that services were provided, billing for the services, and then collecting for the services. The exact set of activities depends on the type of provider and the form of reimbursement. Payment for surgery, for example, may require documents indicating that the provider obtained prior authorization from an insurance company. Healthcare managers often play an important role in the activities of the revenue cycle. For example, the manager of the registration department of a hospital in the United States might be tasked with determining whether prospective patients will be able to pay their bills.

In addition to influencing the revenue cycle, the form of reimbursement may also influence what services are provided. In Australia, for instance, the states and territories pay for hospital care, but nursing home care is paid for by the Commonwealth of Nations. Some researchers have noted that this split in responsibility for payment is in part to blame for problems in transferring patients from hospitals to nursing homes (Willis, Reynolds, and Keleher 2012).

In many instances, the revenue cycle can be flipped, with payment coming before care is delivered. Managed care organizations and governmental agencies often receive payments up front for a defined period and then provide care using those resources. In some settings, the sources of revenue can be mixed and from different sources (some *ex post*, some *ex ante*). Such an arrangement complicates the relationship between revenue, workload, and expenditures and contributes to a complex healthcare delivery environment.

Common Payment Methods

The majority of revenue for healthcare delivery, regardless of the environment, comes through some combination of eight basic payment methods: (1) per time period, (2) per beneficiary, (3) per recipient, (4) per episode, (5) per day, (6) per service, (7) per dollar of cost, and (8) per dollar of charges (Quinn 2015). In many market settings around the world, the links to these categories may not be obvious, but the conceptual links still exist. Exhibit 3.1 provides additional information about each method.

EXHIBIT 3.1
The Basic Payment Methods in Healthcare

Unit of Payment	Common Term	Examples	Incentives Created
Per time period	Budget	Government appropriations, global budgets	Wellness/preventive care, early detection/intervention
Per beneficiary	Capitation	Managed care, per member per month	Wellness/preventive care, early detection/intervention
Per recipient	Contact capitation	Physician specialist services	Wellness/preventive care, early detection/intervention
Per episode	Case rates, bundled payments	Hospital inpatient services (DRG), physician services (RBRVS)	Increase quantity of services provided
Per day	Per diem and per visit	Nursing facilities, ambulatory surgery centers	Increase quantity (longer length of stay or increased number of visits)
Per service	Fee-for-service	Hospital outpatient services (APC), physician services (RBRVS), dentists, medical supplies and equipment	Increase quantity of services provided
Per dollar of cost	Cost-plus reimbursement	Critical access hospitals, nursing facilities	Focus on quality
Per dollar of charges	Discount off charges	Any provider type	Increase quantity of services provided

Note: APC = ambulatory payment classification; DRG = diagnosis-related group; RBRVS = resource-based relative value scale.
Source: Adapted from Quinn (2015).

In most market-based healthcare systems, the per-dollar-of-cost method represents the legacy cost-plus charge system, which has become less prevalent over time. As the costs of healthcare delivery grew, the legacy cost-plus system provided few incentives for healthcare providers to control costs. As a result, the per-dollar-of-cost method has come to be used less frequently by individual payers, institutional payers, and government payers. Today, it is no longer used by most payers of healthcare or is used only in isolated circumstances.

Along the evolutionary path of healthcare delivery systems, new payment models have emerged. Government and private insurance payers have implemented prospective payment system (PPS) models, whereby they determine the prices they will pay for healthcare in advance of the actual delivery of care. This payment approach provides an incentive for healthcare delivery organizations to control costs, because the revenue they receive tied to an episode of care would be capped (unlike in the cost-plus system, where the revenue would always exceed the costs incurred). A PPS approach may include payments for specific services or for specific episodes of care. Prospective payments may cover outpatient services through such systems as the resource-based relative value scale (RBRVS) in the United States or the TarMed (medical tariff) system in Switzerland; they may also cover inpatient services through such systems as diagnosis-related groups (DRGs) in the United States and diagnosis procedure combinations in Japan. The Commonwealth Fund's "International Profiles of Health Care Systems" looked at 19 major countries and found that 17 of them (about 90 percent) used at least some form of PPS to finance healthcare delivery (Mossialos et al. 2017).

Managers in hospital settings must possess a solid understanding of prospective payment systems, and they must have the ability to keep costs under control—in other words, they must be able to effectively manage the budget to ensure organizational success. Moreover, managers at healthcare organizations in competitive market environments must be able to understand what services they can provide in a cost-effective manner, given their revenue streams. The organizations can then choose which services to provide (the ones where they have a cost advantage) and which to eliminate (those where they do not have a cost advantage).

value-based payment (VBP)
An approach in which prospective payments to providers are adjusted based on performance on a set of quality indicators; value-based systems aim to reward quality of care rather than quantity of care.

A recent PPS trend within the United States, driven by provisions of the Affordable Care Act of 2010, is the implementation of **value-based payment (VBP)** systems. Under value-based reforms, prospective payments are adjusted based on a basket of quality indicators. When healthcare delivery organizations perform well on those quality indicators, the payment amounts increase. When organizations perform poorly on those indicators, their payment amounts decrease. These reforms were designed to reward quality of care rather than quantity of care.

For many managed care organizations, payment comes before the delivery of healthcare—meaning they have an inverted revenue cycle. Per-time-period

Vignette: Hospitals in Colombia

In Colombia, high-complexity hospitals use retrospective payment systems—particularly fee-for-service payments, which incentivize the production of services, leading to increased health costs and hospital inefficiency. The financial risk is held by insurers. Colombia's low-complexity hospitals, on the other hand, use capitation payment, with the financial risk assumed by the health service provider.

and per-beneficiary payment methods provide examples of **capitation** and **global budget** systems. In these scenarios, the payments cover patients over a predefined time frame—for instance, a year for global budgets, or a month in per-member-per-month capitation contracts. Those payments cover a predefined set of healthcare services for a predefined population for a specific period.

In this kind of financing environment, organizations are paid in advance and better served financially by keeping patients healthy, with limited need for healthcare services. The organizations, therefore, proactively manage patients' health and focus on patient education, wellness, health screenings, exercise, nutrition, immunizations, and other preventive measures. In instances where patients do need healthcare services, the organizations emphasize early detection and intervention through less-costly means, such as rest, therapy, and pharmaceuticals. Most government-run healthcare organizations operate in this manner. In the Commonwealth Fund's assessment of healthcare systems of 19 countries, 13 of them (about 70 percent) were found to operate on some form of global budget (Mossialos et al. 2017).

Major complications occur when healthcare delivery organizations have multiple payers using multiple payment methods. In environments with a complex "payer mix," payments sometimes come before services, and other times they come after services. For some patients, additional visits will result in additional revenue (because their coverage is paid ex post). Other patients, meanwhile, need to be managed more closely, because additional visits will not result in additional revenue (because their coverage is paid ex ante). Most organizations want to treat every patient equally well, but the form and timing of payment can complicate the way such an approach affects the budget.

capitation
The payment of a fixed amount for a predefined set of services for a predefined population for a specific period.

global budget
The payment of a fixed amount to provide for the healthcare needs of a population for a fixed period of time (typically one year).

Budget Development
Having provided a glimpse of the revenue environments and payment systems used in most countries, we can now address the budget development process, where future operational budgets are forecasted as a means to accommodate the expected healthcare delivery workload. The budget development process

**strategic
management
process**
The ongoing
process by which
an organization
assesses the
environment in
which it operates,
appraises
its current
direction and
market position,
determines the
most appropriate
strategic direction
moving forward,
and develops and
implements goals,
objectives, and
action plans to
accomplish the
strategy.

**balanced
scorecard**
A strategic
planning tool that
places key metrics
on a dashboard
to aid with the
measurement and
assessment of
performance.

is a nested component of the broader organizational strategic management process. The **strategic management process** is the ongoing process by which a healthcare organization (a) assesses the environment in which it operates, (b) appraises its current direction and market position, (c) determines the most appropriate strategic direction moving forward, and then (d) develops and implements goals, objectives, and action plans to accomplish the strategy.

The financial planning process initially assesses the feasibility of proposed strategic goals and objectives, given current financial constraints. Strategy should always drive structure, but the current structure of an organization often constrains its strategic ambition. Once key leaders finalize their "feasible" strategic goals and objectives (i.e., the strategic plan), the budget development process produces a specific financial plan (i.e., budget) for implementing the action plans necessary to accomplish the strategic goals and objectives. Often, organizations will develop financial metrics and track them over time as a means for gauging the ongoing accomplishment of financial and strategic objectives. Financial metrics can be routinely measured and assessed using a tool called a **balanced scorecard**. The most critical financial measures are displayed on a dashboard and kept consistently in front of key leadership.

Healthcare managers play a vital role in the budget development process by providing input on their expected healthcare delivery workload, whether inpatient or outpatient, and the financial resources needed to successfully carry out that workload. These resources include whatever is required to acquire the necessary property, plant, and equipment; to hire sufficient staff; to purchase medical supplies; and to meet other needs. In almost all cases, a direct relationship exists between expected workload and expected costs; however, such a relationship might not be the case between expected workload and expected revenue/funding (market-based or otherwise). The healthcare manager, who is normally much closer to where the workload actually occurs, serves as a valuable source of information to financial planners whenever budgets are developed and finalized.

Most organizations have a periodic budget cycle—often an annual cycle. With an annual cycle, budgets are developed in annual increments, with a planning stage preceding an execution stage (and possibly followed by an ex post assessment stage). The planning stage typically occurs in the year prior to the budget execution stage. Therefore, an annual cycle involves both the execution of the current year's budget (which is short-term financial management, covered later in the chapter) and the planning for the next year's budget. In addition, many organizations (a number of governmental organizations, for instance) also conduct long-range budget development over multiple years into the future.

Exhibit 3.2 provides an illustration of the budget development process. The earliest months are devoted to strategic assessment and guidance from

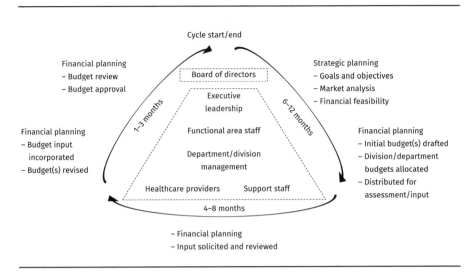

EXHIBIT 3.2
Annual Budget
Development
Process

Source: Data from Cleverley and Cleverley (2018).

senior leadership, clarification of goals and objectives for the upcoming (budget) year, analysis of historical workload and expenditures, and development of the initial draft of the proposed budget for the upcoming year (i.e., the year of execution). Senior leadership then sends out preliminary plans and asks managers how those plans would affect resource requirements and workload expectations for subordinate units within the organization. As the planning year progresses—typically between three and six months out from the start of the execution year—lower-level input is incorporated into the proposed budget. Revisions are made in the final one to three months, and a budget is finalized and approved. The managers of the various subunits of the organization then use the approved budget to develop and implement execution plans for their respective subunits for the new budget year.

Many organizations develop separate budgets for different kinds of requirements, which complicates the budget development process. For instance, separate budgets might exist for construction projects, major capital investments, capital equipment replacement, payroll, and so on. Often, organizations restrict managers from taking resources out of one budget for diversion toward expenditures that should be funded out of another budget. These types of constraints often serve to protect owners, stakeholders, or taxpayers from having their financial resources diverted for unintended use, which may be regarded as waste or abuse.

The important thing for healthcare managers to remember—whether they are at the executive level or closer to the lower levels—is that budgets should not be developed in isolation. Managers should learn about their organization's budget development cycle and then proactively engage in the development process to ensure that they have the resources necessary to accomplish their mission. Most healthcare organizations have some type of a participatory budget development cycle, and participation is the manager's opportunity to provide meaningful input. Long-term perspective is critical to ensuring short-term success.

Budget Execution

Managers are typically expected to play an important role in the execution of the organization's budget. Under the approach of **management by exception**, managers focus attention on items where performance is significantly different from what was planned in the budget, and they analyze the causes of the differences.

management by exception
A managerial approach that focuses attention and analysis on items where performance is significantly different from what was planned in the budget.

variance analysis
A form of analysis in which the manager compares actual revenue and resource use with standards that were developed as part of the budget process.

One type of analysis, **variance analysis**, requires that standards be developed as part of the budget process and used to set expectations for the amount of resources required for a given period. For instance, the budget for a mental health clinic might project as a standard that one hour of clinician time will be required for every two visits; if the estimated volume of visits for the budget period is 80, then 40 hours of clinician time should be budgeted. As the budget is being executed, periodic (perhaps monthly) variance reports are developed. Managers are provided documents that list actual revenue and resource use, and they compare those findings with the budgeted revenue and resource use. In other words, managers are tasked with comparing what actually happened with the standards set forth in the budget.

Variance analysis takes many forms, and they differ from company to company. Some companies look at product lines and begin with revenue variances. In such cases, they may try to figure out how much of the difference between actual and standard revenue is due to price of the services sold and how much of the revenue variance is due to the volume of services sold. Variance analysis can also focus on cost variances, where costs are higher than expected. One possible reason for a cost variance is that output is higher than expected. For example, if a mental health clinic has twice as many appointments as expected, then the total cost of providing care could be higher than budgeted (this type of variance is often called a *volume variance*). A second possible reason for a cost variance is that the clinic has used more inputs than expected, even taking into account the change in volume of services. Continuing our example, the number of mental health visits might be twice the budgeted amount, but the number of hours of a particular type of labor might be more than twice the budget. A third possible reason is that the price of an input is higher than expected. For instance, when the number of mental health visits exceeds expectations, some employees might receive higher wages because of overtime.

Global managers need to recognize that the interpretation of variances depends on the details of the particular situation. For example, in some countries, providers receive an additional payment each time they care for an

Elements of Project Management

Project management processes can be divided into five groups that are applicable to most types of projects: (1) preparation, (2) planning, (3) implementation, (4) monitoring, and (5) delivery. The knowledge involved in project management is based on ten areas: (1) cost, (2) scope, (3) time, (4) integration, (5) quality, (6) management of shareholders, (7) communications, (8) risk management, (9) human resources, and (10) provision.

additional patient. Under such an arrangement, when an unexpectedly large number of patients are treated, a variance analysis might indicate that costs are over budget; however, given that the provider receives additional funds with each patient treated, exceeding the budgeted costs might be acceptable, because revenue is also being generated in excess of the budgeted amount. On the other hand, sometimes providers receive a fixed payment that is supposed to cover the costs of all the care they provide for the entire year. Under this type of arrangement, the treatment of additional patients will not generate additional revenue, so funds to pay for the additional resources necessary to provide services above the budgeted amounts might not be readily available.

Managerial control processes may also be affected by sociocultural factors. Maranz (2001) notes that societies in sub-Saharan Africa have been profoundly affected by the fact that a large proportion of people struggle to meet basic financial needs. Organizations in such settings, even when they have budgets, tend to feel that the financial need that occurs first has priority on available resources, and resources tend to be perceived as available if they are not being actively used. Consequently, budgets and other financial controls are often disregarded.

Vignette: Transition to Value-Based Payment

Imagine you are the chief of a public hospital in the country of Fandango. You have been operating on a global budget allocated by the Ministry of Health for as long as you remember, but you have just left a meeting at which the ministry announced that, as of next year, the country will begin a transition to a value-based payment (VBP) system. Under the new system, your organization will first shift to a diagnosis-related group (DRG) payment methodology. Within the DRG methodology, you will be funded via a

(continued)

mechanism that is directly tied to your level of workload. Subsequently, the Ministry of Health will make adjustments to the size of those DRG payments based on results, outcomes, and quality measures. Achieving higher levels of outcomes/results/quality will result in larger payments, whereas falling short will result in smaller payments. The intent is to transition entirely to a value-based payment system within five years.

Consider the following questions:

- How would you prepare your hospital for the transition?
- How are the workload, quality, and service incentives different under a VBP system, compared to your current budget model?
- How does the new VBP system affect the level of financial risk that your hospital faces?
- How should the budget development and budget execution processes be adjusted under the VBP system?

Capital Project Analysis

Much of the chapter thus far has dealt with short-term financial management issues faced by healthcare managers; however, managers also play an important role in shaping the long-term future direction of their organizations. In this section, we will address the healthcare manager's role in the development, assessment, and implementation of long-term investment projects, or capital projects.

capital project analysis
A formal process that involves the assessment of all the costs and benefits of a potential investment that is large enough to significantly expand the scale or scope of the organization.

Capital project analysis is the most important long-term financial decision-making tool for healthcare managers to understand. It is a formal process that involves the assessment of all the costs and benefits of a potential investment that is large enough to significantly expand the scale or scope of the organization. Capital projects can take many forms. They may involve acquisitions of other healthcare organizations, construction of new healthcare facilities, major expansion of the scale of operations, purchases of major pieces of equipment, and so on. In each of these examples, the size of the project normally exceeds the capability of funding through normal operational budgets.

capital rationing
The process by which potential projects compete for a limited pool of investment capital.

Many long-term investment ideas are generated from the grassroots levels of the organization, and healthcare managers often serve as "champions" for certain projects. Once championed, project ideas are submitted to the top of the organization, vetted for strategic fit, and compared against other potential projects that will compete for a (normally) limited pool of investment capital. This competition between projects is sometimes called **capital rationing**. Scarce investment resources are focused on only those projects that best serve the organization's strategic interests. The size of the pool of investment funds is normally determined by key executives and is often based on the financial health of the organization, the depth of the capital markets, and the anticipated number of projects for a given period.

The goal of capital project analysis is to determine whether the project serves the best interests of your stakeholders. In the case of a for-profit business, the decision to accept or reject the project should be based on maximizing the wealth of the major stakeholder groups, primarily the owners. For a government organization, the decision-making process should focus on maximizing the net benefit to the public at large. For a nonprofit, nongovernmental organization, the focus should be on maximizing the net benefit to the organization's community of focus.

The analysis of a proposed capital project involves multiple steps. This section will provide an overview of those steps; however, we recommend consulting other reference materials for more detailed explanations of the mathematical techniques and applications. The depth is too great to be covered in a single introductory chapter on financial management.

The first step in capital project analysis is determining which projects align with the strategic direction of the organization. Projects that do not serve the long-term interests of the organization tend to be rejected at this early stage, without expending further time and energy on a more thorough analysis. For the investment ideas deemed to have a strategic fit with the organization's future direction, the next stage involves estimating the projected cash flows associated with the project.

Cash flows are broken into cash outflows (i.e., costs) and cash inflows (i.e., benefits). Cash outflows are normally expenditures, though they may also be reduction of revenues (i.e., lowered income). Similarly, cash inflows are normally revenues, though they may also be the reduction of expenditures (i.e., cost savings). Put simply, spending more money and making less money (cash outflows) are bad, and earning more money and spending less money (cash inflows) are good. These cash inflows and outflows are projected over the duration of the project, with the projections based on historical analysis, financial modeling, and, if hard data are not available, realistic assumptions. The cash flows are sorted into separate years over the life of the project and then netted out for each year, producing annual net cash flows. The life of a project can be as short as 3 to 5 years (for a small expansion to the service mix, for instance) or as long as 30 years or more (for a project that involves major construction).

A thorough understanding of the organization's workload, payer mix, payment mechanisms, and payment timing is crucial for effectively measuring a project's cash inflows. Likewise, a thorough understanding of the organization's workload timing and cost structure helps measure a project's cash inflows. Healthcare managers and financial experts add significant value to their organizations when they can reasonably and effectively model a project's expected costs and benefits. Nobody has perfect foresight, but being thorough, methodical, and precise in the estimation phase helps minimize any adverse impact associated with forecasting error.

The next stage of capital project analysis involves calculating a number of financial metrics that are designed to provide key leaders with information about the overall profitability of the project. Certain leaders may prefer one metric over another, but each metric provides distinctly useful information. The metrics quantify time periods, dollar values, percentage rates, and ratios. All of the metrics should be considered when evaluating a project, though managers can choose which metric (or group of metrics) they will emphasize the most.

The **payback period** is a metric that indicates the length of time needed for a project to break even by bringing in sufficient funding to pay back the initial investment. It is normally expressed in number of years. The **discounted payback period** is a closely related metric that takes into consideration the buying power of future cash inflows when adjusted for the time value of money. Future cash flows are adjusted back into present value and then used to calculate the payback period. This calculation results in a more conservative estimate. Because executives will not want the exact same dollar amount recouped but rather the exact same buying power recouped, many prefer the discounted payback period to the traditional payback period. With either metric, a quicker payback is preferable to a longer payback. Healthcare organizations often establish a maximum payback period that acceptable projects must not exceed (e.g., no more than three years).

The most commonly used metric for capital project analysis is the **net present value (NPV)**. This metric represents the overall dollar value of the project to the organization, considering all cash flows over the life of the project. Like the metrics assessing the payback period, NPV takes into account the need to recoup all up-front investment costs. However, NPV also assesses subsequent cash flows accruing to the project, while making an adjustment for the time value of money. Acceptable projects have an NPV greater than zero.

Another commonly used metric is the **internal rate of return (IRR)**, or the closely related modified internal rate of return (MIRR). The IRR and MIRR tell key leaders the percentage rate that the project earns over the course of its life. This rate of return is compared to the investors' rate of return when they provide investment capital (debt or equity) through the capital markets. Acceptable projects have an IRR or MIRR greater than the expected rate of return by debt or equity investors. This concept can be illustrated through a personal finance example. If you are thinking about borrowing money to invest for your retirement, you would not want to borrow money at 10 percent interest and invest the proceeds in something that earned only 5 percent. That would be an unacceptable decision. However, borrowing at 5 percent and investing at 10 percent would be acceptable.

payback period
A metric that indicates the length of time needed for a project to break even by bringing in sufficient funding to pay back the initial investment.

discounted payback period
A metric that indicates the length of time needed for a project to break even, taking into consideration the buying power of future cash inflows when adjusted for the time value of money.

net present value (NPV)
A metric that represents the overall dollar value of a project to the organization, considering all cash flows over the life of the project.

internal rate of return (IRR)
A metric representing the percentage rate that a project earns over the course of its life.

Projects with metrics indicating acceptability—suggesting that the projects pay for themselves quickly, add value, and exceed investor demands—proceed to compete for the pool of investment capital in the capital rationing decision. After projects have been approved and funded, managers are charged with carrying them out in the implementation stage. Once the projects have been implemented, managers continually assess the cash flow realities against the original cash flow projections, and they intervene as soon as possible when adverse deviations arise. Finally, managers and executives continually assess the project's ongoing fit with the strategic direction of the organization. Strategies change over time. Projects implemented in past years might have been a strategic fit when they were conceptualized, approved, and initially implemented, but the new and original strategies may diverge.

The more that managers are involved in the planning, assessment, and implementation of a project, the greater the likelihood that the project will be successful to the organization and continue to add value toward achieving strategic goals. Exhibit 3.3 provides a conceptual visualization of the **capital budgeting** process.

Capital project analysis in nonprofit and governmental settings differs in a number of ways from the type of analysis used at for-profit organizations. The major differences involve (a) where the investment capital is sought and (b) the discount rate that is applied to calculations of some of the metrics. Nonprofit and governmental organizations normally have restricted access to capital markets that are open to for-profit organizations. For-profit organizations have deep access to the equity capital markets, where investors may take an ownership position in the organization in exchange for their investment capital. Nonprofit and governmental organizations do not have this same access and must rely heavily on debt to fund projects.

capital budgeting
The strategic planning process used to evaluate and execute an organization's long-term investments.

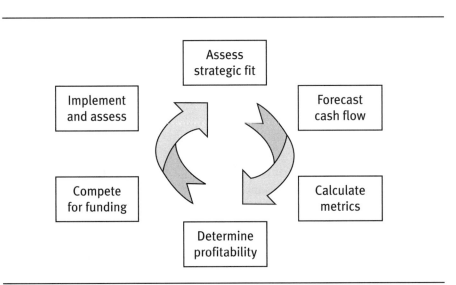

EXHIBIT 3.3
Major Steps in Capital Project Analysis

Pursuing Multinational Operations

Much of the chapter thus far has focused on the types of knowledge and skills that are useful for healthcare managers, regardless of their setting. For the remainder of the chapter, we will focus on issues that are unique to managers at healthcare organizations that operate in two or more countries. These organizations must contend with different healthcare delivery structures, legal systems, currencies, economic conditions, population health concerns, and a host of other issues, all of which affect the financial health of the organization. Given that healthcare delivery on its own is challenging enough, why would an organization choose to pursue other markets around the globe, thereby greatly complicating the scale and scope of its operations?

Health organizations choose to pursue multinational operations for a variety of reasons. Some motivations are the same as those common for businesses outside the health industry, such as the desires to pursue growth opportunities in new markets, to seek new technologies, to find more advantageous regulatory environments, and to pursue lower production costs. Other motivations are more specific to healthcare delivery. For instance, organizations might pursue global operations to address critical population health needs that are unmet in other countries, to pursue faith-based collaborations, to facilitate **medical tourism**, or to defend loss of market share stemming from medical tourism. All of these motivations complicate the standard financial management practices that managers use when operating domestically.

medical tourism The traveling of individuals from one country to another for the purpose of receiving medical treatment.

In this section, we will address these complications from the perspective of an organization wishing to enter a market in a new country, rather than expanding its operations within an existing country. From this perspective, we can focus on the time at which the organization bears the most financial risk and managers face the most complex set of financial considerations. Entry into a new market involves multiple components, and we can address each one sequentially.

When an organization identifies a potential country for expansion, it must assess the financial risks associated with entering the new market, choose the best market entry strategy, identify appropriate sources of new investment capital, and assess the financial net benefits directly associated with the expansion. Because the mechanics of the long-term financial decision-making process are outside the scope of this textbook (they are normally covered in foundational courses preceding a course in global health management), we will focus on how managers make adjustments to the financial decision-making process when considering global investments.

Major Sources of Risk

Major sources of financial risks associated with multinational operations include the following:

- *Regulatory/legal risk.* Governments may regulate industry to protect citizens, national security, or the environment, or to sustain optimal levels of economic activity. The level of government involvement varies significantly around the globe, thereby creating differing levels of regulatory and legal risk. For instance, in 2015, the Vietnamese government gave a major boost to foreign direct investment by lifting its 49 percent foreign-ownership limit, thereby permitting foreign investors to take a majority ownership in Vietnamese publicly traded companies (Peel and Linh 2015). Such a change lowers risk by enabling owners and managers to exert greater control over the company's operations and to have a higher claim on profits. Often, within a country, the level of government control varies by industry. Healthcare is often more highly controlled than other industries; in some countries, this control extends to the point of the government running its own healthcare system.

- *Political risk.* A country's political stability (or lack thereof) may have a significant impact on an organization's operating environment. In some cases, political risk may result in an increase in government control, or even expropriation of assets. Significant political risk has been associated with medical tourism. The medical tourism industry, according to some estimates, is now worth as much as $72 billion annually (Patients Beyond Borders 2017), but many common destinations for the practice (e.g., Singapore, Thailand, Malaysia, Dubai) are in parts of the world associated with heightened risk of terrorist activity.

- *Currency/exchange rate risk.* Any cash flows resulting from operations within a country will be affected by the stability of that country's currency. When an organization repatriates foreign earnings to its home country, the company must convert those earnings to its home currency, and the value of those earnings becomes directly tied to exchange rates. Since 2006, Hospital Corporation of America (HCA) has operated a number of public–private partnerships in England through a subsidiary known as HCA NHS Ventures. In the "Brexit" vote of June 2016, the people of the United Kingdom voted to leave the European Union, which spurred a two-week drop of 13 percent in the value of the British pound against the US dollar. As a result, HCA's foreign earnings in British pounds became significantly less valuable when converted to US dollars.

- *Capital access.* Organizations may choose to transfer investment capital from their home country to a foreign country (and accept any currency exchange implications), or they may seek investment capital in the foreign setting. Some countries have deep capital markets where sufficient investment capital can be acquired within the borders of the new expansion. Many underdeveloped countries, however, do not have deep capital markets. This constrained supply often drives up the cost of investment capital from within undeveloped countries, thereby leading organizations to pursue the transfer of investment capital across borders (and alternatively exposing health organizations to currency/exchange rate risk).

These sources of risk significantly complicate the decisions that managers face when pursuing investment opportunities in foreign countries. When considering new markets, managers must measure the levels of risk and then identify ways to avoid or manage those risks. In many cases, the prospects of expanding into new markets, meeting population health needs, establishing new partnerships, and increasing solvency/profitability make the associated risks worthwhile.

Market Entry Strategies

One of the key decisions an organization will face initially when entering a new market is the selection of an appropriate entry strategy. The most common market entry strategies include (1) the export of goods and services, (2) licensing/franchising agreements, (3) foreign production of goods and services, (4) strategic alliances/partnerships, and (5) joint ventures. Each of these strategies creates unique financial considerations that managers must consider.

Within the field of healthcare, the first entry strategy—exporting goods and services—primarily occurs with the manufacturing and sale of pharmaceuticals and durable medical equipment. In such cases, tangible products can be manufactured within a home country and then exported to another country for sale. The primary source of risk for this strategy is the currency/exchange rate risk associated with repatriating foreign sales revenue back into the domestic market.

licensing/ franchising
A type of agreement in which one organization contracts with another to use its name and business model, normally in exchange for a fee or percentage of profits.

In a **licensing/franchising** agreement, the home organization grants a foreign organization the right to use its intellectual property (license) or its business model (franchise) for a prescribed period, in exchange for a predetermined fee. Licensing/franchising outsources most of the financial risk onto external participants within the new market, in exchange for a licensing/franchising fee. As with exporting, organizations still face currency/exchange rate risk when repatriating licensing/franchising fees that are normally paid in the foreign currency, but sometimes even that risk can be outsourced by requiring fee payments in the organization's home currency. One example of an organization using this entry strategy is the home care organization ComForCare, which has used franchising as a means to establish a global footprint, with locations in the United States, Canada, and the United Kingdom.

Foreign production, strategic alliances/partnerships, and joint ventures all create much higher levels of financial risk, and all require a much larger financial investment. Foreign production occurs when a health organization chooses to directly establish and manage new operations in a foreign country. One way these new operations can be established is through construction of new infrastructure, the hiring of a new workforce, and the direct management of operations. Alternatively, an organization may choose to obtain infrastructure through the acquisition of an existing foreign market participant. An example of an organization establishing new operations occurred in 2014 when Ascension Health, the largest nonprofit health system in the United States, opened Health City Cayman Islands, a tertiary care hospital in a British territory. Two examples of entry through acquisition occurred in 2013 when Bupa, a UK-based international healthcare group, entered the healthcare delivery markets in Poland and Chile (Bupa 2014). Bupa acquired 100 percent of the share capital of LUX MED, an integrated healthcare organization providing both inpatient and outpatient services in Poland, for £165.6 million. Bupa also acquired a 56 percent stake in Cruz Blanca Salud SA (now known as Bupa Chile SA), which primarily focused on outpatient and home care services, for £205.6 million (*International Private Medical Insurance [IPMI] Magazine* 2014).

Strategic alliances/partnerships and joint ventures are entry strategies where two organizations partner to share the risks associated with entering a new market. In alliances and partnerships, organizations collaborate but choose to remain separate entities. An emerging form of strategic alliance/partnership is the **public–private partnership**, in which a private organization partners with a government or government-controlled entity to share financial risk. Sanford Health, a US-based nonprofit integrated delivery system, established a public–private partnership with China in 2014 as part of its International Clinics initiative (Gerszewski 2014; Sanford Health 2014). Under the partnership, Sanford worked with YMCI Calmette Medical Investment & Management Company, a state-owned company in China, to develop a pediatric clinic in China's Yunnan Province. Under the terms of the agreement, YMCI maintained ownership of the facility, but Sanford managed the daily operations of care delivery. This project extended Sanford's global presence to include locations in Asia (China), Africa (Ghana), and Latin America (Mexico).

Joint ventures occur when two or more organizations combine resources to establish a new entity that is jointly owned and controlled. CHRISTUS Health, a US-based Catholic nonprofit health system, and Pontificia Universidad Católica de Chile (UC), a Catholic university in Santiago, Chile, formalized an agreement in 2013 to partner in such a joint venture (CHRISTUS Health 2013). The two organizations established Red de Salud UC–CHRISTUS through joint ownership, operation, and expansion of the former UC health

public–private partnership
A strategic arrangement in which a private organization partners with a government or government-controlled entity to share financial risk.

joint venture
A business enterprise developed and co-owned by two or more parties, which otherwise retain their own distinct identities.

network. This joint ownership arrangement allowed the two entities to finalize a mutually beneficial investment that the sides might not have been able to pursue on their own.

The various market entry strategies provide health organizations with options for mitigating some of the long-term financial risk associated with pursuing operations in foreign markets. In addition to choosing an entry strategy, organizations must also consider the sources of capital financing necessary to implement their global strategy, as well as the capital budgeting processes needed to evaluate the investments made to implement that strategy. Although the same primary sources of investment capital exist globally (debt and equity) and many of the same capital project assessment principles (e.g., net present value, internal rate of return, payback period) can still be applied, some key differences exist for global projects, particularly with regard to **capital access** and the organization's cost of capital. Once managers understand how foreign projects complicate the standard financial decision-making tools, they will be better able to address those complications in their decisions.

Global Capital Markets

When organizations pursue capital projects in foreign markets, obtaining adequate investment capital is an important consideration. As with domestic projects, debt and equity continue to be the two main types of investment capital. However, foreign projects present managers with unique challenges. Internal sources of capital—primarily **retained earnings**—may prove insufficient to fund major projects in foreign markets. Managers may prefer to seek investment capital within their domestic markets, with the intent of shifting capital to the foreign market; however, issuing domestically causes organizations to incur the transaction costs of converting domestic capital into the foreign currency before initiating the project. One way around this up-front cost is to seek investment capital in the country of the new capital project.

Alternatively, healthcare organizations in less developed countries may face a limited investor base and may attract stronger demand by seeking investment capital abroad, where the **capital market depth** is more favorable. Managers may also be able to exploit more advantageous market conditions in foreign capital markets in the form of lower interest rates (for debt) or greater stability in asset prices (equity). Ultimately, managers must seek the source of investment capital that lowers their overall cost of capital for the foreign project and most positively influences the project's cash flows.

The primary means for attracting foreign capital are the foreign bond markets and the foreign equity markets. Bond markets are deep in developed regions around the world—such as North America, Europe, and Asia—where currencies are relatively strong and stable. Such conditions lower borrowing costs for companies that issue debt. Bond markets in less developed regions—such as parts of Africa, Central America, and South America—have experienced

capital access
An organization's ability to obtain investment capital through various sources, such as debt and equity.

retained earnings
Earnings not paid out to an organization's owners but rather retained by the organization to be reinvested in business operations.

capital market depth
The overall level of investment capital collectively made available by investors to organizations for the purpose of strategic investments.

only limited growth, primarily because of unstable currencies and higher levels of inflation. These conditions increase borrowing costs for companies that issue bonds. Exhibit 3.4 shows average long-term lending rates across countries with varying levels of economic development. As the data indicate, the more developed countries provide healthcare organizations with lower interest rates and, therefore, lower borrowing costs.

For taxable organizations, one of the main benefits of using debt instead of equity is the preferential tax treatment of interest expense. Most countries of the Organisation for Economic Co-operation and Development (OECD) allow interest expense to be deducted when calculating taxable business profits, thereby providing a tax shield and reducing the after-tax cost of debt. The value of the debt shield is directly related to business income tax rates. The after-tax cost of debt capital can be calculated using the equation $K_d = r_d \times (1 - T)$, where K_d denotes the after-tax cost of debt capital, r_d denotes the required rate of return on debt, and T denotes the business tax rate. Exhibit 3.5 illustrates the distribution of corporate tax rates around the world.

World Bank Income Group	Average Lending Interest Rate
High (OECD)	4.18%
High (non-OECD)	7.18%
Upper middle	11.57%
Lower middle	12.69%
Lower	20.93%

EXHIBIT 3.4
Lending Interest Rates (2016)

Note: OECD = Organisation for Economic Co-operation and Development.
Source: Data from World Bank (2018a).

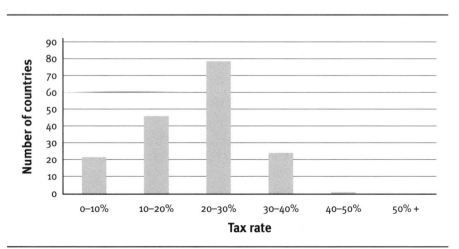

EXHIBIT 3.5
Corporate Tax Rates (2015)

Sources: Data from Pomerlau (2015); World Bank (2018b); KPMG (2018).

As with debt, the depth of the global equity markets is closely linked with a region's level of economic development. A key difference is that, whereas few formal bond exchanges exist, many countries have formal stock exchanges. These formal exchanges greatly facilitate the issuing and trading of equity securities and provide companies with greater access to external equity capital. Exhibit 3.6 provides information about the prevalence of stock exchanges around the world. It should be noted that most companies list their stock on a primary exchange and that, once listed, the stock also trades on additional exchanges that have trading relationships with the main exchanges. These additional exchanges provide investors with additional liquidity for their shares. Exhibit 3.7 shows the total market capitalization of all companies listed within the world regions. By far, most of the equity market depth is concentrated within the developed regions of North America, Asia, and Europe. Organizations in the less developed regions face significant constraints to equity investment capital because of the severe lack of market depth.

Multinational Capital Structure and Cost of Capital Issues

capital structure
The policy for how a firm finances its overall operations and growth, using debt or equity.

With domestic healthcare organizations, the mix of debt and equity used to pursue capital projects depends on the **capital structure** policy of the organization. Whether following an optimal capital structure policy or a "pecking order" policy, the mix of debt and equity, investor expectations (regarding required rates of return), and an organization's tax structure determine the overall cost of capital. With multinational healthcare organizations, these capital structure decisions become significantly more complicated, also taking into account varying levels of economic development, differing expectations of debt and

EXHIBIT 3.6
Prevalence of Stock Exchanges (2016)

World Bank Income Group	Number of Countries	Countries with Exchanges	Total Exchanges	Percent with Exchanges	Exchanges per Country
High (OECD)	32	31	63	96.9%	2.03
High (non-OECD)	46	18	20	39.1%	0.43
Upper middle	46	38	48	82.6%	1.04
Lower middle	52	26	36	50%	0.69
Lower	31	4	4	12.9%	0.13

Source: Data from World Stock Exchanges (2018).

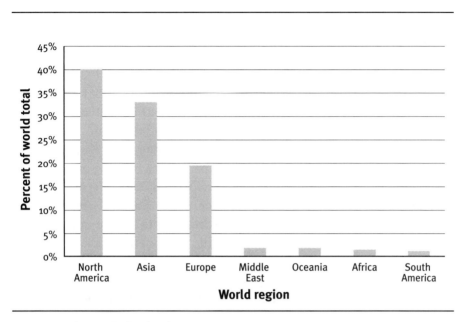

EXHIBIT 3.7
Depth of Equity
Markets (2015)

Source: Data from Desjardins (2016).

equity investors, the depth of debt and equity markets, and the tax regimes in the countries of current operations and planned expansions.

Ultimately, managers must select the mix and location of external investment capital that both meet the organization's strategic planning priorities and optimize the financial viability of any multinational investments. Differences in borrowing rates, investor expectations, tax policies, and the depth of foreign capital markets greatly impact the financial viability of initiating or expanding operations in another country. Managers may consider adjustments to conventional decision making by seeking capital in the foreign country if investor expectations are more favorable, or obtaining capital domestically and shifting resources abroad when foreign capital markets are suboptimal for financing the project. In some cases, regional exchanges provide additional depth across multiple countries. Examples include the Bourse Régionale des Valeurs Mobilières SA, serving West Africa; the NYSE Euronext, serving much of mainland Europe; and Nasdaq OMX Nordic, serving Nordic and Baltic countries.

Multinational Capital Budgeting

Managers of healthcare organizations face unique complexities that influence the cash flows and subsequent profitability of foreign projects. A major complexity for foreign projects is exchange rate fluctuation, which can reduce the value of cash inflows or increase the value of cash outflows. Managers need to evaluate the impact of exchange rate fluctuations on projected cash flows and then adjust where necessary to optimize the project's financial viability.

derivative
A financial asset (such as a stock option or a forward/future contract) whose market value is derived from the value of an underlying asset (such as a stock or commodity).

Significant research in the field of finance has been devoted to forecasting exchange rates and managing potential adverse impacts to the value of foreign projects. Forecasting techniques may involve the use of historical trends (technical analysis), currently observable economic variables and exchange rates (fundamental analysis), and market-based observable data (spot rates and forward rates). Once exchange rates can be reasonably forecasted, organizations can measure their level of exchange rate exposure and then implement strategies to reduce that exposure. The most common strategy is to use **derivative** securities as a means of managing the exchange rate risk (e.g., interest rate swaps, forward/future contracts, currency swaps). Professional financial managers have a number of tools and strategies for minimizing (but not completely eliminating) the unique financial risks associated with operating in multiple countries, but these strategies are beyond the scope of this book.

Short-Term Financial Considerations and Risk Management

Having discussed a variety of long-term planning and strategy considerations, we now turn our attention to more short-term and operational issues that affect the ongoing solvency of the organization. Typically, these issues address financial decisions within the next year, rather than across multiple years. We will pay special attention to a number of considerations that are unique to healthcare organizations operating in multiple countries. Although much of the content in this section would fall under the purview of key executives and functional-area experts (in this case, financial managers), healthcare managers at lower- and mid-level positions should nevertheless have a basic understanding of these concepts. The complexities discussed in this section have a significant impact on the availability of financial resources and the amount of risk borne by the larger organization in multinational settings.

Working Capital Management

working capital management
The area of management concerned with the short-term assets and liabilities used in the day-to-day operations of a firm.

Working capital management is concerned with the short-term assets and liabilities used in the day-to-day operations of a firm. In terms of items on financial statements, this area deals with cash, short-term marketable securities, accounts receivable, inventory, accounts payable, and other short-term debt. For financial managers at US firms, working capital management largely involves a trade-off between liquidity and efficiency. For managers in global settings, it becomes more of a three-way trade-off, with the consideration of risk taking on greater importance. Even in global settings, many working capital management issues can be addressed with information from a standard financial management text (see Gapenski and Pink [2015]). However, the specifics of certain issues will vary from country to country, so country-specific resources are often useful, if not required (e.g., for India, see Mathur [2013]). The cash management process is central to working capital management, so we will begin with that issue.

Cash Management in the Global Context

Whether the organization is focused on operations in a single country or in multiple countries, **cash management** involves procedures that monitor, control, and allocate the firm's cash. However, global health managers should be aware that, for multinational companies (MNCs), the process is much more complex. Whereas all firms must hold cash balances to make normal day-to-day business expenditures, an MNC needs to maintain those balances in multiple countries and in multiple currencies, while dealing with the constraints of multiple legal and tax systems. In addition, firms must have precautionary cash balances to ensure that they have sufficient money for unforeseen events, and managers in global settings must take into account a broader range of possible events. Finally, firms might hold speculative balances because they believe security prices will fall, and they might keep additional cash in a particular country because they expect changes in exchange rates.

> **cash management**
> The set of procedures associated with monitoring, controlling, and allocating a firm's cash.

Another critical portion of any cash management system is the **cash concentration system**. Ideally, a cash manager would like to have all funds combined into a single account. However, even at a stand-alone domestic hospital, separate accounts might exist for the deposits from the cafeteria, gift shop, parking lot, admissions, and so on. To allow for more efficient management, all the cash collected during a day might be concentrated into a single account by "sweeping" across the various accounts each night. In the case of a US hospital system with multiple hospitals, a second sweep most likely occurs across the concentration accounts from each hospital into a single account each night. Sweeps may be set to leave zero balances, or they may leave a target amount in an account—for example, to cover payroll the next day.

> **cash concentration system**
> A system for combining funds from separate accounts into a single account for more efficient management.

For managers at MNCs, the cross-country cash concentration process is more complex. First, the process is shaped by consideration of the best location for a concentration account, given differing tax rules and legal frameworks. One objective is netting of accounts. For example, if one affiliate of the MNC is holding a cash balance and earning a relatively low interest rate while another affiliate is borrowing in the same currency, it makes sense to reduce the borrowing cost by lending the funds within the company by netting the accounts. The banking regulations of some countries allow notional pooling of balances, where a bank pays interest on the overall net balance of a group of accounts but the funds remain separated in the various accounts. This practice contrasts with physical sweeping, where the funds are moved into a sweep account. Sometimes, cross-currency notional pooling is possible, where the netting includes daily calculation of net balances based on exchange rates and also considers the differing interest rates paid on balances of different currencies. Notional pooling can sometimes be extended to involve pooling funds with a cross-border sweeping process. In such cases, an MNC can avoid commingling funds from multiple entities but still benefit from netting balances and liabilities.

Exchange Rate Exposure

A global healthcare manager will likely need to work with multiple currencies. For example, a hospital in India might receive its payments in rupees but have to pay overseas pharmaceutical suppliers with dollars and euros. Although the hospital can convert the rupees into other currencies, the currency transactions have a cost. In addition, the rates at which the currencies may be exchanged vary over time, which creates a risk that the hospital might not be able to convert its rupees into enough dollars to purchase the required pharmaceuticals.

Exchange rates affect a number of working capital management decisions, and they generate three main types of risk for global healthcare managers:

1. *Transaction exposure* occurs when exchange rates fluctuate between the time a transaction is agreed to and the time of payment. One way to mitigate this risk is through forward contracts, as described in the next section.

2. *Translation exposure* occurs when a company reports overseas assets on its balance sheet. If an American company owns a hospital in India, the value of the hospital in rupees is translated to dollars each time the firm reports its balance sheet. If the value of the hospital in rupees stays the same over time but the exchange rate changes, then the value on the balance sheet will also change. One solution to translation exposure is to offset the value of a firm's assets in a particular currency with an equal value of liabilities in the same currency. For example, if a firm held both assets and liabilities valued at $100,000 in a particular currency, a 25 percent decrease in the exchange rate would leave both the assets and liabilities values at $75,000, with no net effect on the firm's net worth.

3. *Economic exposure* occurs because changes in exchange rates influence the value of future cash flows from long-term transactions. For example, an American firm might buy a hospital in India and expect that the cash flows will be sufficient to pay the debt used to buy the hospital. However, fluctuations in exchange rates might result in the cash flows back to the American firm being different than budgeted. One solution is to use flexible sourcing to offset expected cash flows. As a case in point, perhaps the American firm expects $500,000 per year in remittances from the hospital in India; the firm could then plan to source some expense of $500,000 annually in India. For example, the

firm might agree to outsource the coding of claims to India. Because the firm then would have an expense for coding equal to the amount of a revenue stream, any change in exchange rates would result in offsetting effects.

Hedging Risks to Working Capital

Health managers in global settings should recognize that a number of methods are available to reduce the costs of currency transactions and to lower the risk of potential currency fluctuations. The purchasing of a financial investment for the purpose of reducing the risk of adverse price movements in another asset is called **hedging**. One approach to risk hedging involves the use of **forward contracts** to "lock in" an exchange rate. For example, a hospital in India that agrees to pay a supplier in dollars in 60 days might want protection against possible changes in exchange rates that might occur over those 60 days. One solution is to buy a 60-day forward contract at the time the order to the supplier is placed. The forward contract could specify that the hospital will convert a certain number of rupees into a certain number of dollars on that date.

Transfer Pricing

Transfer pricing involves establishing the price at which one unit of an organization transfers a good to another unit of the organization. Global health managers should recognize that the issue of transfer pricing is both important and controversial. For example, consider a case in which an American hospital system purchases supplies and pharmaceuticals in bulk at a central location and redistributes the items to hospitals in multiple countries. The profit that each hospital earns on a particular item—and the corresponding tax on profit—will depend in part on the internal price that the system bills the hospitals for the item. Costs can be assigned to particular items through a variety of methods—for instance, a price might include the amount the system paid for the item as well as a certain amount of overhead allocated to the item. Because different countries have different tax rates, firms have an incentive to transfer at the prices that will result in profit occurring in the country with the lowest taxes. Transfer pricing can also have important effects on managers' incentives. For example, if the transfer price for certain items is relatively high, managers may want to steer customers to other products that generate more profit for their hospital.

Transfer pricing issues can be a major source of conflict between firms and taxing authorities. For instance, from 1989 to 2005, the US Internal Revenue Service (IRS) disputed the method of transfer pricing used by Glaxo-SmithKline Holdings (GSK). At issue was the price that US operations of GSK charged overseas operations for pharmaceuticals. At the resolution of the dispute in 2006, GSK agreed to pay the IRS approximately $3.4 billion—which at that time was the largest settlement agreement in the history of the IRS. In

hedging
The purchasing of a financial investment for the purpose of reducing the risk of adverse price movements in another asset.

forward contract
A type of contract that can "lock in" an exchange rate for a future date to protect against exchange rate fluctuations.

transfer pricing
Establishing the price at which one unit of an organization transfers a good to another unit of the organization.

announcing the settlement, the commissioner of the IRS noted that "transfer pricing is one of the most significant challenges for us in the area of corporate tax administration" (IRS 2006). The use of transfer pricing to avoid taxes is increasingly coming under scrutiny. David Chamberlain, an official of an American accounting firm, has stated that "governments have a very legitimate concern on excessive profit-shifting and they have the right to crack down on it" (Kun 2015).

Short-Term Financing

commercial paper
Debt issued by firms and sold to investors.

Within the United States, managers raise short-term financing through such sources as commercial paper, bank loans, and secured short-term debt. **Commercial paper** is debt issued by firms and sold to investors. Bank loans include notes, which are for a specific amount and period (e.g., 90 days), and lines of credit. Secured short-term debt may involve **factoring receivables**, whereby a lender, at a discount, buys receivables that are owed to another company and then collects the receivables. Global health managers should be aware of the differences between countries in the availability and operation of alternative sources of short-term financing. For example, in some countries, factoring receivables might not be possible.

factoring receivables
An arrangement whereby a lender, at a discount, buys receivables that are owed to another company and then collects the receivables.

Supply Chain Management

Supply chain management, which focuses on coordinating the functions associated with materials and supplies, varies greatly from country to country. Some countries face a severe lack of supplies. In Cuba, for instance, trained healthcare workers are available, but equipment and supplies are scarce. Spooner and Ullmann (2014, 29) have likened the situation to "a well-trained army with no weapons and no ammunition." A second source on Cuba further highlights the country's outdated technologies and lack of supplies, pointing out that, at a time when the United States was spending $4,000 per capita on healthcare, the entire GDP of Cuba was just $2,000 per capita (Whiteford and Branch 2009). The abundance of labor and lack of equipment in Cuba stand in contrast with reports from Russia, which has faced shortages of medical personnel, in part because of low salaries. In 2007, the average physician or nurse in Russia was making $392 per month, compared to $596 for workers in industry (Lovett-Scott and Prather 2014). Such differences between countries create significant complexity for global supply chain managers.

Maranz (2001) notes that, given chronic shortages, parts of Africa have adopted an informal system of sharing resources (including items such as inventory). He cites an example of a physician in Chad who ran a hospital and used resources according to cultural expectations. If the government ran out of gasoline, the physician allowed the government to use gasoline that the hospital held in inventory for the ambulance. Similarly, if the hospital ran out of gasoline, the government allowed the hospital to take from its inventories. At times, both the hospital and the government would be out of gasoline, but this arrangement was considered preferable to the hospital "hoarding" gasoline for its ambulance. Maranz acknowledges that such an informal system would not be appropriate in the West.

The resource and cost differences that exist between countries are not always a disadvantage to the developing countries. For instance, consider India's rapidly developing generic drug industry, which includes more than 120 plants approved by the US Food and Drug Administration (Seshadri 2014). One report states that the price of medication in India is about 20 percent less than the price of the same drugs in the United States. Similarly, at a time when cardiac surgery cost $50,000 in the United States, similar care was estimated to cost just $4,000 in India (Lovett-Scott and Prather 2014). With an increasingly global supply chain, these cost differences are both a threat and an opportunity for global managers.

Financial Reporting and International Accounting

Sharan (2012) suggests that the concept of international accounting should be addressed in three dimensions. First, international accounting considers the wide diversity of practices among the various countries. The second dimension is the related issue of "harmonization," which involves attempts to establish international norms for accounting practices. Third, international accounting deals with issues related to consolidation of an MNC parent and its foreign affiliates.

A number of specific issues also affect international accounting. We have already discussed transfer pricing and the way that exchange rate variability influences the accounting on financial statements. Another key issue is **transparency**, which looks at the degree to which a country's reporting standards lead to full disclosure. Disclosure standards vary by country. Affiliates of American companies, for instance, are required to meet US standards established under the Sarbanes-Oxley Act of 2002. Finally, accounting for inflation plays an important role as well. For several decades, the United States had relatively slow rates of inflation, but during this time many other countries had considerable changes in price levels, with significant implications for international accounting.

transparency
The degree to which a country's reporting standards lead to full disclosure.

Summary

In this chapter, we focused on micro-level considerations unique to the financial decisions that managers face when healthcare organizations operate in complex domestic and multinational environments. We addressed the long- and short-term financial concerns that organizations must adequately address when entering new markets, when expanding the scale or scope of operations within existing markets, and when financing the provision of healthcare in multinational settings. Operational managers should be familiar with the financial complexities that emerge when organizations operate in multiple countries and when they move financial resources across countries and through multiple currencies. These matters might primarily be the responsibility of professional financial managers, but operational healthcare managers should nonetheless be familiar with these challenges and understand how their decisions shape the organization's financial results.

Discussion Questions

1. What are some of the key factors that healthcare organizations might use to identify a foreign country in which to set up new operations? Consider the question both from a financial perspective and from a mission perspective. What types of financial risks must they assess, and how might they go about managing or mitigating those risks to achieve their organization's healthcare mission?

2. What are some of the financial pros and cons of the different market entry methods? Does a trade-off exist between the entry strategy and the ability to achieve the organization's desired mission-related healthcare outcomes?

3. What would be some of the main reasons that healthcare organizations might choose to seek new investment capital domestically and then move the money abroad? What would be some of the main reasons companies might choose to seek new investment capital within the foreign country where they seek to expand operations?

4. In what ways might you treat cash inflows and outflows differently when assessing a new capital project idea that requires investment in a foreign country, as opposed to a purely domestic investment?

5. How does a healthcare organization balance the long-term interests of entering new markets with the need to ensure the short-term financial viability of those initiatives? Should foreign initiatives be evaluated in isolation (i.e., each on its own merit, like an individual stock) or as part of a collection of projects (i.e., as a component of a larger portfolio)?

Case Study: CHRISTUS Health Pursues a Joint Venture with a Large Health System in Chile

In 2012, Pontificia Universidad Católica de Chile (PUC) in Santiago, Chile, chose to pursue negotiations with CHRISTUS Health, a US-based Catholic nonprofit health system, toward a joint venture agreement for the ownership, operation, and expansion of PUC's health network (CHRISTUS Health 2012, 2013). The agreement was finalized in 2013. Under the agreement, CHRISTUS acquired a 50 percent ownership interest in Clínica San Carlos de Apoquindo UC, a full-service hospital based in Santiago. CHRISTUS supplied a local executive team, including a CEO, a chief operating officer, and a chief financial officer.

PUC is a top Chilean university owned by the Catholic Church. Its health network, at the time of the agreement, consisted of two hospital campuses totaling approximately 600 beds, as well as 11 outpatient centers and a large laboratory and imaging services network (CHRISTUS Health 2012). In addition to being one of the largest health systems in Chile, this network serves as the main teaching campus of the university's medical school, which is recognized as the premier school for the training of medical professionals in Chile and one of the best in all of Latin America.

"We are honored to be chosen by PUC as the organization they will work with to form an exclusive partnership," said Ernie Sadau, president and CEO of CHRISTUS Health, at the time of its selection by PUC (CHRISTUS Health 2012). "We believe that our international expansion will help us extend our mission around the world, meeting health care needs that are great and deeply felt in Latin America and complement our strong position in the U.S. . . . The partnership we create in Chile will also help us diversify our operations, increase long-term sustainability and help CHRISTUS lead the development of new, worldwide health care models."

CHRISTUS Health was one of the few American health systems that had a long-standing international presence. Since 2001, CHRISTUS Health had maintained a successful track record in Mexico with Grupo CHRISTUS Muguerza, a seven-hospital system operated as a joint venture. CHRISTUS Muguerza pioneered the development of innovative models of care, including a host of successful outpatient medical clinics. CHRISTUS implemented this strategy in 2001, before these models had found success in the United States. CHRISTUS's long-term experience in Mexico made it an ideal partner to bring management expertise and strategic planning to the network in Santiago (CHRISTUS Health 2012).

(continued)

Banchile Citi Global Markets and Citigroup Global Markets acted as exclusive financial advisers to CHRISTUS Health in the negotiations toward the definitive joint venture partnership agreement. Sadau said, "We look forward to the opportunity to answer this calling in Santiago, following the example of our sponsoring congregations in extending the healing ministry of Jesus Christ and strengthening Catholic health care around the world" (CHRISTUS Health 2012).

Case Study Discussion Questions
1. Why were CHRISTUS Health and the Pontificia Universidad Católica de Chile a good fit to partner on such a venture?
2. How would CHRISTUS Health go about evaluating the financial costs and benefits of such a project?
3. What sources of investment capital would CHRISTUS Health seek to underwrite this joint venture?
4. In terms of risks faced by CHRISTUS Health, how does this international joint venture compare to a similar joint venture within the United States?
5. If the venture proves profitable, what complications might arise for CHRISTUS in financially benefiting from the partnership?

Additional Resources

Basu, S., J. Andrews, S. Kishore, R. Panjabi, and D. Stuckler. 2012. "Comparative Performance of Private and Public Healthcare Systems in Low- and Middle-Income Countries: A Systematic Review." *PLOS Medicine*. Published June 19. http://journals.plos.org/plosmedicine/article?id=10.1371/journal.pmed.1001244.

Jasso-Aguilar, R., H. Waitzkin, and A. Landwehr. 2005. "Multinational Corporations and Health Care in the United States and Latin America: Strategies, Actions and Effects." In *Commercialization of Health Care: Global and Local Dynamics and Policy Responses*, edited by M. Mackintosh and M. Koivusalo, 38–50. London: Palgrave Macmillan.

Karanikolos, M., P. Mladovsky, J. Cylus, S. Thomson, S. Basu, D. Stuckler, and M. McKee. 2013. "Financial Crisis, Austerity, and Health in Europe." *Lancet* 381 (9874): 1323–31.

Mossialos, E., A. Djordjevic, R. Osborn, and D. Sarnak (eds.). 2017. "International Profiles of Health Care Systems." Commonwealth Fund. Published May. www.commonwealthfund.org/~/media/files/publications/fund-report/2017/may/mossialos_intl_profiles_v5.pdf?la=en.

Quinn, K. 2015. "The 8 Basic Payment Methods in Health Care." *Annals of Internal Medicine* 163 (4): 300–6.

Tuohy, C. H., C. M. Flood, and M. Stabile. 2004. "How Does Private Finance Affect Public Health Care Systems? Marshaling the Evidence from OECD Nations." *Journal of Health Politics, Policy and Law* 29 (3): 359–96.

Waitzkin, H., and C. Iriart. 2001. "How the United States Exports Managed Care to Developing Countries." *International Journal of Health Services* 31 (3): 495–505.

Yip, W. C. M., W. C. Hsiao, W. Chen, S. Hu, J. Ma, and A. Maynard. 2012. "Early Appraisal of China's Huge and Complex Health-Care Reforms." *Lancet* 379 (9818): 833–42.

References

Bupa. 2014. *Annual Report 2013: Living Bupa's Purpose Together.* Accessed April 18, 2018. www.bupa.com/~/media/files/site-specific-files/our%20performance/pdfs/financial%20results%20-%20historical%20financial%20info/2013%20group%20financial%20info/annual-report-and-accounts-2013.pdf.

CHRISTUS Health. 2013. "CHRISTUS Health and Pontificia Universidad Católica de Chile Finalize Partnership in Chile." Published December 20. www.christushealth.org/press-releases-html-stripped/christus-health-and-pontifica-universidad-cat_lica-de-chile-finalize-partnership-in-chile.

———. 2012. "CHRISTUS Health Chosen to Pursue Exclusive Negotiations with Large Health System in Chile." Published October 1. www.christushealth.org/press-releases-html-stripped/christus-health-chosen-to-pursue-exclusive-negotiations-with-large-health-system-in-chile.

Cleverley, W., and J. Cleverley. 2018. *Essentials of Health Care Finance*, 8th ed. Burlington, MA: Jones & Bartlett Learning.

Desjardins, J. 2016. "All of the World's Stock Exchanges by Size." Money Project. Published February 16. http://money.visualcapitalist.com/all-of-the-worlds-stock-exchanges-by-size/.

Gapenski, L. C., and G. H. Pink. 2015. *Understanding Healthcare Financial Management*, 7th ed. Chicago: Health Administration Press.

Gerszewski, G. 2014. "Sanford Health Opens Pediatric Clinic in Kunming, China." PRWeb. Accessed April 18, 2018. www.prweb.com/releases/2014/10/prweb12244290.htm.

Internal Revenue Service (IRS). 2006. "IRS Accepts Settlement Offer in Largest Transfer Pricing Dispute." Published September 11. www.irs.gov/newsroom/irs-accepts-settlement-offer-in-largest-transfer-pricing-dispute.

International Private Medical Insurance (IPMI) Magazine. 2014. "Bupa Completes Acquisition of Cruz Blanca Salud, Chile." Published February 27. https://

ipmimagazine.com/medical-health-insurance/en/news/insurance-industry-mergers-acquisitions/item/2597-bupa-completes-acquisition-of-cruz-blanca-salud-chile.

KPMG. 2018. "Corporate Tax Rates Table." Accessed April 18. https://home.kpmg.com/xx/en/home/services/tax/tax-tools-and-resources/tax-rates-online/corporate-tax-rates-table.html.

Kun, L. 2015. "Transfer Pricing Makes Big Splash on Global Taxes." CCTV.com. Published October 28. http://english.cntv.cn/2015/10/28/ARTI1446023289912521.shtml.

Lovett-Scott, M., and F. Prather. 2014. *Global Health Systems: Comparing Strategies for Delivering Health Services.* Burlington, MA: Jones & Bartlett Learning.

Maranz, D. 2001. *African Friends and Money Matters: Observations from Africa.* Publications in Ethnography, vol. 37. Dallas, TX: SIL International.

Mathur, S. B. 2013. *Working Capital Management and Control: Principles and Applications,* 2nd ed. New Delhi, India: New Age International Publishers.

Mossialos, E., A. Djordjevic, R. Osborn, and D. Sarnak (eds.). 2017. "International Profiles of Health Care Systems." Commonwealth Fund. Published May 31. www.commonwealthfund.org/publications/fund-reports/2017/may/international-profiles.

Patients Beyond Borders. 2017. "Medical Tourism Statistics & Facts." Updated December 14. www.patientsbeyondborders.com/medical-tourism-statistics-facts.

Peel, M., and N. P. Linh. 2015. "Vietnam Scraps Foreign Ownership Limits in Investment Push." CNBC. Published June 29. www.cnbc.com/2015/06/29/vietnam-scraps-foreign-ownership-limits-in-investment-push.html.

Pomerlau, K. 2015. "Corporate Income Tax Rates Around the World, 2015." Tax Foundation. Published October 1. http://taxfoundation.org/article/corporate-income-tax-rates-around-world-2015.

Quinn, K. 2015. "The 8 Basic Payment Methods in Health Care." *Annals of Internal Medicine* 163 (4): 300–6.

Sanford Health. 2014. "Sanford Health Opens Pediatric Clinic in Kunming, China." Published October 14. www.sanfordhealth.org/newsroom/2014/10/sanford-health-opens-pediatric-clinic-in-kunming-china.

Seshadri, V. 2014. "The Indian Pharmaceutical Sector: The Journey from Process Innovation to Product Innovation." In *India's Healthcare Industry: Innovation in Delivery, Financing, and Manufacturing,* edited by L. R. Burns, 441–476. Delhi, India: Cambridge University Press.

Sharan, V. 2012. *International Financial Management,* 6th ed. New Delhi, India: PHI Learning.

Spooner, M. H., and S. Ullmann. 2014. *Cuban Health Care: Utopian Dreams, Fragile Future.* Lanham, MD: Lexington.

Whiteford, L. M., and L. G. Branch. 2009. *Primary Health Care in Cuba: The Other Revolution.* Lanham, MD: Rowman & Littlefield.

Willis, E., L. Reynolds, and H. Keleher. 2012. *Understanding the Australian Health Care System*, 2nd ed. Sydney, Australia: Elsevier.

World Bank. 2018a. "Lending Interest Rate (%)." Accessed April 18. https://data.worldbank.org/indicator/FR.INR.LEND.

———. 2018b. "Total Tax Rate (% of Commercial Profits)." Accessed April 18. https://data.worldbank.org/indicator/IC.TAX.TOTL.CP.ZS?end=2017&start=2015&view=chart.

World Stock Exchanges. 2018. "World Stock Exchanges: List of Stock Exchanges Around the World." Accessed April 18. www.world-stock-exchanges.net.

4

HUMAN RESOURCE MANAGEMENT IN A GLOBAL CONTEXT

David Briggs, PhD, Godfrey Isouard, PhD, Leonard H. Friedman, PhD, FACHE, and Myron Fottler, PhD

Chapter Focus

The healthcare sector is essentially a human enterprise, and the connections between people who engage in health work are key to organizational success. This chapter examines human resource principles and effective human resource management practices in a global context. It discusses best practices, sociocultural perspectives, and the impact of culture, while also providing lessons from the global health workforce. It also examines self-management and emotional intelligence in the context of being an effective manager.

Learning Objectives

Upon completion of this chapter, you should be able to

- describe the impact of human resource management and practice in the global context,
- discuss the challenges associated with human resources in healthcare,
- identify the core principles of human resource management in healthcare in global contexts,
- use best-practice human resource management to effectively maximize organizational performance,
- distinguish the health workforce as a global strategic issue for health services, and
- consider the diverse sociocultural perspectives and understand the impact of culture on the global health workforce.

Competencies

- Analyze problems, promote solutions, and encourage decision making.
- Demonstrate the ability to optimize the healthcare workforce and address local workforce issues such as shortages, scope of practice, skill mix, licensing, and fluctuations in service.
- Provide leadership in defining staff roles and responsibilities, developing appropriate job classification/grading systems, and planning the workforce.
- Effectively manage departmental human resource processes, including scheduling; performance appraisals; incentives; recruitment, selection, and retention; training and education; motivation; coaching and mentoring; and use of appropriate productivity measures.

Key Terms

- Capability
- Capacity
- Competence
- Critical reflection
- Emotional intelligence (EI)

- Managerial rounding
- Resilience
- Skill mix
- Staff mix
- Task shifting

Key Concepts

- Best practices
- Communication
- Complex adaptive systems
- Continuous feedback
- Global health workforce
- High, middle, and low performers
- Human resource management (HRM)

- Human resources (HR)
- Leadership
- Organizational culture and behavior
- Self-management
- Sociocultural perspectives

Introduction

Effective human resource management (HRM) in a global context recognizes that the healthcare sector is essentially a human enterprise—one of "people engaging and serving other people" (Briggs 2016, 9). The connections between people who engage in health work have long been recognized as integral to the professionally dominant roles within the sector. Egener and colleagues (2017) espouse this idea in their "Charter on Professionalism for Health Care Organizations," which states that organizational culture is reflected in "the well-being of patients and employees" and that operational and business practices must incorporate "commitment to fair treatment, education, and development" for employees.

Healthcare has traditionally been delivered through relatively large organizations with bureaucratic structures, but the field is becoming increasingly systemized. Boundaries are being redefined to respond to aging populations (and workforce), the increasing burden of chronic disease, the impact of technology, social movements, and socioeconomic determinants (Egener et al. 2017). This struggle to redefine and reform health systems as "professional organizations" has been evident since the work of Brock, Powell, and Hinings (1999) and Brock (2006). Healthcare today is mostly delivered within systems that are complex and adaptive (Best et al. 2012), with networks of practice that cross organizational boundaries in an increasingly global context (Briggs and Isouard 2015). This movement distinguishes healthcare organizations from other types of enterprises, and it presents new challenges for the dynamics of human resources (HR) in the field.

This chapter will discuss the core principles of HRM and consider how we can be more effective as managers and leaders through the use of best practices. The globalized nature of today's workforce presents both internal strategic challenges and strategic opportunities, as organizations seek a competitive advantage in recruiting, training, and retention; the chapter therefore approaches HRM as a global strategic issue. It addresses organizational cultures, sociocultural contexts, interpersonal relationships, and workforce performance, as well as the importance of self-management and emotional intelligence.

Human Resources for Healthcare: Core Principles and Issues

The Society for Human Resource Management (SHRM 2016)—with input from more than 1,200 HR professionals from 33 different nations—created a competency model that describes what might be considered the core principles of HR. This global initiative was developed with four career levels in mind—entry, mid, senior, and executive. The model was intended to serve as a resource and "road map" to help HR professionals develop their proficiencies and those of others and to achieve their goals. (The model's introduction notes that it is for developmental purposes only and not to be used as the basis for selection decisions.) It suggests nine primary competencies (SHRM 2016):

1. HR expertise
2. Relationship management
3. Consultation
4. Leadership and navigation
5. Communication
6. Global and cultural effectiveness
7. Ethical practice
8. Critical evaluation
9. Business acumen

task shifting
The redistribution of tasks among workforce teams.

The SHRM's initiative provides a starting point for considering strategic HR issues for the health sector. Strategic HR approaches in healthcare may involve **task shifting** (i.e., the redistribution of tasks among workforce teams) and extending scopes of practice; placing a concerted emphasis on competency training and workforce development; addressing questions of size, distribution, and composition within an organization or a country's healthcare workforce; carrying out specific agendas for regional, rural, and remote communities; and ensuring organizational readiness for large-scale transformational reform.

The World Health Organization (WHO), in a 2008 report, has expressed concern that the world's health systems may be unable to achieve improved health outcomes without "significant strengthening of human resources for health" and "innovative ways of harnessing and focusing . . . the human resources that already exist" (WHO 2008, 5). The report specifically highlights task shifting and extended scopes of practice as strategic initiatives to address workforce shortages. Advances in technology, e-health, and telemedicine have had a significant impact on workforce readiness and availability, leading to greater consideration of task shifting and the emergence of new roles. The WHO report stresses the need for a framework that supports task shifting, alongside other ways of increasing the supply of skilled workers. It calls for HR analysis incorporating new and existing quality assurance mechanisms; greater definition of roles and associated competencies as the basis for recruitment, training, and evaluation; and competency-based training that is needs driven, accredited, and tied to certification, registration, and career progression mechanisms (WHO 2008). Although the WHO report has a specific focus on HIV/AIDS, it is relevant to the broader HR needs of health systems—particularly in recognizing that "at the heart of every health system is the health workforce" and that "the world is experiencing a chronic shortage of trained health workers" (WHO 2008, 14). The words used in the WHO report resonate with the core SHRM principles described previously.

A group of Canadian researchers has presented a set of key questions and issues pertaining to human resources in healthcare in a global context. The key issues can be summarized as follows (Kabene et al. 2006):

1. The size, distribution, and composition of a country's healthcare workforce are key indicators of the country's capacity to deliver services and interventions.

2. Human resources personnel must consider the composition of the health workforce in terms of both skill categories and training levels.

3. A properly trained and competent workforce is essential to any successful healthcare system.

4. The migration of healthcare workers is a critical issue for global healthcare systems.

5. The movement of healthcare professionals closely follows the migration pattern of professionals in general; the internal movement of the workforce to urban areas is common to all countries.

6. Workforce mobility can create imbalances that require better workforce planning.

7. Evidence suggests that a significant positive correlation exists between a country's level of economic development in and its supply of human resources for health.

8. Aging populations and the aging health workforce have a significant impact on health workforce capacity and sustainability.

9. Cultural and geographical factors affect the supply and demand of human resources for health and therefore must be considered when examining global healthcare systems.

10. Human resources have a significant impact on attempts at health reform, and this impact should not be underestimated.

11. Human resources are one of three main health system inputs, along with physical capital and consumables; they are the hardest of the three inputs to develop, manage, and maintain.

12. The global nature of the health workforce poses challenges to countries in managing and retaining their local health workforce.

Delving further into key issues facing HRM in healthcare, the WHO (2008, 2010) has called for national policies to improve retention of the healthcare workforce in remote and rural areas, where access to healthcare services is often lacking. Meanwhile, Weiner (2009) has focused on readiness for change within organizations and the health workforce. Best and colleagues (2012, 421) have conducted a comprehensive review of large-system transformation in healthcare, and they set forth five simple rules: "(1) blend designated leadership with distributed leadership; (2) establish feedback loops; (3) attend to history; (4) engage physicians; and (5) include patients and families."

The challenges facing healthcare apply equally to HR policy, leadership, and practice. Although designed to facilitate strategic intent, HR practices can

skill mix
The combination of skills available in an organization.

staff mix
The number, qualifications, and experience of people on staff.

at times be inhibitors of progress, and imbalances in HR can result in poor and inadequate use of health personnel (Dubois and Singh 2009). Dubois and Singh (2009) propose an "HR optimization" approach to ensure better congruence between HR practices and organizational and external policy contexts. An examination of HR practices in an organization can start by looking at **skill mix** (the combination of skills available) and **staff mix** (the number, qualifications, and experience of people on staff). In greater detail, the examination can look at the numbers of workers and defined occupational groups; the appropriate ratios of staff members per patient; the number of procedures, prescriptions, and so on; and the implications of the various approaches. Ensuring the proper mix of qualifications and levels of experience is an important dimension of staff planning and workforce development. Additional concerns include skill substitution and replacement, levels of junior and senior staff, the potential need for higher levels of certification, the impact of interprofessional practice, and the fostering of teamwork and collaborative approaches.

Dubois and Singh (2009) suggest that effective HRM in today's healthcare landscape requires more than the traditional approach focused on numbers, types, grades, education, and experience. They recommend a "skill management" approach, with a more adaptive use of workers' knowledge, skills, behaviors, and other attributes. Such an approach emphasizes the capacity to learn and adapt and take on new roles through role enhancement, role enlargement, skill flexibility, role substitution, and role delegation.

The field of HRM is often described in terms of planning and staffing policies, education and training, working conditions, and performance management, but the effectiveness of these approaches often depends on the organizational fit. Research suggests that organizational characteristics likely to contribute to a good fit in healthcare include flat hierarchies with few supervisors, significant worker autonomy, participative management, professional development opportunities, high organizational status for nurses, and collaboration (Dubois and Singh 2009). Teamwork, empowerment, affinity with vision and mission, staff participation in decision making, innovation, career opportunities, and fairness in industrial practice are all considered positive attributes of organizational HR practice.

Effective Human Resource Management

Regardless of where on the globe a healthcare organization is located, optimal patient care cannot be delivered without effective HRM. Healthcare delivery requires large numbers of inputs from multiple clinical practitioners who are supported by a complex infrastructure of managers, technical staff, administrators, and others in key roles. Optimal care requires outstanding staff at all levels. For many healthcare organizations, the HR function is limited to a number of core activities, such as hiring and firing staff, ensuring compliance with HR-related laws, and serving as a resource for managers throughout the organization. In our estimation, these activities are necessary but not sufficient. The HRM function must be explicitly connected with the larger strategic goals of the organization.

This section will discuss the additional considerations that must be factored into operations if an organization intends to move beyond the basics and optimize its HRM. We will carefully consider HR best practices that have proved effective in global contexts, with lessons from a variety of countries. We will also examine key elements of effective HRM, including self-management and emotional intelligence, which research tells us is probably more important for organizational success than traditional intelligence.

HR Best Practices

A major challenge in global HRM in healthcare is identifying best practices—those practices that significantly improve organizational performance and outcomes. A number of studies have shown that effective HRM in business can increase profitability, annual sales per employee, productivity, market value, and growth and earnings per share (Messersmith and Guthrie 2010; Kaufman 2010). Researchers have used surveys to measure the sophistication of organizations' HR practices, assigning organizations scores from 0 to 100, with high scores representing "state-of-the-art" practices. The research has indicated that organizations with better HR practices tend to experience better financial performance (Becker, Huselid, and Ulrich 2001). Further evidence was provided by a survey of 200 chief financial officers, in which 92 percent of respondents believed that managing employees effectively improves customer satisfaction (Mayer, Ehrhart, and Schneider 2009). Customers also report that they are more satisfied when the climate of the organization is positive, employees generally get along well, and turnover is low (Nishii, Lepak, and Schneider 2008).

So, specifically, what types of HR practices can help an organization achieve these positive outcomes? Exhibit 4.1 provides a summary. The practices listed in the exhibit occur repeatedly in studies of high-performing organizations, and they tend to be present in organizations that are effective in managing their human resources. In addition, these practices are interrelated and mutually reinforcing; positive results are difficult to achieve by implementing just one practice on its own.

Although these HR best practices will generally have a positive impact on organizational performance, their relative effectiveness may vary depending on their alignment (or lack thereof) with the organization's mission, values, culture, strategies, goals, and objectives (Ford et al. 2006). Effectiveness may also depend on how well the practices reinforce one another in a particular type of organization.

EXHIBIT 4.1
Effective HR
Practices for
Healthcare
Organizations

Category	Practices	
HR planning / job analysis	• Encourage employee involvement to ensure strong "buy-in" of HR practices and managerial initiatives. • Encourage teamwork so employees are more willing to collaborate. • Provide employment security.	• Use self-managed teams and decentralization as basic elements of organizational design, thereby minimizing management layers. • Develop strategies to enhance employee work–life balance.
Staffing	• Be proactive in identifying and attracting talent. • In selecting new employees, use additional criteria (e.g., attitudes, customer focus, cultural fit) beyond basic skills.	
Training / organizational development	• Invest in training and organizational programs to enhance employee skills related to organizational goals. • Provide employees with future career opportunities by giving promotional priority to internal candidates.	• Include customer service in new employee onboarding and skill development. • Provide opportunities for employee growth so that employees are "stretched" to enhance all their skills.
Performance management and compensation	• Recognize employees through both monetary and nonmonetary rewards. • Offer high compensation contingent on organizational performance, with the aim of reducing employee turnover and attracting high-quality employees.	• Reduce status distinction and barriers such as dress, language, office arrangement, parking, and wage differentials. • Base individual and team compensation on goal-oriented results.
Employee rights	• Communicate effectively with employees and keep them informed about major issues and initiatives. • Share financial, salary, and performance information to develop a high-trust organization. • Give higher priority to internal candidates for promotion, thereby enhancing employee motivation.	• Provide employment security for employees who perform well, protecting them against economic downturns or strategic errors by senior management.

Sources: Bruce (2013); Chuang and Liao (2010); Gomez-Mejia and Balkin (2011); Pfeffer (1995, 1998); Suttapong, Srimai, and Pitchayadol (2014); Wright et al. (2005).

Applying these findings in a global healthcare context has some limitations. First, most of the research deals with organizations in general, not healthcare organizations specifically. Second, the research tends to be focused in the United States, meaning that it might not reflect the prevalent values and cultures of other parts of the world. Often, the major stakeholders for US organizations are the stockholders, so the analysis might not sufficiently address the goals and objectives for other stakeholders in diverse cultures. In addition, it is difficult to prove whether excellent organizational performance leads to effective HR practices or whether good HR practices cause better organizational performance (Wright et al. 2005).

Nonetheless, effective HR practices are clearly associated with excellent organizational performance (Lepak, Smith, and Taylor 2007), and it seems reasonable that healthcare systems should consider the implementation of the HR practices associated with the best-performing organizations. Once the practices have been implemented, the systems can determine whether the practices and their benefits are applicable to a particular global context.

Sociocultural Perspectives and the Impact of Culture: Lessons from the Global Health Workforce

The diverse, multicultural nature of today's global health workforce and the mobility of labor and capital from one part of the world to another carry significant implications, which have been examined in depth by a number of authors. Short, Marcus, and Balasubramanian (2017) and Taylor (2016) have focused their analyses on the healthcare systems in Asia and the Pacific Islands, while Martins (2016) has conducted a comparative analysis of the United Kingdom, the United States, Canada, New Zealand, and Australia, specifically considering the different choices the nations have made with regard to workforce utilization. The United Nations *Human Development Report 2015* makes several key points relevant to the health workforce. It emphasizes that work—including voluntary and creative work, not just jobs—contributes to human progress and enhances the health and wellness of populations (United Nations Development Programme 2015). The report also cautions that globalization and the technological revolution are rapidly changing how we work and what we do. The mobility of the global health workforce has the potential to alleviate workforce shortages and reduce inequalities between countries, yet it can also contribute to shortages and inequality in certain instances. For example, Australian health professionals often work in other countries, and this migration is one of the reasons that Australia has had to rely on doctors trained in other countries to sustain health services in its rural and remote communities.

HR strategy and practices need to recognize the impact of the cultural differences that exist among nations and among communities within the same nation, as well as the differences that exist among various professional groups in the health setting. This intersection of diverse cultures complicates relationships and makes navigation through HR policy and practice more complex. At the same time, however, these attributes can also help us improve the ways we learn, manage, and lead. (See the case study that accompanies this section.)

The distinct cultures, values, legal frameworks, and political systems of various countries and regions shape the way that individual health systems operate. Although the central functions of HR are somewhat similar across the globe—HR planning, job analysis and design, staffing, training, performance appraisal, and labor relations—the prevalence of particular HR practices and their impact on outcomes vary widely. For example, the US healthcare system relies heavily on private, for-profit organizations, whereas many countries of Latin America and Asia have more socialized systems (e.g., universal healthcare) (Lytle et al. 1995). Consequently, US employers tend to place a greater emphasis on individual performance and performance-driven rewards. In a comparison of management priorities in the United States and mainland China, US managers were more concerned about getting the job done, whereas Chinese managers were concerned with maintaining harmony (Ralston et al. 1992).

The social psychologist Geert Hofstede (2018) suggests that societies differ on six dimensions: (1) power distance, (2) individualism, (3) masculinity, (4) uncertainty avoidance, (5) long-term orientation, and (6) indulgence. Of these dimensions, the most relevant for HR practices are individualism, masculinity, and long-term orientation. Detailed information about how various countries compare across these dimensions is available via Hofstede Insights (2018) at www.hofstede-insights.com/product/compare-countries/.

Cultural and legal differences have a powerful influence on HR policies and practices. The American emphasis on individuality, for instance, might explain why managers in the United States have fewer constraints in downsizing employees than managers in other countries do (Brewster 2004). The US concept of employment at will—which gives employers substantial freedom to terminate employees—does not exist in Europe, where firing or laying off workers is often very expensive (Poutsma, Ligthart, and Veersma 2006). Similarly, in India, employers with more than 100 employees must have government approval to lay off or fire workers (Srivastava 2011), and Brazil imposes a fine of 4 percent for employees who are fired without "just cause" (*Economist* 2011). Autocratic countries, meanwhile, often fail to protect "whistleblowers" who divulge negative information about their employers.

Case Study: Sociocultural Perspectives in Researching Healthcare Systems and Developing Health System Managers

The following case study was developed in 2017 through the work of colleagues at the Naresuan University College of Health Systems Management (NUCHSM) in Tha Pho, Phitsanulok, Thailand: D. S. Briggs, P. Tejativaddhana (Thailand), P. Barua (Bangladesh), K. Dorji (Bhutan), S. Hasan (Bangladesh), D. Tshering (Bhutan), and C. Wangmo (Bhutan). It may be used for teaching, research, and referencing purposes with attribution to NUCHSM (http:// chsm.nu.ac.th/en/).

The field of health system management has been relatively unknown in many Asian Pacific countries, where the traditional focus has been on public health, not on acute care health systems. Often, doctors and nurses have taken positions as health managers or hospital directors without having any prior health management education or experience. Still, these countries are embarking on an era of health reform and looking to move from "developing country" status to "developed country."

Thailand has become famous for its successes in health reform, adopting universal healthcare, using health volunteers to influence villages toward better health, and establishing district health systems as the entry point to healthcare (Tejativaddhana, Briggs, and Thonglor 2016). In addition, the College of Health Systems Management at Naresuan University has been established to educate Thailand's health professionals in the concepts and practices of effective health system management. NUCHSM was established with strong strategic initiatives that included establishment of

- learning and research practices based on a global perspective;
- international partnerships in both learning and research;
- networks of learning and research that incorporate collaborative management and leadership practices (VanVactor 2012); and
- comparative learning and research in the subregion, leading to local, sustainable health system practices (Tejativaddhana, Briggs, and Thonglor 2016; Briggs, Tejativaddhana, and Kitreerawutiwong 2010; Taytiwat, Fraser, and Briggs 2006).

The college is already regarded as a success and has been recognized by the country's Ministry of Foreign Affairs as a center for scholarships for foreign students from the subregion. People in other countries have become focused on learning how Thailand and NUCHSM achieved such early success and how that success could be replicated in other settings.

Doctoral and research students predominantly from the countries of Bhutan and Bangladesh have undertaken an analysis of key health management issues, taking into consideration the ways that their national cultures compare to that of Thailand. Bhutan's culture emphasizes a behavior code known as "Driglam Namzha" (order, discipline, custom, rules, and regimen) and loyalty to benevolent superiors. The country has a collectivist, interdependent society that holds equality and solidarity in high regard. The influence of these traits on management reflects strong identity, harmony, and trust, all relevant to teamwork. As a precursor to their research, the students used Hofstede's (2018) six dimensions of culture to develop the comparison

(continued)

shown in exhibit 4.2. In terms of power distance, Bhutan ranks highest, followed by Bangladesh and then Thailand. Collectivism, meanwhile, is higher in Bangladesh and Thailand than in Bhutan. Bangladesh is regarded as a more masculine society, whereas Bhutan and Thailand are more feminine.

Having established the countries' measures across the various cultural dimensions, the students then devoted time to reflection and discussion about how their findings might influence various research topics they had identified within a health management context. Their intended topics included childhood obesity, rehabilitation services, leadership and management competencies in district health services, village health volunteers, and application of the sufficiency economic philosophy to health—an approach based on moderation, reasonableness, and prudence.

Many readers will work in more "developed" countries' health systems and may be thinking, "Well, this is all well and good, but what does it mean for me as an HR manager?" First, we would point out that many of the topics mentioned here are contemporary challenges in advanced health systems, just as they are in developing systems. Second, we would suggest that management, including HR management in healthcare organizations, is often practiced in normative, rational, and mechanistic ways—in planning, leading, sometimes directing, organizing, and controlling. However, organizations and their management often do not truly operate in that manner because they function as complex adaptive systems. Achievement of strategy, alignment of managers to the mission and vision, and successful reform are difficult tasks, and the results are often partial and, at best, layered on existing practice.

Next, we ask: To what extent do you understand organizational culture and behavior? Do you understand the differences, interplay, and tensions

EXHIBIT 4.2
Thailand's Cultural Dimensions, in Comparison with Bangladesh and Bhutan

	Thailand	Bangladesh	Bhutan
Power distance	64	80	94
Individualism	20	20	52
Masculinity	34	55	32
Uncertainty avoidance	64	60	28
Long-term orientation	32	47	N/A
Indulgence	45	20	N/A

Source: Data from Hofstede Insights (2018).

between distinct health professions, and have you analyzed the typology of the archetype of managers in your organization (Briggs, Cruickshank, and Paliadelis 2012)?

Finally, we would ask you to look around and see how many distinct national and cultural groups reside in the communities that you serve, and in your health workforce. The communities likely are multicultural. We would suggest that a greater emphasis on culture in practice and learning, reinforced through training, might create greater value and outcomes for your organizations. The adoption of NUCHSM's four dot points, listed earlier in this case study, might be a good starting point.

Labor relations and labor costs vary widely from one country to another, with the United States and other developed economies having higher compensation levels than less developed nations do. In many European countries, global work councils of employee representatives meet monthly with managers to address such HR issues as layoffs and antidiscrimination policy. Collective bargaining in Western Europe tends to be industrywide, whereas in the United States it tends to occur at the organizational level. In addition, significant intracountry differences in HR practices exist depending on public or private ownership, multinational or national structures, and urban or rural location. Organizations that are large, private, and multinational tend to have more elaborate HR practices (Akhtar, Ding, and Ge 2008; Fox 2006).

Exhibit 4.3 outlines a few of the major cultural differences between the United States and various other countries with regard to values and HR practices. Clearly, the United States has a culture that emphasizes individualism and free enterprise to a greater degree than most other countries across the globe. These values, in turn, influence the types of HR practices that are implemented, as well as the relative success or failure of those practices. The question then becomes, To what degree can we rely on past/present research and our knowledge of institutions to predict the prevalence and success of various HR practices in global healthcare organizations?

A number of challenges arise when assessing the impact of HR practices on organizational performance of global healthcare organizations. One particularly significant challenge is that the components of performance will vary across cultures. For example, US organizations will tend to place a greater focus on financial outcomes, whereas organizations in Western Europe will tend to focus on the satisfaction of a wider variety of stakeholders (employees and customers). However, if countries are converging in a global economy, then cultural distinctions and interindustry differences may become less significant over time.

EXHIBIT 4.3
Prevalence of
Values and HR
Practices in the
United States
and Other
Countries

		Values		HR Practices	
Individualism	US values: • Personal responsibility • Internal focus	Alternative values (Singapore, South Korea): • Employer involvement in employees' personal lives • Loyalty to organization	US practices: • Performance-based pay • Extrinsic motivation • Short-term orientation	Alternative practices (Singapore, South Korea): • Group-based performance evaluation • Seniority-based pay • Intrinsic motivation • Pay related to needs
Masculinity	US values: • Gender stereotyping • Higher power and status of males	Alternative values (Netherlands, Norway, Sweden): • Minimal gender stereotyping • Gender equality	US practices: • Gender inequality • Occupational segregation	Alternative practices (Netherlands, Norway, Sweden): • Gender pay equity • Gender equality of opportunity
Short-term vs. long-term orientation	US values: • Past and present oriented • Immediate gratification	Alternative values (Japan, China): • Future oriented • Delayed gratification • Long-term goals	US practices: • Short-term rewards • Low investment in training and development • Low employment security	Alternative practices (Japan, China): • Long-term rewards • Seniority as a basis for pay • Employment security • Major investments in training and development

Source: Adapted from Gomez-Mejia, Balkin, and Cardy (2012).

Given the paucity of research on this topic, strong empirical evidence is not currently available. However, a comparison of exhibit 4.1 (listing effective HR practices) with exhibit 4.3 (showing prevalence of values and practices) allows for some conclusions. First, little correlation appears to exist between the effectiveness of HR practices and their prevalence. In the United States, for instance, the *most effective* HR practices tend to be the *least prevalent*. Many such practices—such as gender equality and management emphasis on employment security, training, and development—tend to be more prevalent in countries other than the United States. Given the trend of increasing globalization—which could be reversed in the event of a major war or increased trade barriers—we expect to see greater convergence over time in national and economic systems, which would likely make the most effective HR practices more common in the United States and other developed countries.

Managing Others—Competency, Capability, and Capacity

For years, there was "no widespread agreement as to a definitive way to describe, let alone define, the health manager's role and required capabilities" (Briggs, Smyth, and Anderson 2012, 71). However, global healthcare leaders in recent years have begun working toward a better understanding of managerial competence, capability, and capacity. Historically, the HR challenge for healthcare and health management was set forth by Filerman (2003), who asserted that effective organized health programs and systems depended on effective management but that health systems worldwide faced a lack of competent managers at all levels. Filerman's challenge has prompted a variety of responses, though much work remains to be done. In Australia, for instance, reports and research indicate that the country, despite having a highly regarded health system, still has variable utilization, costs, and outcomes—suggesting that it continues to have room for improvement with regard to management (Duckett 2016; Podger 2016).

In 2008, the Society for Health Administration Programs in Education (SHAPE) published the "SHAPE Declaration on the Organisation and Management of Health Services," which aims to explain how health services might best be organized and effectively managed. Its proposed principles include the idea that "health managers should be appropriately qualified, skilled and adept in managing complex health service organisations" (Briggs 2008, 11). The declaration maintains that managers, to be effective, must be able to manage "out" and "down" to staff and other stakeholders, as well as "up" to central authorities, while at the same time being accessible to multidisciplinary clinical teams and capable of delivering environments, cultures, and systems "to support the delivery of safe, quality care" (Briggs 2008, 11). The declaration states that "health managers need to be capable in a number of areas," including the following (Briggs 2008, 12):

1. Being trained and experienced to lead and manage in a range of differing health system and organisational arrangements.

2. Possessing a deep contextual understanding of health systems, public policy, professional cultures and politics.

3. Having competency in organisational sensemaking as negotiators of meaning, active participants, constructors, organisers and persuaders within health systems.

4. Being drawn from a range of backgrounds including those with clinical and non-clinical experience and qualifications who can demonstrate broad contextual health knowledge that demonstrates more than one logic.

5. Understanding how clinical work should be structured and managed and work actively with clinicians and others to deliver coherent, well-managed health services.

In 2009, at the First International Conference of Health Service Delivery Management, held in Phitsanulok, Thailand, some 450 delegates from 17 countries and 14 organizations adopted a declaration espousing five principles (Briggs, Tejativaddhana, and Kitreerawutiwong 2010):

1. Priority in resourcing and policy implementation should be given to developing leadership, management and governance as the means to strengthen health systems development;
2. Successful management of health services requires leadership and teamwork from managers who have positive personal and professional values and self-perceptions and are empowered to engage with individuals and communities and to respond to the needs of the poor and to marginalised groups;
3. Leadership for health systems, public health and PHC [primary healthcare] requires that managers have access to high quality education, training and experiential health context and knowledge that equips them to operate effectively in health systems;
4. A research culture is required that networks and engages in collaborative research to develop health management capacity and evidence as a basis for decisions, to guide policy development and that both challenges and aligns researchers and operational health systems professionals, citizens and communities.
5. Outcomes identified from this conference for leadership and health management education training and research be conveyed to health organizations, professional bodies, local government, Ministry(s) of Health and Education and research funding bodies.

Filerman (2003) asserts that "management competence is the essential precondition for program success" and that "HR is the advocate for making the investment in managerial competence." He states that, to serve this role, HR must "start with a solid assessment of the need," analyzing every position at every level to "identify the specific management competencies required to meet the objectives of the position."

Liang and colleagues (2013) have responded positively to Filerman's challenge through their ongoing research in Australia, New Zealand, Thailand, and China, in which they have identified competencies from actual managers occupying positions at various levels. Isouard and Martins (2014), meanwhile, have taken a strategic and evidence-based approach to identifying health management skills and competencies, basing their work on real-world health management issues.

The International Hospital Federation (IHF) Global Consortium, in a report titled *Leadership Competencies for Healthcare Services Managers*, has identified six critical areas for professionalizing healthcare management (IHF 2015):

1. Accountability and transparency
2. Service improvement
3. Educational standards
4. Integrity
5. Commitment to sharing leading practices
6. Equity in access to and delivery of care

Building on the Global Consortium's work, the Australasian College of Health Service Management (ACHSM) has adopted a competency framework with five domains (ACHSM 2016):

1. Leadership
2. Health and healthcare environment
3. Business skills
4. Communications and relationship management
5. Professional and social responsibility

These domains, presented in exhibit 4.4, represent five areas in which healthcare managers should demonstrate competence.

    The terms *competence*, *capability*, and *capacity* are sometimes used interchangeably, but they are distinct concepts. **Competence** refers to the knowledge,

competence
The knowledge, skills, and attitudes that people possess; what people know and do.

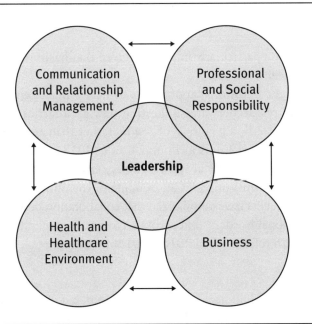

EXHIBIT 4.4
Five Competency Domains

Source: Reprinted with permission from IHF (2015).

capability
The abilities reflected in the breadth of a role, usually expressed in strategic, tactical, operational, and transactional terminologies.

capacity
The amount and variety of work that a workforce can accomplish.

skills, and attitudes that people possess; it is typically expressed in terms of what people know and do. **Capability**, for a manager, is usually expressed in strategic, tactical, operational, and transactional terminologies that reflect the breadth of the role. Finally, **capacity** is the amount and variety of work that a workforce can accomplish (Vincent 2008). Essentially, competence and capability—together with curriculum, workplace learning, formal education, and ongoing professional development—help develop the capacity of the health workforce to operate in complex systems that are experiencing continuing health reform. Any discussion of health management competence needs to recognize that health is "a complex, adaptive, professionally dominated, politically driven system, experiencing constant change" (Briggs, Smyth, and Anderson 2012, 71).

In evolving organizations in complex systems, we need to do more than just enhance competence; we need to educate for the capability to work in uncertain contexts. Thus, Briggs, Smyth, and Anderson (2012, 77) pose the following questions:

1. How do we move the debate from capability and competence of managers and leaders working in traditional, rational and mechanistic organizational forms toward the capabilities required in organizational forms that are focused on delivering services through collaborations in networked services across the health, human and community service sectors?
2. How do we link up workplace learning, education and ongoing professional development—what do we each have to do to get some real, innovative partnering happening?
3. How do we select for capability?

These questions are particularly important given that health managers have a leading role in health reform.

Increasingly, traditional approaches to health management are being questioned, and researchers are suggesting new approaches toward health services delivery based on a culture of *health*, rather than a culture of *healthcare*. The Robert Wood Johnson Foundation's (2018) "Building a Culture of Health" website (available at www.rwjf.org/en/how-we-work/building-a-culture-of-health.html) provides an example of this shift. A number of US authors and researchers have emphasized that collaboration between providers, across organizational borders, and across sectors is an imperative for cultural change and health reform (Weil 2016a, 2016b; Chandra et al. 2016).

Managing Self

Managing others is an important aspect of leadership, but effective management of oneself cannot be overlooked. Leadership roles often require a high level of performance in difficult circumstances, and people in those positions typically serve as role models, mentors, and educators of others. In addition, in any setting where tenure is not a given, management of one's own performance largely determines the individual's likely career outcomes. Thus, leaders must constantly manage themselves and the ways they behave, lead, and respond to various situations. Self-management is closely related to mindfulness, resilience, and critical reflection, all of which tie into the broader concept of emotional intelligence.

Emotional Intelligence

The human dimension of management—which includes relationship building, communication, conflict resolution, decision making, teamwork, and collaboration—is critical to an organization's overall performance in the delivery of services. For an organization to function effectively in those areas, **emotional intelligence (EI)** needs to be recognized, practiced, and enhanced at every level. Renowned organizational psychologist Daniel Goleman (1998, 317) defines *emotional intelligence* as "the capacity for recognizing our own feelings and those of others, for motivating ourselves, and for managing emotions well in ourselves and in our relationships." Research has shown that the ways we feel and engage within organizations affect the quality of our decisions, our behavior, and our responses toward others. Clearly, managers within healthcare organizations must be able to drive peoples' emotions in the right direction. However, not all managers have developed the appropriate emotional competencies and strengths.

Key aspects of emotional intelligence include resilience and critical reflection. **Resilience**, simply put, is the ability to withstand or rebound from adversity, to overcome difficult circumstances, and to add new capabilities and opportunities. Resilient individuals possess a range of personal attributes and are adaptable to change. Resilience can be learned and is an important part of self-management. **Critical reflection** is a well-recognized professional practice that involves identifying and assessing the underlying assumptions and values that influence one's performance. Critical reflection is imperative in times of rapid change, when practitioners and organizations are facing increased demands with fewer resources (Gardner 2014). Astute HR managers will see the value of critical reflection as an organizational learning approach, and health managers will appreciate employees who are reflective in their decision making.

Managers constantly face challenges rooted in poor communication and engagement among healthcare professionals and the people receiving care. For a system to function well, managers and employees must demonstrate a capability for engaging and communicating with one another. They must also have the EI to contend with the emotional pressures and strains of the job. Failure to manage EI can have a considerable impact on the effectiveness of the overall system.

emotional intelligence (EI)
The capacity for recognizing, understanding, and managing emotions in oneself and in one's relationships.

resilience
The ability to withstand or rebound from adversity, to overcome difficult circumstances, and to add new capabilities and opportunities.

critical reflection
The practice of identifying and assessing the underlying assumptions and values that influence one's performance.

Emotional intelligence, therefore, should be regarded as an essential management competency. Effective healthcare managers need more than just cognitive and technical skills; they need to be able to control emotions and apply them to everyday work. Successful managers generally possess self-awareness, self-regulation, motivation, empathy, and social skill (Goleman 2004). They have a highly stable mind and disciplined nature, are adaptable to change, and can manage problematic situations through careful decision making. Managers need to be conscious of their own state of mind, and they need to know what is happening with their workers and the people with whom the workers engage. Essentially, effective managers lead the way for building an engaging workplace that thrives on the ways people are feeling, communicating, and building working relationships together; such a setting leads to positive interactions, high-quality decisions, and improved performance (Goleman 1998).

The attainment of a high level of EI enhances managers' competency for handling the key issues confronting them and the wider organization, and it provides a foundation of reassurance and confidence for the management of a team. At the other end of the spectrum, poor EI management often leads to communication deficiencies, mistrust, uncertainty, reluctance to engage, low productivity, and reduced job satisfaction. Managers who lack EI often "shoot from the hip" rather than thoughtfully considering the needs and wants of the people they manage, which contributes to poor attitudes among team members. Managers must maintain a degree of emotional independence so that they can deal with emotions at all levels and assess how these emotions might affect their decision-making processes.

Impact on Organizational Behavior

Today's healthcare managers are tasked with continuously improving the development, organization, and delivery of health services in the face of increasing workloads and a high-pressure, results-driven climate. Effective managers use their emotional intelligence to establish a harmonious working environment for an enthusiastic group of people who are motivated to get work done. In the ideal situation, all levels of employees work toward being connected and engaged. People generally perform better when they feel supported, understood, valued, and trusted. Senior management must make sure that all employees are aware of management's commitment to achieving better outcomes for patients and other clients, as well as for them as valued employees.

Within a team structure, emotional status is generally a good indicator for evaluating group effectiveness. Emotions tend to grow out of social interactions, and they have a significant impact on work group behavior. One management practice known to create emotional stability is dispersed decision making, in which people directly involved with a particular task are empowered to make their own decisions within the organization. When people feel empowered, they can be creative, communicate widely, voice constructive criticism, and develop new ideas; the likelihood of emotional conflicts and negative reactions is reduced.

Leading-Edge HR Practices

Arguably, the most important function of HRM for any healthcare organization is making sure that the right people are hired and that they are a good fit for the organization. This function may sound straightforward, but it is perhaps the most difficult task an HR department must accomplish. Too often, healthcare organizations are so eager to fill a vacant position that they focus only on the requisite qualifications with regard to licensure, education, and experience, without taking the time to see how well a person fits within the culture of the organization. Furthermore, at the same time these organizations are rushing to fill vacancies, they often are reluctant to terminate the employment of workers who are underperforming.

We encourage readers to examine existing practices at their organizations and reflect on how effective those practices might be. Consider the range of HR practices described in exhibit 4.3 earlier in the chapter. See if you can obtain data on the rate at which new staff members at your organization voluntarily leave during the first 18 months of employment. How satisfied are you and your colleagues with new staff members? What sort of effort is being made to determine the likely work behaviors of a prospective employee before an offer of employment is made? Astute HR practitioners recognize that every occasion of disengagement or recruitment incurs a cost, as do the strategies adopted to retain staff.

By now, it has become clear that most healthcare organizations do a poor job both in getting the right staff on board and in removing low-performing employees. What can be done to correct this dual problem? In this section, we will examine the approaches of "hiring slow" and "firing fast," along with the concept of high, middle, and low performers. We encourage readers to challenge well-established beliefs and practices and develop their own conceptions of what might be considered "leading edge."

Hire Slow

Without question, staff vacancies can create significant problems in both clinical and administrative areas, and such problems are exacerbated when multiple vacancies exist or when an opening has gone unfilled for an extended period. Thus, the common temptation is to quickly fill an open position with someone who meets the minimum qualifications and then hope that that person will be able to work effectively with current staff members. Such an approach might be an adequate short-term solution, but it is probably not the approach organizations should take to ensure retention and continued outstanding performance.

We recommend that, in addition to making sure applicants meet any minimum requirements in terms of education, experience, and licensure, HR departments and hiring managers take into account the following attributes:

- *Talent.* According to Buckingham and Coffman (1999) in their book *First, Break All the Rules,* great managers define *talent* as a recurring pattern of thought, feeling, or behavior that can be productively applied. The job of the hiring manager is to determine what talents the candidate possesses and whether these talents are the most appropriate for the position at hand.
- *Cultural fit.* Every healthcare organization has an overall culture, as well as a set of "microcultures" specific to particular teams and work groups. Given that cultures are unlikely to change quickly, the hiring manager should prioritize finding new staff members who will fit within the existing culture. As part of this task, the hiring manager must be able to verbalize the critical parts of the culture that are tied to organizational success.
- *Corporate citizenship.* An important question to ask of all prospective new employees is how willing they are to go above and beyond the basic elements of the job description. Are they willing to participate in projects, committees, and other activities that are not directly linked to their specific job? This willingness to pitch in cannot be measured by simply looking at a resume.

These three attributes are essential if a new employee is to grow to full capacity, but they are not readily apparent in a resume or application. Thus, applicants should be engaged in a series of behavior-based interview questions that indicate how they will perform under a variety of conditions and situations. Furthermore, we recommend that prospective employees be interviewed by a group of high-performing members of the current work team. Workers who are already performing at a high level will want only other high performers to join them.

Proper consideration for these attributes might require an organization to slow down the hiring process somewhat. However, taking this time can help make sure that the candidate possesses the requisite talent, is a good fit for the organization, and will bring value to the organization at every turn.

Fire Fast

Healthcare organizations exist for the purpose of taking care of sick people and helping to make them well, and in serving this purpose, we are in the mind-set of taking whatever time is needed to work with patients to assist them to a full recovery. Unfortunately, we too often approach underperforming staff members the same way. For instance, we might treat low-performing staff members as though they have some sort of problem and that, if we give them time and support, they will finally achieve what we expect them to deliver. However, this patience with workers often does a disservice to the organization and its patients.

How many organizations can afford for their clinicians to deliver substandard care? Is it OK for front-office staff to be chronically late or to treat patients and visitors with a dismissive or uncaring attitude? How many mistakes can be made by back-office personnel, leading to lost revenue, improper coding, or disrespectful behavior, before others recognize that there is a problem?

One common approach for a low-performing worker is, first, to ignore the problem and hope it resolves itself. When that approach fails, the manager asks the staff member to come in for a chat. The supervisor discusses the problem and the expectations going forward, and the employee responds with a long list of problems that are affecting work. The manager often will walk out of that meeting feeling sorry for the employee and wishing that more could be done to help. In many instances, there may be no other option but to discipline or even terminate the employee. Even then, managers often will stall, delay, and otherwise put off the difficult conversations until work conditions deteriorate so badly that action becomes absolutely necessary.

The question here is, Why do managers wait so long to deal with underperforming staff and individuals whose behavior negatively affects the quality of work done by others? Assuming the staff member has the requisite skills to do the job (and if not, the worker should not have been hired in the first place), the issue is one of behavior. All staff members, regardless of rank or seniority, must be made aware of the sorts of behaviors that are expected in the organization, and behaviors that are inconsistent with those expectations must be addressed. Bad behavior that goes unnoted or uncorrected is assumed to be acceptable. In the words of Quint Studer (2009), "What you permit, you promote."

We are not suggesting that staff be disciplined or terminated at the first instance of a behavior that is out of line with standards or expectations. However, if problematic behavior has been brought to an employee's attention and the behavior does not change, the manager must be prepared, without delay, to have a frank and honest conversation with the employee. If low-performing employees either cannot or will not change, and if no suitable options exist for moving them to another role in the organization, their employment should be terminated. In other words, fire fast, and do not delay the inevitable.

Distinguish Between High, Middle, and Low Performers

All organizations are populated by employees who can be categorized as performing at high, middle, or low levels. Ideally, everyone in a healthcare organization would be a high performer; unfortunately, however, that is not always the case. Each of the three types of employees brings a particular set of challenges and opportunities to the healthcare organization. Exhibit 4.5 provides a summary of the attributes of high, middle, and low performers.

Simply stated, high performers are those staff members who consistently perform their work at an optimal level. They come to work with a good attitude and display the sort of professionalism that you wish everyone would exhibit; thus, they serve as role models for others in the organization. High performers help solve problems and seek out opportunities to continually improve. Middle performers are usually those staff members whose work is generally good but who need more experience. They might need coaching to improve their work, but their hearts are in the right place and they want to do a good job. Low performers are those staff members who come to work with a poor attitude and tend to have an excuse for everything that goes wrong. They make up a minority of the workforce but require a large percentage of the manager's time. Managers must continually try to get them to perform in ways that are in alignment with the goals of the work unit.

Given the critical nature of patient care, it is reasonable to ask why managers spend so much time tolerating low performers, especially when their performance can suck the life out of the organization. Typically, coworkers know who the low performers are and are waiting for managers to act. Managers, however, often have excuses and reasons of their own for not acting. They might be aware of a workforce shortage and concerned about the difficulty of finding a replacement, or they might be hopeful that low performers will improve with time and guidance. Sometimes, managers simply feel that removing the low performer will be too difficult, so they choose to ignore the problem and hope it goes away. Often, problems in the organization grow worse when high performers take notice of the permissiveness and special attention that low performers are receiving; these high performers may then choose to reduce their own job performance or, sadly, leave the organization.

The most important thing to remember is that, wherever you are in the world, healthcare delivery is too important to be left to low performers. Nurture and grow your high performers, coach and develop your middle performers, and deal quickly and efficiently with your low performers.

Exhibit 4.5, which was developed by the Studer Group based on findings from its national learning lab, can be used as a worksheet for staff assessment. When performing the assessment, the most difficult decisions for leaders tend to involve employees who have four or five good qualities but who have one quality that holds them back and actually hurts the performance of the department. A good question to ask during the assessment is, Knowing what I know, would I hire them again? We encourage readers to customize the questionnaire's characteristics based on the standards and expectations within their specific organizations.

	High	Middle	Low	
Definition	Comes to work on time. Good attitude. Problem solver. You relax when you know they are scheduled. Good influence. Use for peer interviews. Five Pillar ownership. Brings solutions.	Good attendance. Loyal most of the time. Influenced by high and low performers. Wants to do a good job. Could just need more experience. Helps manager be aware of problems.	Points out problems in a negative way. Positions leadership poorly. Master of We/They. Passive aggressive. Thinks they will outlast the leader. Says manager is the problem.	**EXHIBIT 4.5** High, Middle, and Low Performers
Professionalism	Adheres to unit policies concerning breaks, personal phone calls, leaving the work area, and other absences from work.	Usually adheres to unit policies concerning breaks, personal phone calls, leaving the work area, and other absences from work.	Does not communicate effectively about absences from areas. Handles personal phone calls in a manner that interferes with work. Breaks last longer than allowed.	
Teamwork	Demonstrates high commitment to making things better for the work unit and organization as a whole.	Committed to improving performance of the work unit and organization. May require some coaching to fully execute.	Demonstrates little commitment to the work unit and the organization.	
Knowledge and Competence	Eager to change for the good of the organization. Strives for continual professional development.	Invested in own professional development. May require some coaching to fully execute.	Shows little interest in improving own performance or the performance of the organization. Develops professional skills only when asked.	
Communication	Comes to work with a positive attitude.	Usually comes to work with a positive attitude.	Comes to work with a negative attitude. Has a negative influence on the work environment.	
Safety Awareness	Demonstrates the behaviors of safety awareness in all aspects of work.	Demonstrates the behaviors of safety awareness in all aspects of work.	Performs work with little regard to the behavior of safety awareness.	

Source: Reprinted with permission from Studer (2009).

Provide Continuous Feedback

Another leading-edge HR practice involves ongoing communication and the provision of continuous feedback to staff members throughout the year. Too often, the only time an employee receives feedback from a direct supervisor is during the annual performance evaluation. Annual performance evaluations are necessary to meet internal organizational policies, but they are not enough to ensure optimal performance. When employees receive continuous feedback, they are able to modify their performance and correct their behaviors without delay. Furthermore, they know exactly how they are doing, so they are not surprised by any of the information conveyed during the annual evaluation.

managerial rounding
A practice in which a manager visits employees at their workstations on a weekly basis to provide feedback, discuss work-related issues, and address employee concerns.

One widely used method for providing continuous feedback is **managerial rounding** (Hotko 2018). The principle is simple: On a weekly basis, managers "round" on their direct reports, visiting them at their workstations to discuss work-related issues. During each visit, the manager asks a short list of questions that are pertinent to the job being done by the staff member. If a staff member requests an action, the manager acts on the request and reports back, making sure all employees know their concerns are being addressed. No matter how busy a manager might be, rounding must take priority. The practice can contribute to higher staff and patient satisfaction, and it can help ensure that managers know firsthand and in real time what is happening in their workplace. This practice is similar to long-standing rounding approaches that emphasize the need for managers to be seen around and about their organization and to engage with staff through discourse.

Be Mindful of Gender and Generational Considerations

Leaders in modern global health systems must also be mindful of gender and generational concerns, which present significant challenges in both developing and developed countries. Gender equity is essential for maximizing the health workforce, and a lack of such equity is widely regarded as a failure of HR leadership (Newman 2014). Newman (2014) points out that gender inequalities are "systems inefficiencies that contribute to clogged health worker educational pipelines, recruitment bottlenecks, attrition, and worker maldistribution." Other gender-related considerations include the need to eliminate workforce violence, to equalize career opportunities, and to ensure fairness with regard to pay. Such concerns are commonly incorporated into policies at the health system level and at the national and international levels (Newman 2014). HR managers addressing these concerns should be aware that they often must take into account long-held values and beliefs both within the workforce and within management (Briggs and Isouard 2015).

In recent years, the health workforce has been a mix of at least four distinct generations: (1) Veterans, or Traditionalists, born between approximately 1922 and 1943; (2) Baby Boomers, born between 1943 and 1960; (3) Generation X, born between 1960 and 1980; and Generation Y, or Millennials, born between 1980 and 2000 (Smith 2012). Each of these generations has distinctive values and attitudes toward work. Typically, older generations are more likely to value long-term commitments with organizations, whereas younger generations are more interested in short-term commitments, progression across organizations, and the possibility for casual, part-time, or contracted roles. Younger generations tend to place a greater emphasis on work–life balance. In the past, members of older generations often were "jettisoned" by organizations after they reached age 50, but today they are regarded as highly valuable in the face of workforce shortages.

Today's health professionals are ready travelers, and the health workforce has become fully globalized and multicultural. Thus, today's HR managers must be able to understand and address the needs of diverse groups through effective policy, data collection, and system procedures (Briggs and Isouard 2015; Isouard and Martins 2014; Short, Marcus, and Balasubramanian 2017).

Summary

This chapter has highlighted the importance of human resource management for healthcare delivery organizations across the globe. The HRM function is too important to be minimized or pushed to the sidelines. High-functioning healthcare organizations depend on equally high-functioning HR departments to attract and retain the best employees possible.

Healthcare services are delivered by skilled clinical, technical, and support staff. Without capable people serving these roles, healthcare would not be possible. This chapter has examined core HR principles and discussed a variety of issues affecting HR in healthcare across the globe, with key concepts supported by lessons from specific countries. Effective HRM requires cooperation with senior organizational leadership to ensure that HR structures and practices are aligned with larger strategic goals and objectives. Much HR activity centers on managing others, but self-management—supported by a high degree of emotional intelligence—is also crucial. Managers and leaders who have a good sense of their emotions and the emotions of others have a much better chance of fostering an environment conducive to motivation, teamwork, and high performance.

This chapter has also explored "leading-edge" HR practices that can help organizations achieve better outcomes and avoid common pitfalls. Among other things, it has discussed the benefits of hiring slow, firing fast, and distinguishing between high, middle, and low performers. Finally, the chapter has stressed the importance of providing staff with continuous feedback and taking into account gender, generational, and other sociocultural considerations in a global context.

Discussion Questions

1. What do you consider to be the key challenges for human resource leadership, management, and practice in the global context?
2. What impact has the current global health workforce crisis had on access to high-quality healthcare and improved health outcomes? How

has it affected attainment of the Millennium Development Goals (see www.un.org/millenniumgoals/)?

3. What aspects of good leadership and management make a difference in achieving improved global health outcomes?

4. Human resource management systems in a global health context aim to provide an environment in which the health workforce can function effectively. However, a variety of factors—such as HRM functions being fragmented across too broad a range of stakeholders—can impede an otherwise smooth HRM operation. What are some other factors that might prevent HRM systems from operating at an optimal level?

References

Akhtar, S., D. Z. Ding, and G. L. Ge. 2008. "Strategic HRM Practices and Their Impact on Company Performance in Chinese Enterprises." *Human Resource Management* 47 (1): 15–32.

Australasian College of Health Service Management (ACHSM). 2016. *Master Health Service Management: Competency Framework.* Accessed April 24, 2018. http:// achsm.org.au/Documents/Education/Competency%20framework/2016_ competency_framework_A4_full_brochure.pdf.

Becker, B. E., M. A. Huselid, and D. Ulrich. 2001. *The HR Scorecard: Linking People, Strategy, and Performance.* Boston: Harvard Business School Press.

Best, A., T. Greenhalgh, S. Lewis, J. E. Saul, S. Carroll, and J. Bitz. 2012. "Large-System Transformation in Health Care: A Realist Review." *Milbank Quarterly* 90 (3): 421–56.

Brewster, C. 2004. "European Perspectives of Human Resources Management." *Human Resource Management Review* 14 (4): 365–82.

Briggs, D. S. 2016. "What Problem Is Being Solved? Critical Issues in Health Systems Management." *Asia Pacific Journal of Health Management* 11 (3): 6–9.

———. 2008. "SHAPE Declaration on the Organisation and Management of Health Services: A Call for Informed Public Debate." *Asia Pacific Journal of Health Management* 3 (2): 10–13.

Briggs, D. S., M. Cruickshank, and P. Paliadelis. 2012. "Health Managers and Health Reform." *Journal of Management & Organization* 18 (5): 644–62.

Briggs, D. S., and G. Isouard. 2015. "Managing and Leading Staff." In *Leading and Managing Health Services: An Australasian Perspective,* edited by G. E. Day and S. Leggat, 204–15. Melbourne, Australia: Cambridge University Press.

Briggs, D. S., A. Smyth, and J. A. Anderson. 2012. "In Search of Capable Health Managers: What Is Distinctive About Health Management and Why Does It Matter?" *Asia Pacific Journal of Health Management* 7 (2): 71–78.

Briggs, D. S., P. Tejativaddhana, and N. Kitreerawutiwong. 2010. "Health Declarations." *Asia Pacific Journal of Health Management* 5 (1): 25–30.

Brock, D. M. 2006. "The Changing Professional Organization: A Review of Competing Archetypes." *International Journal of Management Reviews* 8 (3): 157–74.

Brock, D. M., M. J. Powell, and C. R. Hinings (eds.). 1999. *Restructuring the Professional Organization: Accounting, Health Care, and Law*. New York: Routledge.

Bruce, S. 2013. "Top 10 Best Practices in HR Management in 2013." HR Daily Advisor. Published January 27. https://hrdailyadvisor.blr.com/2013/01/27/top-10-best-practices-in-hr-management-for-2013/.

Buckingham, M., and C. Coffman. 1999. *First, Break All the Rules: What the World's Greatest Managers Do Differently*. New York: Pocket Books.

Chandra, A., C. E. Miller, J. D. Acosta, S. Weilant, M. Trujillo, and A. Plough. 2016. "Drivers of Health as a Shared Value: Mindset, Expectations, Sense of Community, and Civic Engagement." *Health Affairs*. Published November. https://www.healthaffairs.org/doi/abs/10.1377/hlthaff.2016.0603.

Chuang, C.-H., and H. Liao. 2010. "Strategic Human Resource Management in Service Concept: Taking Care of Business by Taking Care of Employees and Customers." *Personnel Psychology* 63 (1): 153–96.

Dubois, C.-A., and D. Singh. 2009. "From Staff-Mix to Skill-Mix and Beyond: Towards a Systematic Approach to Health Workforce Management." *Human Resources for Health*. Published December 19. http://human-resources-health.biomedcentral.com/articles/10.1186/1478-4491-7-87.

Duckett, S. 2016. "What Problem Is Being Solved: 'Preventability' and the Case of Pricing for Safety and Quality." *Asia Pacific Journal of Health Management* 11 (3): 6–9.

Economist. 2011. "Employer, Beware; Brazil's Labour Laws." March 11, 43.

Egener, B. E., D. J. Mason, W. J. McDonald, S. Okun, M. E. Gaines, D. A. Fleming, B. M. Rosof, D. Gullen, and M. L. Andersen. 2017. "The Charter on Professionalism for Health Care Organizations." *Academic Medicine*. Published January 10. https://journals.lww.com/academicmedicine/Fulltext/2017/08000/The_Charter_on_Professionalism_for_Health_Care.26.aspx.

Filerman, G. L. 2003. "Closing the Management Competence Gap." *Human Resources for Health*. Published October 8. http://human-resources-health.biomedcentral.com/articles/10.1186/1478-4491-1-7.

Ford, R. C., S. A. Sivo, M. D. Fottler, D. Dickson, K. Bradley, and L. Johnson. 2006. "Aligning Internal Organizational Factors with a Service Excellence Mission: An Exploratory Investigation in Healthcare." *Health Care Management Review* 31 (4): 259–69.

Fox, A. 2006. "China: Land of Opportunity and Challenge." *HR Magazine*, September, 38–44.

Gardner, F. 2014. *Being Critically Reflective: Practice Theory in Context*. New York: Palgrave MacMillan.

Goleman, D. 2004. "What Makes a Leader?" *Harvard Business Review* 82 (1): 82–91.

———. 1998. *Working with Emotional Intelligence.* New York: Bantam Books.

Gomez-Mejia, L. R., and D. B. Balkin. 2011. *Management: People, Performance, Change.* Upper Saddle River, NJ: Prentice Hall.

Gomez-Mejia, L. R., D. B. Balkin, and R. L. Cardy. 2012. *Managing Human Resources,* 7th ed. Upper Saddle River, NJ: Prentice Hall.

Hofstede, G. 2018. "The 6D Model of National Culture." Accessed April 24. https:// geerthofstede.com/culture-geert-hofstede-gert-jan-hofstede/6d-model-of-national-culture/.

Hofstede Insights. 2018. "Compare Countries." Accessed April 24. www.hofstede-insights.com/product/compare-countries/.

Hotko, B. 2018. "Rounding for Outcomes: How to Increase Employee Retention and Drive Higher Patient Satisfaction." Studer Group. Accessed April 24. www.studergroup.com/hardwired-results/hardwired-results-01/rounding-for-outcomes.

International Hospital Federation (IHF). 2015. *Leadership Competencies for Healthcare Services Managers.* Accessed May 14, 2018. www.ihf-fih.org/resources/pdf/ Leadership_ Competencies_for_Healthcare_Services_Managers.pdf.

Isouard, G., and J. M. Martins. 2014. "Health Service Managers in Australia: Progression and Evolution." *Asia Pacific Journal of Health Management* 9 (2): 35–52.

Kabene, S. M., C. Orchard, J. M. Howard, M. A. Soriano, and R. Leduc. 2006. "The Importance of Human Resources Management in Health Care: A Global Context." *Human Resources for Health.* Published July 27. http://human-resources-health.biomedcentral.com/articles/10.1186/1478-4491-4-20.

Kaufman, B. E. 2010. "SHRM Theory in the Post-Huselid Era: Why It Is Fundamentally Misspecified." *Industrial Relations* 49 (2): 286–313.

Lepak, D. P., K. G. Smith, and M. S. Taylor. 2007. "Value Creation and Value Capture: A Multilevel Perspective." *Academy of Management Review* 32 (1): 180–94.

Liang, Z., S. G. Leggat, P. F. Howard, and L. Koh. 2013. "What Makes a Hospital Manager Competent at the Middle and Senior Levels?" *Australian Health Review* 37 (5): 566–73.

Lytle, A. L., J. Brett, Z. I. Barsness, C. H. Tinsley, and M. Janssens. 1995. "A Paradigm for Confirmatory Cross-Cultural Research in Organizational Behavior." In *Research in Organizational Behavior,* vol. 17, edited by L. L. Cummings and B. M. Staw, 167–214. Greenwich, CT: Jai Press.

Martins, J. M. 2016. "Health Systems in Australia and Four Other Countries: Choices and Challenges." *Asia Pacific Journal of Health Management* 11 (3): 45–57.

Mayer, D., M. G. Ehrhart, and B. Schneider. 2009. "Service Attribute Boundary Conditions of the Service Climate–Customer Satisfaction Link." *Academy of Management Journal* 52 (5): 1034–47.

Messersmith, J. G., and J. P. Guthrie. 2010. "High Performance Work Systems in Emergent Organizations: Implications for Firm Performance." *Human Resource Management* 49 (2): 241–64.

Newman, C. 2014. "Time to Address Gender Discrimination and Inequality in the Health Workforce." *Human Resources for Health.* Published May 6. https://human-resources-health.biomedcentral.com/articles/10.1186/1478-4491-12-25.

Nishii, L. H., D. P. Lepak, and B. Schneider. 2008. "Employee Attributions of the 'Why' of HR Practices: Their Effects on Employee Attitudes and Behaviors, and Customer Satisfaction." *Personnel Psychology* 61 (3): 503–45.

Pfeffer, J. 1998. *The Human Equation: Building Profits by Putting People First.* Boston: Harvard Business School Press.

———. 1995. "Producing Sustainable Competitive Advantage Through Effective Management of People." *Academy of Management Executive* 9 (1): 55–72.

Podger, A. 2016. "Federalism and Australia's National Health and Health Insurance System." *Asia Pacific Journal of Health Management* 11 (3): 28–37.

Poutsma, E., P. E. M. Ligthart, and U. Veersma. 2006. "The Diffusion of Calculative and Collaborative HRM Practices in European Firms." *Industrial Relations* 45 (4): 514–46.

Ralston, D. A., D. J. Gustafson, P. M. Elsass, F. Cheung, and R. H. Terpstra. 1992. "Eastern Values: A Comparison of Managers in the United States, Hong Kong, and the People's Republic of China." *Journal of Applied Psychology* 71 (5): 664–71.

Robert Wood Johnson Foundation. 2018. "Building a Culture of Health." Accessed April 25. www.rwjf.org/en/how-we-work/building-a-culture-of-health.html.

Short, S. D., K. Marcus, and M. Balasubramanian. 2017. "Health Workforce Migration in the Asia Pacific: Implications for the Achievement of Sustainable Development Goals." *Asia Pacific Journal of Health Management* 11 (3): 58–64.

Smith, R. 2012. "Overview of the Generations—Generation Y, Generation X, Boomers, and Veterans (Part 4)." Society for Human Resource Management. Published April 25. https://blog.shrm.org/blog/overview-of-the-generations-generation-y-generation-x-boomers-and-veterans.

Society for Human Resource Management (SHRM). 2016. "SHRM Competency Model." Accessed April 25, 2018. www.shrm.org/learningandcareer/competency-model/pages/default.aspx.

Srivastava, M. 2011. "In India, 101 Employees Poses Big Problems." *Bloomberg Businessweek*, January 23, 13–14.

Studer, Q. 2009. *Results That Last: Hardwiring Behaviors That Will Take Your Company to the Top.* Pensacola, FL: Fire Starter Publications.

Suttapong, K., S. Srimai, and P. Pitchayadol. 2014. "Best Practices for Building High Performance in Human Resource Management." *Global Business and Organizational Excellence* 33 (2): 39–50.

Taylor, R. 2016. "The Tyranny of Size: Challenges of Health Administration in Pacific Island States." *Asia Pacific Journal of Health Management* 11 (3): 58–64.

Taytiwat, P., J. Fraser, and D. S. Briggs. 2006. "The Thai-Australian Health Alliance: A Case Study of Inter-Organisational Collaboration." *Asia Pacific Journal of Health Management* 1 (1): 38–44.

Tejativaddhana, P., D. S. Briggs, and R. Thonglor. 2016. "From Global to Local: Strengthening District Health Systems Management as Entry Point to Achieve Health-Related Sustainable Development Goals." *Asia Pacific Journal of Health Management* 11 (3): 81–86.

United Nations Development Programme (UNDP). 2015. *Human Development Report 2015: Work for Human Development.* Accessed April 25, 2018. http://hdr.undp.org/sites/default/files/2015_human_development_report.pdf.

VanVactor, J. D. 2012. "Collaborative Leadership Model in the Management of Health Care." *Journal of Business Research* 65 (4): 555–61.

Vincent, L. 2008. "Differentiating Competence, Capability and Capacity." *Innovating Perspectives.* Published June. www.innovationsthatwork.com/images/pdf/June08newsltr.pdf.

Weil, A. R. 2016a. "Building a Culture of Health." *Health Affairs* 35 (11): 1953–58.

———. 2016b. "Defining and Measuring a Culture of Health." *Health Affairs* 35 (11): 1947.

Weiner, B. J. 2009. "A Theory of Organizational Readiness for Change." *Implementation Science.* Published October 19. http://implementationscience.biomedcentral.com/articles/10.1186/1748-5908-4-67.

World Health Organization (WHO). 2010. "Increasing Access to Health Workers in Remote and Rural Areas Through Improved Retention: Global Policy Recommendations." Accessed April 25, 2018. www.who.int/hrh/retention/guidelines/en/.

———. 2008. *Task Shifting: Rational Redistribution of Tasks Among Health Workforce Teams: Global Recommendations and Guidelines.* Accessed April 25, 2018. http://apps.who.int/iris/handle/10665/43821.

Wright, P. M., T. M. Gardner, L. M. Moynihan, and M. R. Allen. 2005. "The Relationship Between HR Practices and Firm Performance: Examining Causal Order." *Personnel Psychology* 58 (2): 409–46.

INFORMATION TECHNOLOGY FOR HEALTHCARE

Mark Gaynor, PhD, Alice Noblin, PhD, Martin Rusnák, MD, PhD, Viera Rusnáková, MD, PhD, MBA, and Feliciano (Pele) Yu Jr., MD, MSHI, MSPH

Chapter Focus

This chapter seeks to provide healthcare managers a basic understanding of information technology (IT) in healthcare. It provides an introduction to electronic health records (EHRs), the ways data can be exchanged between EHRs, and the ways EHR data can be used in clinical support systems to improve patient care. The chapter continues with a discussion about privacy, security, and the protection of patient information. Finally, it addresses system selection, with a focus on EHRs.

Learning Objectives

Upon completion of this chapter, you should be able to

- demonstrate an understanding of health information technology (HIT);
- justify the use of standards to encode and transmit healthcare data;
- evaluate the relationship between EHRs and clinical support systems;
- assess how HIT can provide innovative approaches to important health management issues, such as quality and evidence-based management; and
- analyze examples of how HIT can provide a strategic advantage to a healthcare organization.

Competencies

- Understand the major features of the information revolution; the role of knowledge workers; data analysis and reporting; and major trends in IT, particularly as they relate to HIT. This competency includes the use of data sets to assess performance, establish targets, monitor indicators and trends, and determine when and if deliverables are met.

- Use information and trend analysis within the organization (with regard to business intelligence, information management, and clinical and business systems) to guide decision making and analyze health trends.
- Examine the modern EHR, and assess its current and potential value. This competency involves understanding the importance of interoperable EHR/HIT systems and knowing how to pick between centralized or distributed architecture.
- Understand the role of standards and protocols in HIT, the principal systems of protocols applicable to HIT, and the responsible parties for HIT standards, policies, and development.
- Evaluate health information classification systems and terminologies.
- Explore innovative uses for existing and emerging technologies to optimize and improve healthcare delivery and efficiency.
- Advocate for and participate in innovative healthcare policies that may have an impact on national or global healthcare delivery systems.
- Assess and implement policies related to the security of systems to protect data integrity, validity, and privacy.
- Identify threats to data integrity and validity.
- Understand the purpose, use, and key functions of various clinical information systems and the factors that might influence adoption.
- Take part in new or upgraded system selection processes, including designing and planning for the selection and acquisition.

Key Terms

- Best-of-breed (BoB) approach
- Big data
- Clinical support system
- Cloud computing
- Computerized provider order entry (CPOE)
- Data governance
- Data integrity
- Diagnosis-related group (DRG)
- E-health
- Electronic health record (EHR)
- Electronic medical record (EMR)
- Health informatics (HI)
- Health information and communication technologies (HICT)
- Health information governance (IG)
- Health information management (HIM)
- Internet of things
- Interoperability
- Meaningful use
- Monolithic approach
- Personal health record (PHR)
- Request for information (RFI)
- Request for proposal (RFP)
- Request for quote (RFQ)

Key Concepts

- Clinical decision support
- Data repositories
- EHR architecture
- EHR system assessment, selection, and implementation
- Health Insurance Portability and Accountability Act (HIPAA) regulations

- Innovation
- Security and privacy of medical information
- Standards for encoding and exchanging medical data

Introduction

Health informatics (HI) is the application of information and computer science to all levels and settings of healthcare, including health-related research. It requires knowledge and skills in technical, clinical, and administrative domains. One limiting factor in the effective implementation of technology is the intersection between human resources and business policies. Lack of an adequately trained workforce often hampers HI adoption and use. Standards for education and training—such as the inclusion of human–computer interaction into informatics programs—are necessary to elevate the HI professions.

According to estimates, the global healthcare IT market will grow to $280 billion (US dollars) by 2021 (Markets and Markets 2018). As it has in other industries, IT in healthcare has changed from a support service to a strategic driver. Just as online package tracking created new advantages in the shipping industry, the introduction of **electronic health records (EHRs)**, combined with **clinical support systems**, offer significant improvements for the delivery of healthcare. Today, many hospitals order medications for patients electronically while checking for adverse drug events, such as allergic reactions and harmful interactions with other medications. Often, online patient portals allow patients to access lab results and communicate securely with their providers. Despite these benefits, even the most advanced HIT systems have problems. As Dr. Robert Wachter (2015) has pointed out in an American Medical Informatics Association keynote speech and in his book, *The Digital Doctor*, mistakes do happen, and interoperability between EHRs from different vendors is challenging.

In Europe, **e-health** (often written eHealth) and digital health projects have been available for more than a decade, supported by European Union (EU) grants. The World Health Organization (WHO) Regional Office for Europe (2016, 7) defines *e-health* as "a broad group of activities that use electronic means to deliver health-related information, resources and services." It covers a

health informatics (HI)
The application of information and computer science to all levels and settings of healthcare, including health-related research.

electronic health record (EHR)
A digital version of a patient's records from healthcare providers.

clinical support system
An information technology system that uses patient information to help guide clinical decision making.

e-health
The use of electronic methods to deliver health-related information and services; often written as *eHealth*.

variety of domains—including EHRs, mobile health, and health analytics—and functionalities that aim to deliver information at the right place at the right time and provide services to a wider population in a personalized manner. Evidence suggests that appetite for e-health capabilities is growing and that tangible progress is being made in the mainstreaming of technology solutions. However, ambitious e-health strategies have only been partially implemented in most EU member states. Denmark has been a leader in e-health in Europe.

The increasing use of HI requires a significant emphasis on education and workforce preparation. The International Medical Informatics Association (IMIA) has recommended a competency-based model of HI with four domains (Mantas et al. 2010): (1) biomedical and health informatics core knowledge and skills; (2) medicine, health and biosciences, and health system organization; (3) informatics/computer science, mathematics, and biometry; and (4) optional modules in biomedical health informatics and related fields. The European Federation for Medical Informatics has endorsed the IMIA model, as have professional organizations in Japan, Australia, and elsewhere.

The American Health Information Management Association (AHIMA), together with the Global Health Workforce Council (GHWC), has published a detailed report titled *Global Academic Curricula Competencies for Health Information Professionals* that serves as a practical guide for developing and implementing academic programs in three health information professions (AHIMA and GHWC 2015): (1) **health information management (HIM)**, focused on the acquisition, analysis, and protection of information; (2) health informatics (HI), broadly focused on technology-based innovations across the continuum of care; and (3) **health information and communication technologies (HICT)**, focused on the technological aspects of health information and systems. The intersection of HIM, HI, and HICT defines a new area of professional interest: **health information governance (IG)**, which "focuses on information as a strategic asset that requires high-level oversight" (AHIMA and GHWC 2015, 3). The road map provided through the AHIMA/GHWC structure allows for customization of academic programs to account for the specific needs of regions or countries. The report provides competency summaries, linkages to levels of Bloom's taxonomy, and curricular considerations on several levels (foundational, entry, intermediate, advanced) for the defined professions.

The Association of University Programs in Health Administration (AUPHA 2016) provides another set of curriculum guidelines for an area it calls Health Information Management Systems Technology and Analysis (HIMSTA). The HIMSTA curriculum consists of 14 modules spread across 8 domains: (1) information management; (2) strategy and planning; (3) assessment, system selection, and implementation; (4) management of information systems and resources; (5) assessment of emerging technologies; (6) assessment

health information management (HIM)
The professional area dealing with the acquisition, analysis, and protection of health information.

health information and communication technologies (HICT)
The professional area dealing with the technological aspects of health information and systems.

health information governance (IG)
The professional area dealing with health information as a strategic asset requiring high-level oversight.

of the value of IT; (7) security and privacy; and (8) systems and standards. The full list of HIMSTA domains and competencies is available via the AUPHA Network at http://network.aupha.org/himstacurriculum.

This chapter will examine current informatics trends in the United States, Europe, Asia, and the other parts of the globe. The first section focuses on innovation through IT in healthcare, with a discussion about the "internet of things" as a driver of innovation. The chapter then looks at EHRs and the ways they provide the building blocks for clinical support systems and population-based health information. The discussion then moves to standards for the exchange of data and a definition of *interoperability*. The chapter explores the architecture of EHRs, along with their international adoption and performance. Additional topics include clinical decision support systems and how they integrate with data from EHRs; standards for clinical coding; privacy and security from the policy and management perspectives; and selection and implementation of HIT systems. The chapter ends with a discussion about international sources of healthcare data.

Innovation in Information Technology

Innovative use of technology is essential in the global health market, where organizations often are geographically dispersed and consist of members from diverse cultural, educational, and language backgrounds. The internet has had a profound impact on all areas of management, and it has enabled continued innovations that aid in overcoming language barriers (e.g., translating software), dictating and transcribing documents (e.g., voice recognition software), and communicating with groups (e.g., Skype, WhatsApp). News, information, and multimedia content can be followed globally, documents can be easily shared and edited by multiple users, and mobile devices allow the easy transport of technologies worldwide. New technologies continue to emerge, and global managers need to stay abreast of new innovations as they are introduced.

Given the rapid pace of change, staying abreast of innovation requires significant time and effort. Technology innovation award events, such as those presented by Ventana Research (2016), can help leaders remain aware of developments that can potentially improve their work. Ventana's award categories for 2016 are shown in exhibit 5.1. One Ventana award winner was the Business Cloud, by Domo, which combined **big data** with analytics and **cloud computing** in biomedical research, medical practice, and healthcare system management. In the early days of cloud computing, the main area for application was associated with laboratories (Rosenthal et al. 2010). Today, however, we see the potential in sharing biomedical information through commercial cloud products almost everywhere.

big data
Huge collections of information that can be mined from various sources.

cloud computing
Computing through remote servers that provide resources on demand via the internet.

EXHIBIT 5.1
Categories
of Business
Technology
Innovation
Awards (2016)

Overall Business Technology Innovation Award	
Business Technology Innovation Awards	**Information Technology Innovation Awards**
• Big Data	• Overall Information Technology
• Business Analytics	• Analytics and Business Intelligence
• Collaboration	• Cybersecurity
• Cloud Computing	• Information Optimization
• Internet of Things	• Information Management
• Mobile Technology	• IT Analytics
• Social Media	• Location Analytics
• Wearable Computing	• Operational Intelligence
	• Predictive Analytics

Source: Ventana Research (2016).

The adoption of cloud computing practices has not been as rapid in healthcare as it has in other areas of business, but it is increasing. Griebel and colleagues (2015) conducted a literature review focused on the topic and identified results in six categories: (1) telemedicine/teleconsultation, (2) medical imaging, (3) public health and patient self-management, (4) hospital management and clinical information systems, (5) therapy, and (6) secondary use of data. Applications for hospital management were found in 13 papers.

Some award-winning innovations combine multiple technologies. The Wearable Sensing and Smart Cloud Computing for Integrated Care to Chronic Obstructive Pulmonary Disease Patients with Comorbidities (WELCOME) system, for instance, is described as "an innovative European Union telehealth project that aims to develop a wearable vest with sensors for the monitoring of physiological signals using cloud-computing technology. The system uses a number of patient-held devices, such as a blood glucose metre and an inhaler adherence monitoring device to assess the patient's inhaler technique. This is accompanied by a patient support system through a mobile phone application providing life-style advice, mental health assessment and other functions" (Kayyali et al. 2016).

Applications of big data and data mining have changed the way we acquire new information for early warnings of infectious disease outbreaks. The EU supports MedISys, a monitoring and analysis system that provides event-based surveillance to rapidly identify potential threats to the public health using information from the internet. It displays articles with interest to public health, grouped by disease or disease type, and it warns users with automatically generated alerts. The system screens publicly available web sources using multilingual keywords in more than 40 languages (Mantero et al. 2014).

internet of things
The vast network of everyday objects and devices connected via the internet.

The "**internet of things**"—the various devices and everyday objects connected via the internet—is becoming increasingly prevalent in healthcare.

The growing interest in the topic—as reflected by search results on the PubMed database—is illustrated in exhibit 5.2. The earliest result returned by PubMed, dating back to 2004, describes a demonstration of future technologies for the White House/Smithsonian millennium events. These technologies included a smart bathroom shelf that could detect pill bottles, remind people when to take their medication, let pharmacists know when refills were needed, and help doctors supervise care (Gershenfeld, Krikorian, and Cohen 2004).

In another application of the internet of things, automated monitoring systems can be used to provide healthcare workers with feedback regarding their hand hygiene compliance, encouraging self-awareness and more hygienic actions. Such a system may rely on an indoor positioning component to collect data about workers' positions, leading to assumptions about the use of alcohol-based hand-rub dispensers and sinks (Marques et al. 2016). As new applications continue to emerge, the potential for global health seems to be enormous. Bhagade, Kanawade, and Nikose (2016, 683) describe an innovation in which "wearable sensors recognize anomalous and unforeseen conditions by examining physiological parameters along with the symptoms and transfer the vital signs for medical evaluation. Hence, prompt provisional medication can be done immediately to avoid severe conditions."

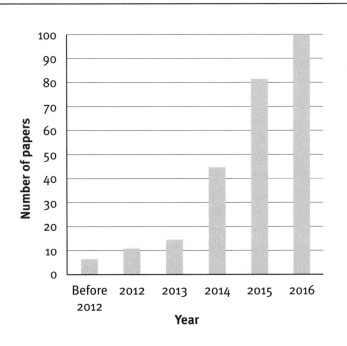

EXHIBIT 5.2
Search Data for "Internet of Things" in Title and Abstract of Papers Referenced in PubMed by Year

Note: 2016 data are through September 14.
Source: Data from PubMed (2016).

The Modern Electronic Health Record

The earliest EHRs were created in the 1960s and 1970s at academic medical centers. Those EHRs had separate components to track different aspects of the patient experience, such as patient information, billing, and progress notes. As technologies evolved, some early EHRs failed. Cedars-Sinai, for instance, spent $34 million building an EHR that their clinical care providers refused to use (Connolly 2005).

Since that time, however, the EHR has become a central component of the infrastructure driving the delivery of healthcare. The EHR provides demographic information about the patient as well as the patient's medical history, all of which can be used by clinical support systems to assist in diagnosis and treatment (Cimino 2013). Furthermore, aggregated data from EHRs can determine optimal treatments for evidence-based medicine and also help monitor for population health. Nonetheless, problems remain with the emerging EHR infrastructure in the global health context. For instance, how do we exchange data from disparate EHR systems in different countries and in different languages? The HIMSTA modules provide guidance to organizations looking to adopt EHR systems and facing decisions relating to quality improvement, cost effectiveness, or regulatory requirements.

A basic EHR contains the patient's medical and treatment histories, whereas an advanced EHR system goes beyond standard clinical data to provide a broader view and offer additional capabilities. An advanced EHR system might incorporate such elements as the following:

- The patient's medical history, diagnoses, medications, treatment plans, immunization dates, allergies, radiology images, and laboratory and test results
- Access to evidence-based tools and clinical support systems that providers can use to make decisions about the patient's care
- The ability to report to public agencies to aid in monitoring population health
- A portal through which patients may view their medical information and communicate with providers

To be effective, EHRs must enable the secure sharing of information among healthcare providers and organizations—such as laboratories, specialists, medical imaging facilities, pharmacies, emergency facilities, and school and workplace clinics—so that the records contain information from all the clinicians involved in the patient's care.

Establishing the Terminology

As we begin this discussion, we need to distinguish between electronic health records, electronic medical records, and personal health records. An **electronic** medical record (EMR) contains the standard medical and clinical data gathered for a patient in a particular provider's office (Garrett 2011). It is a digital version of the paper chart that contains the patient's medical history at one practice. An EHR, by contrast, is a digital version of the patient's paper charts from *all* their care providers (HealthIT.gov. 2018). EHRs are real-time, patient-centered records that make information securely available to authorized users. Finally, a **personal health record (PHR)** is a web or computer application used by patients to maintain and manage their health information in a private, secure, and confidential environment (HealthIT.gov 2016). PHRs are different from portals that simply allow patients to communicate with providers or view provider information in their EHRs.

Basic EHRs with Clinical Notes Versus Comprehensive EHRs and Clinical Support Systems

According to the Office of the National Coordinator for Health Information Technology (ONC), an EHR is considered *basic* if it has implemented the following computerized functions in at least one clinical unit of the hospital (Adler-Milstein et al. 2014):

- Electronic maintenance of patient demographic information, physician notes, nursing assessments, patient problem lists, patient medication lists, and discharge summaries
- Electronic viewing of laboratory reports, radiologic reports, and diagnostic test results
- Electronic ordering of medications

An EHR is considered *comprehensive* if it performs those functions plus an additional set of functions related to testing and imaging results, **computerized provider order entry (CPOE)**, and clinical decision support.

Providers using a CPOE system make selections from drop-down menus for the medications, treatments, and tests they prescribe. For medications, they also must select dose and frequency. To take advantage of best-practice protocols, many facilities develop order sets for specific diagnosis care and postoperative care. These standardized order sets are developed and maintained with input from the specialists who will be using the orders, as well as from nurses, pharmacists, physical and occupational therapists, and others. The development of the order sets requires that providers agree on specific medications, rehabilitation protocols, and so on, and that clinical workflows be taken into account (Ayatollahi, Roozbehi, and Haghani 2015).

Once the streamlined standard order sets are in place, providers using CPOE see focused drop-down menus associated with the protocols that were agreed upon by the subset of the medical staff as appropriate for the specific needs of the patient. These focused menus can save providers both time and

electronic medical record (EMR)
A digital record containing the standard medical and clinical data gathered for a patient in a particular provider's office.

personal health record (PHR)
A web or computer application that patients use to maintain and manage their health information in a private, secure, and confidential environment.

computerized provider order entry (CPOE)
An application that allows providers to enter patient orders via a computer system.

frustration, as they receive fewer alerts based on medication selection. In addition, selection errors are minimized. For maximum benefit, however, physicians need to be trained on a broader range of CPOE functionalities, including how to find and use specific order sets (Khajouei et al. 2011).

To gain the full benefits of EHR systems, providers must access the records in real time while patients are undergoing care, and they must properly take any notifications into account. When providers enter orders into EHRs, they may receive a variety of alerts warning them about drug interactions associated with certain medication orders. Over time, some providers experience alert fatigue, causing them to pay less attention to the alerts or skip over them altogether (Khajouei and Jaspers 2010).

Clinical decision support provided through comprehensive EHRs may also include standardized protocols for diseases, such as HIV/AIDS, in areas of the world where resources are constrained, such as sub-Saharan Africa or the Caribbean (Oluoch et al. 2012). Treatment guidelines have proved beneficial to providers even when challenges exist with regard to infrastructure and computer literacy.

Meaningful Use

meaningful use
Use of certified electronic health record technology in a meaningful manner, consistent with government guidelines.

The US government has set standards for the **meaningful use** of EHR technology, and it has instituted an incentive payment system to encourage providers to comply with those standards. The concept of meaningful use was introduced as part of the Health Information Technology for Economic and Clinical Health (HITECH) Act of 2009, with further details given in section 3002, part 7, of the Affordable Care Act (ACA) of 2010 (Government Publishing Office 2010). Given that the United States spent 17.6 percent of its 2010 gross domestic product on healthcare (Kane 2012), the overarching goal of meaningful use was to drive down the cost of care by improving efficiency and quality outcomes through the use of EHRs.

The concept of meaningful use rests on five "pillars" of health outcomes (Centers for Disease Control and Prevention 2017):

1. Improve quality, safety, and efficiency, and reduce health disparities
2. Engage patients and families
3. Improve care coordination
4. Improve population and public health
5. Ensure the privacy and security of personal health information

The meaningful use requirements were arranged into three stages, intended to be phased in as shown in exhibit 5.3. However, many of the details of meaningful use have evolved in response to various problems and changes in leadership at the ONC. The concept has also been modified through the

Stage	Main Ideas	Examples
1	Data capture and sharing (2011–2012)	Data stored in standardized fields
2	Advanced clinical processes (2014)	Computerized provider order entry with adverse drug event checking
3	Improved outcomes (2017)	Meeting metrics for better patient outcomes, such as hospital readmission rates

EXHIBIT 5.3
The Stages of Meaningful Use

Source: Data from Gálvez et al. (2015); Centers for Disease Control and Prevention (2017).

introduction of the Medicare Access and CHIP Reauthorization Act (MACRA) of 2015, which includes meaningful use in its "Advancing Care Information" category, dealing with EHRs and other HIT tools (ONC 2018). Today, many EHR systems still fall short of standards that were supposed to be achieved by 2014 (Gálvez et al. 2015).

EHR Standards and Data Exchange

The ability of EHRs to improve efficiency and coordination of care depends in large part on the degree to which data can be shared from one provider to another. Thus, **interoperability**—the ability of systems and devices to exchange and interpret data—is a key concern. As technology changes and EHR systems develop differently, the goal of interoperability can be like trying to hit a moving target. However, a number of international organizations have been working for years to develop standards.

interoperability
The ability of systems and devices to exchange and interpret data.

Health Level Seven (HL7) International is a standards-developing organization that promotes the global interoperability of health data (HL7 International 2018c). Its standards allow for the transferability of both clinical and administrative data between hospital and information systems. The standards are grouped into seven reference categories: (1) primary standards, (2) foundational standards, (3) clinical and administrative domains, (4) EHR profiles, (5) implementation guides, (6) rules and references, and (7) education and awareness.

HL7 was founded in 1987 and introduced its Version 2 standards in 1989 (HL7 International 2018a, 2018b). Version 2 has been used in more than 35 countries and in 95 percent of US healthcare organizations (HL7 International 2018d). Version 3, introduced in 2005, aims to improve Version 2 with a stricter standard and new capabilities (Corepoint Health 2018). An expanded scope includes community medicine, epidemiology, veterinary medicine, clinical genomics, and other areas (HL7 International 2018b).

Health information exchange usually focuses on transferring specific documents that provide a summary of patient care. HL7 provides standards for documents relating to discharges, admission histories, and physicals through its Clinical Document Architecture (CDA) (Ferranti et al. 2006). Use of the CDA is well established in the United States and in Finland, Greece, and Germany. The Mayo Clinic produces thousands of CDAs per week and sees the use of this standardized document as an investment in the future (HL7 International 2018b).

Fast Healthcare Interoperability Resources (FHIR) is the most current standards framework created by HL7. FHIR is applicable in many settings other than EHRs, including mobile phone applications, cloud-based communications, and server communications in large healthcare systems (HL7 International 2017a, 2017b). FHIR provides flexibility for incorporating variability from diverse healthcare processes, which eliminates the need for custom solutions. Like other versions of HL7, FHIR includes both administrative and clinical concepts. As FHIR becomes a more finalized product, it will provide a viable solution to interoperability challenges currently faced by healthcare organizations.

The International Organization for Standardization (ISO 2018) has more than 22,000 published international standards across a variety of industries. ISO/TC 215 includes the consistent interchange of health-related data in its scope, whereas ISO/TR 14639 targets low- and middle-income countries with guidance on the implementation of HIT (Naden 2014). ISO/HL7 10781:2015 was created to provide a common understanding of functions in EHR systems in a variety of settings, such as intensive care, cardiology, and office practice (ISO 2015).

EHR Architecture

A variety of EHR architecture types are available, and organizational management must make key decisions between best-of-breed and monolithic approaches, as well as between cloud-based and local-based systems.

Best-of-Breed Versus Monolithic

best-of-breed (BoB) approach
An approach to electronic health record (EHR) architecture that involves building or buying the best available option for each component of the EHR while adhering to standards that allow interoperability.

Some healthcare organizations, such as the Harvard hospitals, started with a **best-of-breed (BoB) approach**. The BoB method involves building or buying the best available option for each component of the EHR (e.g., clinical documentation, CPOE) while adhering to standards that allow interoperability between the different modules (Elion 2016). This approach allows organizations to have the best EHR system for each aspect of care, with the components able to communicate throughout the hospital and with other systems that comply with the HL7 standards (Atherton 2011). The key drawbacks of the BoB approach involve technical problems with HL7 and the complexity and expense of having disparate EHR components exchanging data. Significant barriers are created if various department systems cannot work together.

Because of the drawbacks associated with the BoB method, the market has shifted in the direction of a **monolithic approach**, where a single vendor, such as Epic or Cerner, provides all aspects of the EHR for all departments of the healthcare system (Koppel and Lehmann 2015). Many organizations favor the monolithic approach because it ensures uniform data standards and interoperability across the healthcare system. In addition, paying one price for centralized architecture for an entire system is generally expected to be less expensive than paying numerous providers in a distributed system (Gaynor and Bradner 2004). Given the potential for monolithic EHRs to improve interoperability, some vendors believed they could easily take their systemwide interoperable systems and make them nationally interoperable. However, the different needs of various organizations have led to the customization of EHRs, making standardization difficult (Tripathi 2012).

> **monolithic approach**
> An approach to electronic health record architecture in which all the aspects and components are provided through a single vendor.

FHIR enables a hybrid architecture where monolithic EHRs allow third-party vendors to create applications that run seamlessly within the EHR. These third-party vendors may have application expertise and data access that other EHR vendors do not. Models allowing third-party application integration vary in the degree to which they are open or closed. Athena Health has one of the most open models. Any vendor can look up Athena's published Application Program Interface and write third-party applications that work with Athena's cloud-based EHR. Epic takes a more closed approach, in which the third-party vendor must work with individual healthcare providers for a particular implementation. We believe that the more open approach is more conducive to innovative applications.

Cerner has opened its EHR architecture to third-party innovations through an "open sandbox" for FHIR applications (Conn 2016; Cerner 2018). A clinical support application called RxCheck, for instance, operates in the Cerner sandbox and helps providers make optimal prescription decisions. Such collaborations are becoming common as EHR vendors race to develop third-party app ecosystems based on FHIR (Francisco 2016).

Cloud-Based Versus Local-Based

An additional architectural choice is whether the EHR system should be centralized via the cloud or arranged according to the more traditional distributed setup, with each organization owning and managing its own EHR. Traditional vendors such as Epic, Cerner, Meditech, McKesson, and Allscripts sell software that is to be owned and managed by the care provider. Such software can be extremely expensive. For example, the Mayo Clinic in Minnesota planned to spend about $1.5 billion on its new Epic infrastructure (*Becker's Health IT & CIO Report 2016*), and a contract Cerner established with the US Department of Defense had an initial payout of $4.3 billion (Miliard 2017). Vendors such as Athena, Practice Fusion, and eClinicalWorks offer cloud-based EHRs that use web-based interfaces and a centralized server that runs EHRs for many clients. Such systems are sometimes called *software-as-a-service* EHRs.

The distinction between centralized and distributed servers and databases for EHRs is illustrated in exhibit 5.4. The right side of the exhibit has two hospital systems (HS1 and HS2), each with two hospitals, along with two independent hospitals (H1 and H2). They all share a centralized server and database accessed over the internet. On the left side are a third hospital system (HS3) and an independent hospital (H3), each with its own distributed server and database.

Both of these options have advantages and disadvantages (Gaynor and Bradner 2004). The traditional model is more expensive but gives the organization control over the EHR and patient data. The centralized cloud-based model is less expensive from a capital point of view and is relatively easy to manage. Some cloud-based EHRs, such as Practice Fusion, are free because they are based on a marketing business model. Smaller organizations that lack technical expertise may find the cloud-based approach very attractive.

EHR Adoption Rates and Top Vendors

In developed countries, EHR adoption rates range from 41 to 98 percent, with the Netherlands having the highest rate (Schoen et al. 2012). In less developed countries, EHR adoption lags, due in large part to socioeconomic conditions and the cost of EHR adoption (Douglas 2009; Healy 2008; Mugo and Nzuki

EXHIBIT 5.4
Centralized
Compared to
Distributed
Architecture for
EHRs

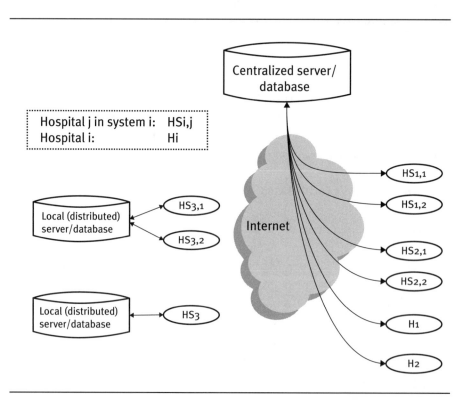

2014). In the United States, 96 percent of hospitals reported adoption of an EHR (Henry et al. 2016). Adoption rates vary by hospital type, as shown in exhibit 5.5, but the increase is apparent across all types. All the hospital categories shown in the exhibit reached 80 percent adoption by 2015 (ONC 2016b).

Exhibit 5.6 breaks down the US EHR adoption rate by vendor for hospitals participating in the Medicare EHR incentive program. (Vendors must offer certified EHRs to qualify for the incentive program.) The top five vendors account for most of the market (ONC 2016a). The top US vendor, Cerner, will implement the Cerner Millennium EHR platform in Department of Veterans Affairs Administration and Department of Defense healthcare facilities over a ten-year period (Slabodkin 2018).

Several reports by the WHO (2012a, 2012b) have discussed EHR adoption, regulations and policies, and privacy and security. These reports indicate that high-income countries have increasingly adopted EHRs and that emerging

EXHIBIT 5.5
Adoption Rate of EHRs in the United States

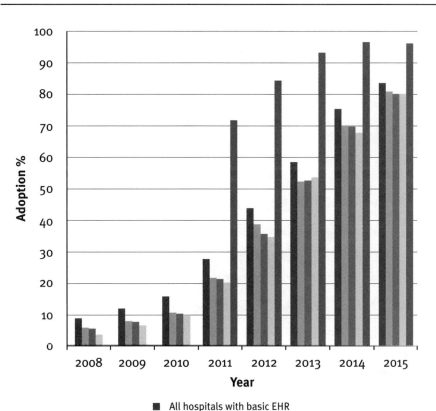

- All hospitals with basic EHR
- All small hospitals with basic EHR
- All rural hospitals with basic EHR
- All critical access hospitals with basic EHR
- All hospitals with certified EHR

Source: Adapted from ONC (2016b).

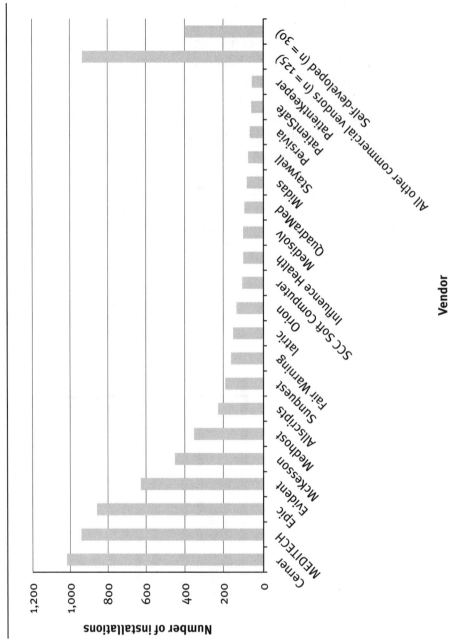

EXHIBIT 5.6
EHR Adoption
Rate by Vendor
for Hospitals
Participating
in the EHR
Incentive
Program (2016)

Source: Data from ONC (2016a).

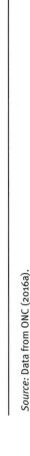

economies such as Brazil, China, and India are developing national EHR infrastructures. Low-income countries, however, continue to have difficulty building integrated EHR systems and developing policies and regulations to protect patient information.

Industrialized countries such as Australia, Canada, China, Denmark, England, France, Germany, India, Israel, Italy, Japan, the Netherlands, New Zealand, Norway, Singapore, Sweden, Switzerland, Taiwan, and the United States have national strategies to promote the use of HIT and EHRs (International Health Care System Profiles 2018). In the United Arab Emirates, the Ministry of Health (MoH) launched an EHR system called Wareed that links all MoH hospitals and clinics in Dubai and the northern emirates (Emery 2017). Exhibit 5.7 shows the leading EHR vendors for parts of the world outside the United States.

Standards for Clinical Coding

Classification of diseases and health conditions is a fundamental procedure for the surveying of health worldwide, but approaches to classification vary. One system might be based on anatomical localization, whereas others might be based on causes of disease or injury or the etiology of pathological processes. The basic criterion for classification reflects the purpose for which the classification should serve. Thus, a number of classification systems for diseases and health disorders exist today (Rusnák, Rusnáková, and Psota 2013).

International Classification of Diseases
The International Statistical Classification of Diseases and Related Health Problems (ICD) is a worldwide classification system maintained by the WHO (2007). Its tenth revision, known as ICD-10, was adopted at the 43rd World Health Assembly in 1990 and has been used in WHO member countries since 1994. The ICD-10 contributes to global patient safety by providing detailed

	Epic	Cerner	InterSystems	Allscripts	MV	Philips
Europe (above-average EHR adoption)	91	80	69			
Middle East (deepest EHR adoption)		72	89			
Asia/Oceania (lightest EHR adoption)	74	81	80			
Latin America (average EHR adoption)					79	79

EXHIBIT 5.7
Adoption Rate and Performance Score for International EHRs

Source: Data from Goff, Christensen, and Paxman (2016).

information about diseases, complications, and global causes of death and by facilitating the identification of medical errors and methods for preventing them. The ICD-10 also contributes to the development of global public health policies and the formulation of global program priorities, and it supports and accelerates innovation transfer between clinical research and practice with a global dimension (Rusnák, Rusnáková, and Psota 2013).

The National Center for Health Statistics in the United States initiated a Clinical Modification of the ICD-10 (ICD-10-CM), which was implemented in 2015. The ICD-10-CM contains more than 68,000 codes, and it helps address insufficiencies of the ICD-9-CM in the coding of clinical measures. However, despite significant progress, the ICD-10-CM is still insufficient for clinical use. It is primarily used for healthcare quality, reimbursement, and outcomes evaluations (Barta et al. 2008).

The WHO has also used other classification systems to facilitate national and international comparisons. The International Classification of Primary Care (ICPC) might be the most promising for understanding global trends in health and health services (Hofmans-Okkes and Lamberts 1996). Developed by a committee of the World Organization of Family Doctors (WONCA), the ICPC is intended to serve as an epidemiological tool for the collection and analysis of patient data and clinical activity in primary care (WONCA 2015).

Systemized Nomenclature of Medicine—Clinical Terms

Systematized Nomenclature of Medicine—Clinical Terms (SNOMED-CT) is a clinical standard maintained by the International Health Terminology Standards Development Organization (IHTSDO). Used in more than 50 countries, it provides standard multilingual healthcare terminology for the clinical content of EHRs. SNOMED-CT was developed to ensure consistent, reliable, and comprehensive records of clinically relevant data in EHR systems (SNOMED International 2018). Codes, or unique identifiers, represent concepts, and they are created pursuant to the principle of "one code one meaning," and vice versa. The codes consist of a chain of 6 to 18 digits, and they have corresponding descriptions and relations, allowing for a hierarchy of terms and correlations to be built (Rusnák, Rusnáková, and Psota 2013; Bhattacharyya 2016). Unlike ICD-10, this system is suitable for use in day-to-day clinical practice. In addition, SNOMED's diagnostic categories can be reliably mapped with the ICPC, which facilitates the use of both systems for a common purpose (National Library of Medicine 2016). Thus, it has significant potential for global research on primary care services and health outcomes.

diagnosis-related group (DRG)
A category of patients whose diagnoses share certain common properties.

Diagnosis-Related Groups

Diagnosis-related groups (DRGs), another classification system, were established with the aim of reducing the great number of details in patients' records, mainly diagnoses, to a limited number of groups with certain common properties (Fetter et al. 1980; Goldfield 2010). DRGs have gradually evolved to a language that allows for the merging of financial and clinical aspects of care for hospitalized patients. Use of DRGs in payment reform efforts has the potential to create significant savings. DRG coding may also be applied to assessments of quality and efficiency (Scheller-Kreinsen, Geissler, and Busse 2009).

Sources of Routine Statistics

The effective application of HIT and clinical support systems depends on the availability of valid, reliable, and comparable health information. Furthermore, when managers consider expanding their activities abroad, they need to possess, at minimum, a crude understanding of the health and healthcare situation in the expansion area. International sources of data provide a broad overview and allow for comparisons across a variety of countries. Local statistical data, often available online, enables a more detailed understanding.

Language differences are often an issue when accessing international data, but services such as Google Translate can help with the translation of data labels. If only printed materials are available, optical character recognition (OCR) software, available from for-profit companies as well as from free internet resources, can help identify printed characters for translation. If a manager needs the service only occasionally, an online service might be the best option. If internet access is limited, as is frequently the case in developing countries, the purchase of a professional OCR tool might be most advisable.

International Organizations
Most international organizations share data from their members, and the majority of those organizations active in health and healthcare provide their data online with unrestricted access. However, most health providers (e.g., hospitals, primary care providers) and purchasers (e.g., insurance companies, private businesses) keep their data confidential.

The World Health Organization collects, maintains, and shares health-related statistics across a broad range of topics, though its focus is primarily on causes of death, illness rates, health conditions, service coverage, and risk factors. The WHO's (2018a) Global Health Observatory (GHO) provides its member states with access to health-related "country data and statistics with a focus on comparable estimates," together with the "WHO's analyses to monitor global, regional and country situations and trends." Through the GHO's interactive repository of statistics, users can view data for selected indicators, topics, countries, and regions, and they can download customized tables in Microsoft Excel format. The GHO also issues analytical reports on important health issues and distributes an annual *World Health Statistics* publication that compiles data for key health indicators.

The WHO (2018b) Mortality Database compiles mortality data by country, age, sex, and cause of death, based on figures reported to the WHO by authorities of the countries involved. The data are classified into groups by year. Working with the data requires consideration of international differences in death registration and coding procedures, mainly in the usage of codes for incorrectly defined and unknown death causes. Raw data files are available for research purposes, together with required instructions, file structures, and code reference tables. People using them, however, need database tools, because the files are too large and complicated for common office programs.

Regional WHO offices also maintain their own databases. The WHO's European Health Information Gateway "Health for All" explorer provides access to a broad spectrum of basic health statistics for 53 European WHO member countries (WHO Regional Office for Europe 2018). The data are collected from various sources, including official registers and surveys. Some of the data are collected annually directly in the member countries, whereas other data come from WHO technical units that acquire respective statistical information within particular areas of specialization. The "Health for All" database contains hundreds of indicators arranged into such categories as demographics, socio-economic conditions, lifestyle factors, healthcare utilization and expenditure, morbidity and disability, maternal and child health, and mortality.

The Pan-American Health Organization (PAHO 2017) maintains health-related information in its database of Core Health Indicators. This comprehensive set of health indicators is organized into categories of demographic-socioeconomic, health status, risk factors, services coverage, and health systems. Data can be explored, filtered, and downloaded for further analysis.

Eurostat, an EU statistical office based in Luxembourg, provides statistics to enable comparisons of the countries and regions of the EU (Eurostat 2018). It offers a wealth of data that can be used by governments, businesses, educational sectors, journalists, and the public during work and daily life. Because Eurostat functions at the EU level rather than at a national level, it seeks to establish a common statistical "language" of terms, methods, structures, and technical standards. In other words, it seeks to ensure comparability through harmonized methodology. The majority of Eurostat's data can be obtained in various formats (e.g., XLS, CSV, HTML, PDF, PC-AXIS, SPSS, TSV) commonly used in the science and research. Eurostat also offers metadata describing particular items. A Eurostat service called the Geographical Information System of the Commission (GISCO) provides access to geographical information and related services, including maps, spatial analyses, and user support (Eurostat 2017).

In the United States, the Agency for Healthcare Research and Quality (AHRQ) maintains the Healthcare Cost and Utilization Project (HCUP), a collection of databases providing inpatient and outpatient visit data, regardless of payer. The databases enable health-related research from a variety angles— whether focused on policy, access to services, treatment outcomes, or medical practice patterns—at national, state, and local levels. The HCUP databases include the National Inpatient Sample, the Kids' Inpatient Database, the Nationwide Emergency Department Sample, the Nationwide Readmissions Database, the State Inpatient Databases, and the State Emergency Department Databases. Access to these databases is purchased through the HCUP Central Distributor (AHRQ 2018).

Data Repositories

Often, accessing data that are dispersed across multiple databases can be extremely difficult, but a number of efforts have aimed to facilitate this type of access. In Norway, for instance, the MacroDataGuide serves as "a user's guide for researchers and students worldwide in search of high quality data for social science research" (Norwegian Centre for Research Data 2018). It provides information on data availability and quality assessments of sources, and its web portal presents information from diverse sources in a uniform manner.

Gapminder is a nonprofit web service that combines easy access to data with analytical tools that are available both on- and off-line (Rosling and Zhang 2011). Based in Sweden, it serves as a sort of modern "museum" on the internet, with the aim of promoting sustainable global development and the achievement of the United Nations Millennium Development Goals. Features of the service can present time series statistics and global development trends through colorful graphics, videos, flash presentations, and interactive animations.

A variety of other international data sources are also available, though they vary in quality. Users should approach sources with caution and carefully consider **data integrity**—that is, the degree to which the completeness, accuracy, consistency, and timeliness of data are maintained (Teslow 2016). Efforts to protect data integrity and foster accurate data exchange through standardization are central to the concept of **data governance**. The WHO provides a Data Quality Review Toolkit (available at www.who.int/health-info/tools_data_analysis/dqr_modules/en/) to help users understand issues of data quality.

data integrity
The completeness, accuracy, consistency, and timeliness of data.

data governance
Efforts to protect data integrity and foster accurate data exchange.

Ensuring the Security and Privacy of Medical Information

The security and privacy of patient information is a serious concern in global healthcare, and lapses and violations are widespread. The *HIPAA Journal* (2017) estimated that, in 2016, more than 16 million patients had their records exposed in data breaches in the United States. In August of 2016, for instance, Banner Health revealed that hackers may have gained access to health plan information of up to 3.7 million patients. That same month, a Blue Cross Blue Shield breach might have exposed the personal information of 3.3 million individuals (Davis 2016). Organizational threats related to accidental and intentional breaches are addressed in the HIMSTA modules.

The privacy and security of healthcare information depend on a combination of technology, policy, and managerial processes. The technology part is easy. We know how to encrypt data to keep it private, how to authenticate where a message came from, and how to ensure that information has integrity (i.e., has not been altered). Unfortunately, the managerial and policy aspects are not so easy and well defined, particularly in the international context.

Healthcare organizations must be vigilant in protecting the health and financial information of patients. A security plan should include access audits and other ongoing review processes, along with consistent backup of all data. Countries vary in the policies and laws that deal with protection of patient information, and these frameworks drive managerial procedures.

HIPAA Regulations

In the United States, the main law dealing with the privacy and security of medical data is the Health Insurance Portability and Accountability Act (HIPAA) of 1996 (US Department of Health and Human Services 2018). A list of the HIPAA security standards, assembled from various Centers for Medicare & Medicaid Services (CMS) sources, is provided in exhibit 5.8. HIPAA regulations define the rights of a patient with regard to protection of their medical information. The list of standards includes administrative safeguards, physical safeguards, technical safeguards, organizational requirements, and policies and procedures and documentation requirements, with "implementation specifications," or specific requirements, provided for the various categories (CMS 2007a, 2007b, 2007c, 2007d).

EXHIBIT 5.8
HIPAA
Standards and
Implementation
Specifications

Administrative (A) Safeguards (CMS 2007a)

1 Security Management Process
Implementation specifications: Risk analysis, risk management, sanction policy, information system activity review

2 Assigned Security Responsibility

3 Workforce Security
Implementation specifications: *Authorization, workforce clearance procedure, termination procedures*

4 Information Access Management
Implementation specifications: Isolating clearinghouse functions, *access authorization, access establishment and modification*

5 Security Awareness and Training
   Implementation specifications: *Security reminders, protection from malicious software, log-in monitoring, password management*

6 Security Incident Procedures
   Implementation specification: Response and reporting

7 Contingency Plan
   Implementation specifications: Data backup plan, disaster recovery plan, emergency mode operation plan, *testing and revision procedures, application and data criticality analysis*

8 Evaluation

9 Business Associate Contracts and Other Arrangements
   Implementation specification: Written contract or other arrangement

Physical (P) Safeguards (CMS 2007c)

1 Facility Access Controls
   Implementation specifications: *Contingency operations, facility security plan, access control and validation procedures, maintenance records*

2 Workstation Use

3 Workstation Security

4 Device and Media Controls
   Implementation specifications: Disposal, media reuse, *accountability, data backup and storage*

Technical (T) Safeguards (CMS 2007d)

1 Access Control
   Implementation specifications: Unique user identification, emergency access procedure, *automatic logoff, encryption and decryption*

2 Audit Controls

3 Integrity
   Implementation specification: *Mechanism to authenticate electronic protected health information*

4 Person or Entity Authentication

5 Transmission Security
   Implementation specifications: *Integrity controls, encryption*

Organizational (O) Requirements (CMS 2007b)

1 Business Associate Contracts or Other Arrangements

2 Requirements for Group Health Plans

Policies and Procedures and Documentation (D) Requirements (CMS 2007b)

1 Policies and Procedures

2 Documentation
   Implementation specifications: Time limit, availability, updates

---

Note: Implementation specifications shown in italics are classified as "addressable" implementation specifications, meaning that they have "particular stipulations related to their implementation" (Gaynor, Bass, and Duepner 2015).

Sources: Data from CMS (2007a, 2007b, 2007c, 2007d).

EXHIBIT 5.8
HIPAA Standards and Implementation Specifications *(continued)*

Chris Bennington, a HIPAA specialist at a law firm in Cincinnati, Ohio, points out that HIPAA rules are difficult to discern, even for healthcare workers, because of their vagueness and lack of detail (Rhea 2007). The focus of the regulations is not on the mandates themselves but rather on the thought process used to address information security. This mind-set leads to an emphasis on what to do, but explanations of how to adhere to specific standards are largely absent. Requirements are generally presented without recommendations or guidance for implementation.

Stephen Stewart, chief information officer of the Henry County Health Center in Southeast Iowa, has stated that, "in health care, the only time anybody does things is if there is a mandate" (Conn 2011). Although HIPAA defines specific requirements, the addressable specifications only require that the organization document that it has examined the standard in terms of its necessity and applicability to the organization. Thus, organizations have some ability to interpret standards as they see fit and decide whether the standards are relevant to information security. Because the standards are inconsistently applied, they are not "standardized" in the classic sense of the term. Two organizations using the same standards could produce quite different solutions for a single security or privacy issue.

PCI DSS Requirements

Most healthcare providers in the United States and throughout the world accept payment by credit card, and any organization that does so must follow the Payment Card Industry (PCI) Data Security Standard (DSS). The PCI Security Standards Council (2018) states that the PCI DSS "applies to all entities that store, process, and/or transmit cardholder data" and "covers technical and operational practices for system components included in or connected to environments with cardholder data." The number and size of transactions conducted by an entity determine the requirements for demonstrating compliance. The PCI DSS goals and requirements are summarized in exhibit 5.9. The second column of the exhibit

EXHIBIT 5.9
PCI DSS Goals and Requirements

Rule Number	Corresponding HIPAA Rule	Requirements
Goal 1: Build and Maintain a Secure Network		
1		Install and maintain a firewall configuration. Establish firewall and router standards that restrict inbound and outbound communication with the cardholder data. Document protocols and configurations.
2		Do not use vendor-supplied defaults for security parameters. Always change vendor-supplied defaults, including passwords and protocol community strings. Eliminate superfluous accounts prior to installation on a network.

Rule Number	Corresponding HIPAA Rule	Requirements
Goal 2: Protect Cardholder Data		
3	P4, T3	Protect stored data. Minimize storage of data, including authentication data, by developing a data retention and storage policy consistent with industry regulations.
4	T5	Encrypt the transmission of data across open, public networks. Use strong encryption and security protocols to protect sensitive data during transmission. Never send unencrypted data over public messaging.
Goal 3: Maintain a Vulnerability Management Program		
5		Use and regularly update antivirus software. Deploy antivirus software on all systems that could be afflicted by malicious software, and ensure that antivirus mechanisms are current, running, and capable of generating audit logs.
6		Develop and maintain secure systems and applications. Ensure that all systems are up-to-date, and establish a process for vulnerability identification within all systems. Develop change control procedures, and document their use.
Goal 4: Implement Strong Access Control Measures		
7	A3, A4, T1	Restrict access to data on a need-to-know basis. Limit data/system access to only those individuals who require such access. Establish an access control system that restricts access based on developed criteria.
8	A3, A4, T1	Assign a unique identification (ID) to each person who has access to data/system. Assign the unique ID before allowing access. Also employ at least one authentication method for local access and multiple levels for remote access.
9	A3, P1, P2, P3, T4	Restrict physical access to data/system. Use appropriate facility controls to limit and monitor physical access, including procedures designed to distinguish between employees and visitors (e.g., a visitor log).
Goal 5: Regularly Monitor and Test Networks		
10	T2	Track and monitor all network resource and data access. Establish a process for linking system components to individual users and for automating audit trails with respect to those components. Secure audit trails and review component logs daily; retain logs for at least one year.
11	A7	Regularly test security systems and processes. Test for the presence of wireless access points at least quarterly, and run internal and external vulnerability scans after any significant network change. Use intrusion-detection systems to monitor all traffic, and alert personnel to any security compromises.
Goal 6: Maintain Information Security Policy		
12	A1, A2, A4, A5, A6, A7, P1, D1, D2	Maintain a policy that addresses information security. Establish and maintain a policy addressing daily operational security procedures, technology usage policies, information security responsibilities, employee security awareness training, employee screening, and an incident response plan.

Source: Adapted from PCI Security Standards Council (2016).

EXHIBIT 5.9
PCI DSS Goals and Requirements *(continued)*

links the PCI DSS rules with the HIPAA standards (as listed in exhibit 5.8) that cover similar topics. For instance, rule 3 of the PCI DSS (under goal 2) is related to HIPAA's physical (P) safeguard rule 4 and technical (T) safeguard rule 3.

ENISA Recommendations

The European Union Agency for Network and Information Security (ENISA) is a center of network and information security expertise for the EU, its 28 member states, the private sector, and Europe's general population (ENISA 2018). ENISA works with various groups to develop recommendations for good practice in information security, assists EU member states in implementing relevant EU legislation, and works to improve the resilience of Europe's critical information infrastructure and networks (Liveri, Sarri, and Skouloudi 2015). The organization seeks to enhance existing expertise in member states by supporting the development of cross-border communities committed to improving network and information security throughout the EU. One ENISA initiative involves providing evaluations of member states' national cybersecurity strategies, to help minimize risks to economic and social programs.

Authors' Recommendation

We believe that using the PCS DSS framework to develop standards based on an international consortium of vendors is an effective approach to protecting patient information across international borders. The standards would be similar to those protecting the information of people who use credit cards internationally. Effective implementation of this approach will likely require (1) an international certification body, (2) rules that are accessible and clear, and (3) appropriate deterrents.

Concerns about data privacy and security can potentially slow the spread of valuable innovations in healthcare. For instance, cloud-based systems may offer significant benefits, but patients will be reluctant to use them if they are not assured that their personal information is safe. A systematic review of published literature suggests that the most applied techniques for addressing patients' data privacy concerns in the healthcare cloud are public/private key identity-based encryption (IBE) and attribute-based encryption (ABE) (Sajid and Abbas 2016). In IBE, a private encryption key is based on who the person is, whereas, in ABE, the key is based on the person's attributes. As more healthcare information moves to the cloud, we need balanced solutions that are able to protect patients' data privacy while considering all the cloud system's various aspects (Sajid and Abbas 2016).

System Assessment, Selection, and Implementation

The benefits of EHRs are well documented, but they accrue only with the proper adoption and implementation across the clinical information system

(Jha et al. 2009). One of the most important steps in EHR adoption is the selection of a system that is appropriate for a specific clinical setting (Krisik 2013). For example, some EHR systems are aimed at supporting large integrated healthcare systems, whereas others cater to niche settings, such as smaller clinical practices. Still other EHR systems support specialty-specific settings, such as dental practices or pediatric offices. Choosing the right scope and fit of the EHR functionality may determine the complexity and cost of the EHR adoption and implementation. Given the size of the EHR industry, a host of EHR vendors and pricing models are available to choose from.

Choosing the right vendor is key to a successful EHR adoption process (Wright 2014). However, before reaching that point, one must first ensure that the organization, at all levels, has appropriate buy-in and an understanding of the pros and cons of EHR implementation. Regardless of the size of the clinical practice, the reasons for purchasing and adopting the EHR should be clearly stated and well vetted, and cost, workforce, and other resources must all be taken into consideration. More importantly, the clinicians and ancillary staff need to be onboard. Clinical subject matter experts should be well represented in the process and actively involved in the implementation plans.

The road to the selection of an appropriate EHR tends to follow a series of key steps:

1. Define functional requirements.
2. Identify EHR vendors.
3. Narrow down the choices.
4. Select the vendor.
5. Manage the implementation.

These steps are described in the sections that follow.

Define Functional Requirements

A key step in the EHR selection process involves defining the project's functional requirements. Functional requirements are a common concern in software design, and they relate to the way a system functions, behaves, and performs. In seeking to define functional requirements, one might ask a series of questions. For instance, how does the EHR system support prescribing medications, writing notes, or reviewing laboratory tests? How do clinicians interact with the EHR system? Do they interact via laptop or desktop, or perhaps by mobile phone?

Key concerns at this stage include the following:

- *Stakeholder representation.* Functional requirements are best gathered when the organization engages the end users of the systems, as well other stakeholders. For instance, the project team must be able to engage and obtain support from clinical leadership, as well as from the individuals who will be paying for and supporting the EHR system (e.g., financial stakeholders, IT staff). Gathering all the key contributors of the project is important, as doing so can help identify a common set of problems, priorities, goals, and requirements that need to be addressed.

- *Financial considerations.* Any limitations in cost and financial resources need to be presented and identified up front, so that the project team knows what the organization can consider. Organizations with very limited funds often do not have the luxury of choosing from a wide variety of vendors.

- *System assessment.* Is the organization moving from paper to electronic? Or is it moving from electronic to a new EHR system? What system do we need to replace? Should we replace the revenue cycle system? Or the radiology system? Perhaps we would replace all clinical systems, except for the laboratory system. A clear understanding of the areas where the new EHR will be implemented can help guide the selection of an appropriate system.

Identify EHR Vendors

After defining its set of functional requirements, the organization can begin exploring the vendor space for likely candidates. Two common ways of exploring the market are the following:

request for information (RFI) A process for gathering information across a broad range of vendors.

- *Gathering information.* A **request for information (RFI)** is a process for gathering information across a broad range of vendors. An RFI helps the organization learn about vendors, their product offerings, their existing clients, their market penetration, and other concerns (e.g., initial public offering status, ownership, longevity). Although elements may later be used in contract negotiations, the RFI is primarily for the purpose of information gathering and discovery.

- *Peer consultation.* An organization can also learn about what is available in the market by asking similar organizations or practices about their preferred EHR systems. One can often get candid comments and evaluations from existing clients about their degree of satisfaction.

request for proposal (RFP) A document in which a potential purchaser invites a vendor to present a proposal tailored to specific project requirements.

Narrow Down the Choices

The narrowing down of vendor choices involves a number of aspects:

- *Obtaining proposals.* A **request for proposal (RFP)** is a document that purchasers of EHRs will produce to request a proposal from an EHR product vendor. The document informs the vendor that the organization is in the market for an EHR system, and it specifies essential functions, products, or services that the system will need to have. Vendors typically respond to an RFP with their best effort to convince the buyer that they have the best set of services and functionality to fit the customer's system requirements.

- *Comparing bids.* A **request for quote (RFQ)** is a process wherein the buyer invites the EHR vendor to bid for the system. This step allows the buyer to compare the potential cost of EHR systems across various vendor options. When selecting the final product, buyers need to consider the total cost of ownership of the system, including both the upfront cost and any ongoing expenses or staffing required to support the product.

- *Demonstration of the product.* One of the essential steps in choosing the right EHR product is to have an actual demonstration of the system's functionalities, whether online or through a visit from the vendor. The demonstration typically occurs after the organization has narrowed down the choice to a select few vendors, based on price and functionality. Clinicians, support staff, and others who will use the EHR system should be present for the demonstration and involved in the decision-making process. The organization must also engage the organization's thought leaders (e.g., leaders of clinical, financial, and ancillary departments) as applicable, allowing them to participate in the demonstration, ask questions, and test day-to-day cases to help envision how the EHR system might improve workflow. Some organizations schedule a visit to other sites that are using the same EHR system. Although this approach is more logistically complicated, it enables the purchasing organization to see the system "in action," to observe and interact with users, and to assess whether the current users are satisfied. After learning about the system's functionality and capability, the organization must have an evaluation mechanism that weighs functionality, configurability, ease of use, and cost, leading to the right decision.

request for quote (RFQ)
A process wherein a potential purchaser invites a vendor to submit a bid (typically, the upfront cost plus any ongoing expenses), allowing for a comparison of bids across vendors.

Select the Vendor

Organizations typically choose the EHR vendor that best fits the organization's criteria. At the selection stage, key decision makers will review the informative documents from the vendor (e.g., the RFP, the RFQ), as well as the comments from the demonstration or any site visits that occurred. The evaluation matrix also considers the vendor's reputation, longevity, financial stability, and customer service. Importantly, comments from the end users need to be taken into account. Finally, the total cost of ownership of the product needs to be estimated, including any costs associated with the archiving of legacy data (paper or electronic), the sun-setting of the systems being replaced, and the procurement of interfaces that will need to be connected to the new system. Contract negotiations typically occur after a vendor has been selected. Organizations work with their finance, legal, administrative, and clinical stakeholders to arrive at a high-level budget for the project, which will help guide the negotiations.

Manage the Implementation

Once the contract has been vetted, the organization prepares to implement the EHR system. Typically, the organization works with the vendor to plan the deployment and define the scope of the implementation—particularly, the specific services, modules, and functionality to be implemented at the product launch. After the scope has been defined, the next step is to determine the human resource requirements for implementing the new system and supporting the system being replaced. As in the selection process, the involvement of end users is essential during implementation. Clinicians, ancillary staff, and other support staff should be part of the project team and governance, and they should have input into the design, build, and training. The involvement of end users encourages buy-in, ensures that current workflows are considered, and increases the likelihood of a successful launch.

Summary

This chapter has sought to provide a broad overview of the topic of health information technology. It has discussed the development and current architecture of electronic health record systems, examined the concepts of interoperability and meaningful use, and explored how HIT has become a strategic driver for healthcare providers worldwide. Later sections discussed standards for clinical coding, sources of reliable statistical data, and concerns related to the security and privacy of medical data. The chapter's final section walked through the basic steps by which an organization assesses, selects, and implements an appropriate EHR system.

Discussion Questions

1. Describe the emerging standards for encoding and exchanging healthcare information.
2. What are the core areas of HIT applications in your specific areas of interest? Select one or two areas, and describe their value for global health.
3. How do the standards discussed in this chapter (e.g., ICD-10, ISO, DRGs, SNOMED) help improve the quality of information sharing in your area of interest?
4. What are the technical, political, and business impediments to the sharing of medical information across international borders?

5. How do organizations decide which vendor to use when buying expensive HIT systems, such as the modern integrated EHR?

6. Why is HIT important for innovation in the delivery and management of healthcare?

7. What is the future of HIT in healthcare?

8. Discuss the threat of internal and external security breaches to healthcare information, including ransomware. How might this threat influence an organization's decision to adopt HIT?

9. What are the most useful HIT innovations you have used in your daily practice? What are the most outstanding features?

10. What factors impede the full use of HIT innovations (e.g., cloud-based systems, big data) in business settings and in global health?

Additional Resources

Organization Websites
- American Academy of Family Physicians, "EHR Product Select & Implement": www.aafp.org/practice-management/health-it/product.html
- American Hospital Association, "Health Information Technology Advocacy—Meaningful Use": www.aha.org/aha/issues/HIT/100226-hit-meaningful.html (available for AHA members only)
- Centers for Medicare & Medicaid Services, "Promoting Interoperability": www.cms.gov/EHRIncentivePrograms
- Health Information and Management Systems Society: www.himss.org
- Health Level Seven International: www.hl7.org
- Office of the National Coordinator for Health Information Technology: www.healthit.gov/topic/about-onc

HIT-Related Videos
- Cerner, "Background of HL7 FHIR Standard": www.youtube.com/watch?v=PbiNZqGX5Yw
- Population Health, "Introduction to HL7 FHIR": www.youtube.com/watch?v=oSqISJw_nv0
- AAPC, "What Is ICD-10?": www.youtube.com/watch?v=ZPDgtDDTc8k

HIT Text books
- Glandon, G. L., D. H. Smaltz, and D. J. Slovensky. 2013. *Information Systems for Healthcare Management*, 8th ed. Chicago: Health Administration Press.

- Sayles, N. B. 2012. *Health Information Management Technology: An Applied Approach*, 4th ed. Chicago: American Health Information Management Association.
- Wager, K. A., F. W. Lee, and J. P. Glaser. 2013. *Health Care Information Systems*, 3rd ed. San Francisco: Jossey-Bass.

Recommended Readings
- Al-Hablani, B. 2017. "The Use of Automated SNOMED CT Clinical Coding in Clinical Decision Support Systems for Preventive Care." *Perspectives in Health Information Management*. Published January 1. www.ncbi.nlm.nih.gov/pmc/articles/PMC5430114/.
- Bauchner, H., D. Berwick, and P. B. Fontanarosa. 2016. "Innovations in Health Care Delivery and the Future of Medicine." *JAMA* 315 (1): 30–31.
- Fernandes, L., and M. O'Connor. 2015. "Accurate Patient Identification—A Global Challenge." *Perspectives in Health Information Management*. Published May. http://bok.ahima.org/doc?oid=301182#.Wus-PaQvxhE.
- Gaynor, M., C. Bass, and B. Duepner. 2015. "A Tale of Two Standards: Strengthening HIPAA Security Regulations Using the PCI-DSS." *Health Systems* 4 (2): 111–23.
- Mandel, J. C., D. A. Kreda, K. D. Mandl, I. S. Kohane, and R. B. Ramoni. 2016. "SMART on FHIR: A Standards-Based, Interoperable Apps Platform for Electronic Health Records." *Journal of the American Medical Informatics Association* 23 (5): 899–908.
- Page, T. 2014. "Notions of Innovation in Healthcare Services and Products." *International Journal of Innovation and Sustainable Development* 8 (3): 217–31.
- Roomaney, R. A., V. Pillay-van Wyk, O. F. Awotiwon, E. Nicol, J. D. Joubert, D. Bradshaw, and L. A. Hanmer. 2017. "Availability and Quality of Routine Morbidity Data: Review of Studies in South Africa." *Journal of the American Medical Informatics Association* 24 (e1): e194–e206.

References

Adler-Milstein, J., C. M. DesRoches, M. F. Furukawa, C. Worzala, D. Charles, P. Kralovec, S. Stalley, and A. K. Jha. 2014. "More Than Half of US Hospitals Have at Least a Basic EHR, but Stage 2 Criteria Remain Challenging for Most."

Health Affairs. Published September. www.healthaffairs.org/doi/full/10.1377/hlthaff.2014.0453.

Agency for Healthcare Research and Quality (AHRQ). 2018. "Healthcare Cost and Utilization Project (HCUP)." Reviewed April. www.ahrq.gov/research/data/hcup/index.html.

American Health Information Management Association (AHIMA) and Global Health Workforce Council (GHWC). 2015. *Global Academic Curricula Competencies for Health Information Professionals.* American Health Information Management Association. Published June 30. www.ahima.org/about/~/media/AHIMA/Files/AHIMA-and-Our-Work/AHIMA-GlobalCurricula_Final_6-30-15.ashx?la=en.

Association of University Programs in Health Administration (AUPHA). 2016. "Health Information Management Systems Technology and Analysis: A Curriculum for Graduate Education Programs in Health Administration." Accessed May 2, 2018. http://network.aupha.org/himstacurriculum.

Atherton, J. 2011. "Development of the Electronic Health Record." *Virtual Mentor* 13 (3): 186–89.

Ayatollahi, H., M. Roozbehi, and H. Haghani. 2015. "Physicians' and Nurses' Opinions About the Impact of a Computerized Provider Order Entry System on Their Workflow." *Perspectives in Health Information Management.* Published November 1. www.ncbi.nlm.nih.gov/pmc/articles/PMC4632876/.

Barta, A., G. McNeill, P. Meli, K. Wall, and A. Zeisset. 2008. "ICD-10-CM Primer." *Journal of AHIMA* 79 (5): 64–66, quiz 67–68.

Becker's Health IT & CIO Report. 2016. "5 Epic Contracts—and Their Costs—So Far in 2016." Published March 8. www.beckershospitalreview.com/healthcare-information-technology/5-epic-contracts-and-their-costs-so-far-in-2016.html.

Bhagade, P., S. Kanawade, and M. Nikose. 2016. "Emerging Internet of Things in Revolutionizing Healthcare." In *Proceedings of the International Conference on Data Engineering and Communication Technology*, vol. 2, edited by C. S. Satapathy, V. Bhateja, and A. Joshi, 683–90. Singapore: Springer.

Bhattacharyya, S. B. 2016. *Introduction to SNOMED CT.* Singapore: Springer.

Centers for Disease Control and Prevention (CDC). 2017. "Meaningful Use." Updated January 18. www.cdc.gov/ehrmeaningfuluse/introduction.html.

Centers for Medicare & Medicaid Services (CMS). 2007a. "Security Standards: Administrative Safeguards." HIPAA Security Series. Revised March. www.hhs.gov/sites/default/files/ocr/privacy/hipaa/administrative/securityrule/adminsafeguards.pdf.

———. 2007b. "Security Standards: Organizational, Policies and Procedures and Documentation Requirements." HIPAA Security Series. Revised March. www.hhs.gov/sites/default/files/ocr/privacy/hipaa/administrative/securityrule/pprequirements.pdf.

———. 2007c. "Security Standards: Physical Safeguards." HIPAA Security Series. Revised March. www.hhs.gov/sites/default/files/ocr/privacy/hipaa/administrative/securityrule/physsafeguards.pdf.

———. 2007d. "Security Standards: Technical Safeguards." HIPAA Security Series. Revised March. www.hhs.gov/sites/default/files/ocr/privacy/hipaa/administrative/securityrule/techsafeguards.pdf.

Cerner. 2018. "Welcome to Code." Accessed May 2. https://code.cerner.com.

Cimino, J. J. 2013. "Improving the Electronic Health Record—Are Clinicians Getting What They Wished for?" *JAMA* 309 (10): 991–92.

Conn, J. 2016. "Cerner Opens Sandbox for SMART on FHIR Interoperability Development." *Modern Healthcare.* Published February 10. www.modernhealthcare.com/article/20160210/NEWS/160219988.

———. 2011. "HIPAA at 15: Some Provisions Still a Work in Progress." *Modern Healthcare.* Published August 22. www.modernhealthcare.com/article/20110822/MAGAZINE/308229962.

Connolly, C. 2005. "Cedars-Sinai Doctors Cling to Pen and Paper." *Washington Post.* Published March 21. www.washingtonpost.com/wp-dyn/articles/A52384-2005Mar20.html.

Corepoint Health. 2018. "Versions of the HL7 Standard." Accessed May 8. https://corepointhealth.com/resource-center/hl7-resources/hl7-standard-versions.

Davis, J. 2016. "10 Worst Health Data Breaches of 2016." Published December 22. www.healthcareitnews.com/slideshow/10-worst-health-data-breaches-2016.

Douglas, G. 2009. "Engineering an EMR System in the Developing World: Necessity Is the Mother of Invention." PhD diss., University of Pittsburgh. Accessed May 2, 2018. http://d-scholarship.pitt.edu/7744/.

Elion, J. 2016. "Best of Breed or Monolithic: The Pendulum Swings." Chartwise. Published November 9. www.chartwisemed.com/best-of-breed-or-monolithic-the-pendulum-swings/.

Emery, C. 2017. "What Is the UAE Doing Right with Healthcare That the Rest of the World Can Learn from?" Future Health Index. Published January 24. www.futurehealthindex.com/2017/01/24/uae-right-healthcare-rest-world-can-learn/.

European Union Agency for Network and Information Security (ENISA). 2018. "About ENISA." Accessed May 11. www.enisa.europa.eu/about-enisa.

Eurostat. 2018. "Eurostat: Your Key to European Statistics." Accessed May 10. http://ec.europa.eu/eurostat/about/overview.

———. 2017. "Geographical Information System of the Commission (GISCO)." Updated November 29. http://ec.europa.eu/eurostat/statistics-explained/index.php/Geographical_information_system_of_the_Commission_(GISCO).

Ferranti, J. M., R. C. Musser, K. Kawamoto, and W. E. Hammond. 2006. "The Clinical Document Architecture and the Continuity of Care Record: A Critical Analysis." *Journal of the American Medical Informatics Association* 13 (3): 245–52.

Fetter, R. B., Y. Shin, J. L. Freeman, R. F. Averill, and J. D. Thompson. 1980. "Case Mix Definition by Diagnosis-Related Groups." *Medical Care* 18 (2 suppl.): iii, 1–53.

Francisco, S. 2016. "RxREVU Embedded App for Prescription Decision Support Receives Cerner Validation." iReach. Published November 14. www.ireach content.com/news-releases/rxrevu-embedded-app-for-prescription-decision-support-receives-cerner-validation-601089306.html.

Gálvez, J. A., B. S. Rothman, C. A. Doyle, S. Morgan, A. F. Simpao, and M. A. Rehman. 2015. "A Narrative Review of Meaningful Use and Anesthesia Information Management Systems." *Anesthesia and Analgesia* 121 (3): 693–706.

Garrett, P. 2011. "EMR vs EHR: What Is the Difference?" *HealthIT Buzz*. Published January 4. www.healthit.gov/buzz-blog/electronic-health-and-medical-records/emr-vs-ehr-difference/.

Gaynor, M., C. Bass, and B. Duepner. 2015. "A Tale of Two Standards: Strengthening HIPAA Security Regulations Using the PCI-DSS." *Health Systems* 4 (2): 111–23.

Gaynor, M., and S. Bradner. 2004. "A Real Options Framework to Value Network, Protocol, and Service Architecture." *ACM SIGCOMM Computer Communication Review* 34 (5): 31–38.

Gershenfeld, N., R. Krikorian, and D. Cohen. 2004. "The Internet of Things." *Scientific American* 291: 76–81.

Goff, J., J. Christensen, and E. Paxman. 2016. "Global EMR Adoption 2016: Who Is Driving EMR Adoption and Satisfaction?" KLAS. Published July 21. https://klasresearch.com/report/global-emr-adoption-2016/1143.

Goldfield, N. 2010. "The Evolution of Diagnosis-Related Groups (DRGs): From Its Beginnings in Case-Mix and Resource Use Theory, to Its Implementation for Payment and Now for Its Current Utilization for Quality Within and Outside the Hospital." *Quality Management in Health Care* 19 (1): 3–16.

Government Publishing Office. 2010. "The Patient Protection and Affordable Care Act." Accessed May 2, 2018. www.gpo.gov/fdsys/pkg/BILLS-111hr3590enr/pdf/BILLS-111hr3590enr.pdf.

Griebel, L., H.-U. Prokosh, F. Köpcke, D. Toddenroth, J. Christoph, I. Leb, I. Engel, and M. Sedlmayr. 2015. "A Scoping Review of Cloud Computing in Healthcare." *BMC Medical Informatics and Decision Making*. Published March 19. https://bmcmedinformdecismak.biomedcentral.com/articles/10.1186/s12911-015-0145-7.

HealthIT.gov. 2018. "What Is an Electronic Health Record (EHR)?" Accessed May 2. www.healthit.gov/providers-professionals/faqs/what-electronic-health-record-ehr.

———. 2016. "What Is a Personal Health Record?" Reviewed May 2. www.healthit.gov/providers-professionals/faqs/what-personal-health-record.

Health Level Seven (HL7) International. 2018a. "About HL7." Accessed May 2. www.hl7.org/about/index.cfm.

———. 2018b. "HL7 Frequently Asked Questions." Accessed May 2. www.hl7.org/about/FAQs/index.cfm.

———. 2018c. "Introduction to HL7 Standards." Accessed May 2. www.hl7.org/implement/standards/index.cfm.

———. 2018d. "Section 3: Clinical and Administrative Domains. HL7 Version 2.7 Standard: Chapter 03—Patient Administration." Accessed May 8. www.hl7.org/implement/standards/product_brief.cfm?product_id=193.

———. 2017a. "FHIR Overview." Accessed May 2, 2018. www.hl7.org/fhir/overview.html.

———. 2017b. "Introducing HL7 FHIR." Accessed May 2, 2018. www.hl7.org/fhir/summary.html.

Healy, J.-C. 2008. *Implementing e-Health in Developing Countries: Guidance and Principles*. International Telecommunication Union. Published September. www.itu.int/ITU-D/cyb/app/docs/e-Health_prefinal_15092008.PDF.

Henry, J., Y. Pylypchuk, T. Searcy, and V. Patel. 2016. "Adoption of Electronic Health Record Systems Among US Non-Federal Acute Care Hospitals: 2008–2015." Office of the National Coordinator for Health Information Technology. Published May. https://dashboard.healthit.gov/evaluations/data-briefs/non-federal-acute-care-hospital-ehr-adoption-2008-2015.php.

HIPAA Journal. 2017. "Largest Healthcare Data Breaches of 2016." Published January 4. www.hipaajournal.com/largest-healthcare-data-breaches-of-2016-8631/.

Hofmans-Okkes, I. M., and H. Lamberts. 1996. "The International Classification of Primary Care (ICPC): New Applications in Research and Computer-Based Patient Records in Family Practice." *Family Practice* 13 (3): 294–302.

International Health Care System Profiles. 2018. "What Is the Status of Electronic Health Records?" Accessed May 3. http://international.commonwealthfund.org/features/ehrs/.

International Organization for Standardization (ISO). 2018. "About ISO." Accessed May 2. www.iso.org/iso/home/about.htm.

———. 2015. "Health Informatics—HL7 Electronic Health Records-System Functional Model, Release 2 (EHR FM)." Published August. www.iso.org/iso/home/store/catalogue_tc/catalogue_detail.htm?csnumber=57757.

Jha, A. K., C. M. DesRoches, E. G. Campbell, K. Donelan, S. R. Rao, T. G. Ferris, A. Shields, S. Rosenbaum, and D. Blumenthal. 2009. "Use of Electronic Health Records in US Hospitals." *New England Journal of Medicine* 360 (16): 1628–38.

Kane, J. 2012. "Health Costs: How the US Compares with Other Countries." PBS News Hour. Published October 22. www.pbs.org/newshour/rundown/health-costs-how-the-us-compares-with-other-countries/.

Kayyali, R., V. Savickas, M. A. Spruit, E. Kaimakamis, R. Siva, R. W. Costello, J. Chang, B. Pierscionek, N. Davies, A. W. Vaes, R. Paradiso, N. Philip, E. Perantoni, S. D'Arcy, A. Raptopoulos, and S. Nabhani-Gebara. 2016. "Qualitative Investigation into a Wearable System for Chronic Obstructive Pulmonary Disease: The Stakeholders' Perspective." *BMJ Open*. Published August 31. http://bmjopen.bmj.com/content/6/8/e011657.

Khajouei, R., and M. W. M. Jaspers. 2010. "The Impact of CPOE Medication Systems' Design Aspects on Usability, Workflow and Medication Orders." *Methods of Information in Medicine* 49 (1): 3–19.

Khajouei, R., P. C. Wierenga, A. Hasman, and M. W. M. Jaspers. 2011. "Clinicians Satisfaction with CPOE Ease of Use and Effect on Clinicians' Workflow, Efficiency and Medication Safety." *International Journal of Medical Informatics* 80 (5): 297–309.

Koppel, R., and C. U. Lehmann. 2015. "Implications of an Emerging EHR Monoculture for Hospitals and Healthcare Systems." *Journal of the American Medical Informatics Association* 22 (2): 465–71.

Krisik, K. M. 2013. "Lessons Learned: How to Smooth Your EHR Implementation." *Health Management and Technology* 34 (3): 8.

Liveri, D., A. Sarri, and C. Skouloudi. 2015. *Security and Resilience in eHealth: Security Challenges and Risks.* Heraklion, Greece: European Union Agency for Network and Information Security.

Mantas, J., E. Ammenwerth, G. Demiris, A. Hasman, R. Haux, W. Hersh, E. Hovenga, K. C. Lun, H. Marin, F. Martin-Sanchez, and G. Wright. 2010. "Recommendations of the International Medical Informatics Association (IMIA) on Education in Biomedical and Health Informatics. First Revision." *Methods of Information in Medicine* 49 (2): 105–20.

Mantero, J., E. Szegedi, L. Payne Hallstrom, A. Lenglet, E. Depoortere, B. Kaic, L. Blumberg, J. P. Linge, and D. Coulombier. 2014. "Enhanced Epidemic Intelligence Using a Web-Based Screening System During the 2010 FIFA World Cup in South Africa." *Euro Surveillance* 19 (18): 1–9.

Markets and Markets. 2018. "*Healthcare IT Market Worth 280.25 Billion USD by 2021.*" Accessed May 2. www.marketsandmarkets.com/PressReleases/healthcare-it-market.asp.

Marques, R., J. Gregório, M. Mira Da Silva, and L. V. Lapão. 2016. "The Promise of the Internet of Things in Healthcare: How Hard Is It to Keep?" *Studies in Health Technology and Informatics* 228: 665–69.

Miliard, M. 2017. "How Cerner Won the Biggest EHR Deal Ever, Twice." *Healtcare IT News.* Published June 6. www.healthcareitnews.com/news/how-cerner-won-biggest-ehr-deal-ever-twice.

Mugo, D. M., and D. Nzuki. 2014. "Determinants of Electronic Health in Developing Countries." *International Journal of Arts and Commerce* 3 (3): 49–60.

Naden, C. 2014. "Building Better National Health Systems with a New ISO Roadmap." International Organization for Standardization. Published October 23. www.iso.org/iso/home/news_index/news_archive/news.htm?refid=Ref1888.

National Library of Medicine. 2016. "New SNOMED CT International Release Downloads Available." *NLM Technical Bulletin.* Published May. www.nlm.nih.gov/pubs/techbull/mj16/brief/mj16_umls_snomed_ct_releases.html.

Norwegian Centre for Research Data. 2018. "About the MacroDataGuide." Accessed May 3. www.nsd.uib.no/macrodataguide/about.html.

Office of the National Coordinator for Health Information Technology (ONC). 2018. "Fact Sheet: Quality Payment Program and Health Information Technology." Accessed May 2. www.healthit.gov/sites/default/files/macra_health_it_fact_sheet_final.pdf.

———. 2016a. "Hospital Health IT Developers." Accessed July. http://dashboard.healthit.gov/quickstats/pages/FIG-Vendors-of-EHRs-to-Participating-Hospitals.php.

———. 2016b. "Non-federal Acute Care Hospital Electronic Health Record Adoption." Published May. http://dashboard.healthit.gov/quickstats/pages/FIG-Hospital-EHR-Adoption.php.

Oluoch, T., X. Santas, D. Kwaro, M. Were, P. Biondich, C. Bailey, A. Abu-Hanna, and N. de Keizer. 2012. "The Effect of Electronic Medical Record–Based Clinical Decision Support on HIV Care in Resource-Constrained Settings: A Systematic Review." *International Journal of Medical Informatics* 81 (10): e83–e92.

Pan American Health Organization (PAHO). 2017. "Health Situation in the Americas: Core Health Indicators 2016." Updated May. www.paho.org/hq/index.php?option=com_content&view=article&id=2470&Itemid.

PCI Security Standards Council. 2018. "Frequently Asked Questions." Accessed May 3. www.pcisecuritystandards.org/merchants/.

———. 2016. *PCI DSS Quick Reference Guide: Understanding the Payment Card Industry Data Security Standard, Version 3.2.* Published May. www.pcisecuritystandards.org/documents/PCIDSS_QRGv3_2.pdf.

PubMed. 2016. "Search." Accessed September. www.ncbi.nlm.nih.gov/pubmed/.

Rhea, S. 2007. "Clooney and Hospital Prying Eyes: Experts Wonder if Incident Will Expose HIPAA Weakness." *Modern Healthcare* 37 (41): 10.

Rosenthal, A., P. Mork, M. H. Li, J. Stanford, D. Koester, and P. Reynolds. 2010. "Cloud Computing: A New Business Paradigm for Biomedical Information Sharing." *Journal of Biomedical Informatics* 43 (2): 342–53.

Rosling, H., and Z. Zhang. 2011. "Health Advocacy with GapMinder Animated Statistics." *Journal of Epidemiology and Global Health* 1 (1): 11–14.

Rusnák, M., V. Rusnáková, and M. Psota. 2013. *Statistics of Health.* Accessed May 3, 2018. http://rusnak.truni.sk/ucebne_texty/Statistika%20zdravia/Health%20Statistics.pdf.

Sajid, A., and H. Abbas. 2016. "Data Privacy in Cloud-Assisted Healthcare Systems: State of the Art and Future Challenges." *Journal of Medical Systems* 40 (6): 155.

Scheller-Kreinsen, D., A. Geissler, and R. Busse. 2009. "The ABC of DRGs." *Euro Observer* 11: 1–5.

Schoen, C., R. Osborn, D. Squires, M. Doty, P. Rasmussen, and S. Applebaum. 2012. "A Survey of Primary Care Doctors in Ten Countries Shows Progress in Use of Health Information Technology, Less in Other Areas." *Health Affairs* 31 (12): 2805–16.

Slabodkin, G. 2018. "Trump Budget for VA Includes \$4.2B to Modernize IT Infrastructure." *Health Data Management*. Published February 13. www.healthdatamanagement.com/news/both-the-va-and-dod-will-implement-cerners-millennium-ehr-platform.

SNOMED International. 2018. "SNOMED CT: The Global Language of Healthcare." Accessed May 3. www.ihtsdo.org/snomed-ct.

Teslow, M. 2016. "Health Data Concepts and Information Governance." In *Health Information: Management of a Strategic Resource*, 5th ed., edited by M. Abdelhak and M. A. Hanken, 88–144. St. Louis, MO: Elsevier.

Tripathi, M. 2012. "EHR Evolution: Policy and Legislation Forces Changing the EHR." *Journal of AHIMA* 83 (10): 24–29.

US Department of Health and Human Services. 2018. "Health Information Privacy." Accessed May 3. www.hhs.gov/hipaa/index.html.

Ventana Research. 2016. "Ventana Research Announces the Technology Innovation Award Winners for 2016." Published October 12. www.ventanaresearch.com/press-release/ventana-research-announces-the-technology-innovation-award-winners-for-2016.

Wachter, R. 2015. *The Digital Doctor: Hope, Hype, and Harm at the Dawn of Medicine's Computer Age*. New York: McGraw-Hill.

World Health Organization (WHO). 2018a. "Global Health Observatory (GHO) Data." Accessed May 3. http://who.int/gho/about/en/.

———. 2018b. "WHO Mortality Database." Accessed May 3. www.who.int/health info/mortality_data/en/index.html.

———. 2012a. *Legal Frameworks for eHealth*. Global Observatory for eHealth series, vol. 5. Accessed May 3, 2018. www.who.int/goe/publications/ehealth_series_vol5/en/.

———. 2012b. *Management of Patient Information: Trends and Challenges in Member States*. Global Observatory for eHealth series, vol. 6. Accessed May 3, 2018. www.who.int/goe/publications/ehealth_series_vol6/en/.

———. 2007. "International Statistical Classification of Diseases and Related Health Problems, 10th revision." Accessed May 3, 2018. http://apps.who.int/classifications/icd10/browse/2010/en.

World Health Organization (WHO) Regional Office for Europe. 2018. "European Health Information Gateway: Health for All Explorer." Accessed May 3. http://data.euro.who.int/hfadb/.

———. 2016. *From Innovation to Implementation: eHealth in the WHO European Region*. Accessed May 2, 2018. www.euro.who.int/en/publications/abstracts/from-innovation-to-implementation-ehealth-in-the-who-european-region-2016.

World Organization of Family Doctors (WONCA). 2015. "From the CEO's Desk—WONCA's Global Reach." Published September. www.globalfamilydoctor.com/News/FromtheCEOsDesk-WONCAsGlobalReach.aspx.

Wright, L. 2014. "Thinking Holistically About EHR Selection and Implementation." *Behavioral Healthcare Executive*. Published January 24. www.behavioral.net/article/thinking-holistically-about-ehr-selection-and-implementation.

LEADERSHIP, ORGANIZATIONAL DESIGN, AND CHANGE

11

PRINCIPLES OF EFFECTIVE LEADERSHIP

Daniel J. West Jr., PhD, FACHE, FACMPE, Zhanming Liang, PhD, FCHSM, and Vladimir Krcmery, MD, PhD, ScD, FRCP

Chapter Focus

Competent leadership is essential for improving healthcare outcomes and quality of care. Global leaders need to possess knowledge, skills, and competencies to develop and modify systems of care and drive continuous change and improvement. In this chapter, we examine leadership qualities, traits, and characteristics, along with issues of responsibility and professional identity. We also discuss contemporary leadership issues, while allowing for country-specific and regional variation. Applied examples of leadership concepts help underscore the importance of managing resources wisely, ensuring sustainable projects, and meeting the needs of vulnerable populations. Discussion questions, vignettes, and exercises further enable application and integration of key concepts and ideas.

Learning Objectives

Upon completion of this chapter, you should be able to

- understand traditional and contemporary concepts, theories, and thinking about leadership;
- analyze approaches for managing people, resources, and organizational change;
- describe the skills, traits, and characteristics needed by global healthcare leaders;
- use competency models to identify appropriate leadership behaviors, knowledge, and skills;
- employ effective leadership while addressing issues of cost, access, and quality and building partnerships, projects, and networks; and
- apply knowledge about leadership to issues affecting low-income countries and emerging economies.

Competencies

- Demonstrate problem solving, decision making, and critical thinking.
- Demonstrate effective interpersonal relationships and the ability to work with marginalized persons.
- Understand and demonstrate the importance of listening and communication skills.
- Promote ethical conduct, professionalism, self-development, and life-long learning.
- Use reflection, discernment, and feedback to improve leadership performance.
- Establish goals and objectives for improving health outcomes.
- Recognize the importance of global health events and their impact on population health.
- Maintain personal and professional accountability, transparency, integrity, and social commitment.
- Understand leadership styles, techniques, and theory.
- Identify and discuss current leadership issues facing healthcare professionals.
- Reflect upon and assess leadership values, abilities, and competencies.
- Understand the importance of cultural diversity, cultural sensitivity, and cultural disparities.
- Identify and discuss issues of social justice.
- Demonstrate the importance of effective interpersonal relationships.

Key Terms

- Andragogy
- Contingency theory
- Cultural proficiency
- Globalization
- Hierarchy of needs
- Job analysis
- Job design
- Leadership
- Management by objectives (MBO)
- Organizational culture
- Path–goal theory
- Professionalism
- Servant leadership
- Situational leadership
- SMART objectives
- SWOT analysis
- Transformational leadership
- Triple aim
- Value-based healthcare

Key Concepts

- Diversity and inclusion
- Emergency response
- Ethics
- Evidence-based management
- Implementing change
- International collaboration and coordination
- Leadership competencies
- Leadership development
- Leadership research
- Mentoring and coaching
- Motivation
- Nongovernment organizations
- Nurse leadership
- Organizational governance
- Organizational performance
- Partnership building
- Physician leadership
- Professional development
- Reflection
- Self-understanding
- Strategic planning
- Talent management
- Team leadership
- Theories of leadership
- Vision
- Vulnerable populations
- Work design

Introduction

Today's healthcare leaders function in an increasingly interconnected world, where events in one region or country have significant effects and implications elsewhere. The concept of **globalization**—the increased interconnectedness across international boundaries—comes up frequently in discussions of public health, infectious disease, health systems, and financing of care. Globalization is driven by individual and collective actions through social groups, and it is further enhanced through personal mobility, consumer consumption patterns, and technological advances. All of these considerations, and more, are central to the context within which today's healthcare leaders operate.

> **globalization**
> Interconnectedness and interdependency across people and cultures, stemming from increased transportation, distribution, communication, and economic activity across international boundaries.

Healthcare leaders must ensure that the resources dedicated to healthcare are used appropriately and effectively, and they must be prepared to deal with significant obstacles and limitations. In many countries, healthcare expenditures represent a large percentage of the gross national product, and the use of public funds for healthcare is the subject of close scrutiny. Furthermore, the demand for healthcare services is constantly changing and increasing; often, resources are unavailable, causing demand to go unmet.

Emergencies, disasters, and conflicts raise additional concerns for global healthcare leaders. Natural disasters such as floods, volcanic eruptions, and earthquakes can cause direct harm and loss of life, while also having significant long-term effects on health and life expectancy. Similarly, world events such as the civil wars in Syria and Iraq, the plight of internally displaced people in

Afghanistan, and humanitarian crises in other parts of the world affect large numbers of people and have a dramatic impact on global health. Disasters and crises can place enormous strain on health systems both locally and internationally. In recent years, hurricanes have caused significant damage and loss of life, often in low- and middle-income countries where the poor tend to be the most vulnerable. In addition to their direct effects, such disasters can have a significant impact on a country's infrastructure, affecting food and water supply, sewage systems, roads, and the health infrastructure, in terms of hospitals, health centers, and clinics. Many disasters and emergencies create refugees and displaced persons who have been forced to migrate to other countries, inevitably placing pressures on the healthcare systems in those countries.

Today's healthcare leaders must be able to prepare for and respond to such emergencies, addressing both direct and indirect health effects, while also providing day-to-day health services in a complex, ever-changing context. This chapter will examine many of the skills, competencies, models, and practices that can help global leaders succeed in this endeavor.

Leadership in an Era of Change

In global health management, change is constant and accelerating. It occurs in every country, and it is typically complex and difficult to navigate. Change can carry significant risk, and it can lead to tension and conflict, particularly if managers and leaders lack sufficient skills. However, when managed effectively, change can create excitement and positive energy, spur new models of service delivery, and produce meaningful organizational benefits.

Change and reform have been constant features of the healthcare sector in recent decades. However, many major reforms and initiatives have not been successful, causing not only financial losses but also cynicism, diminished morale, and change fatigue among healthcare professionals. Navigating this environment is one of the biggest challenges facing healthcare managers in the twenty-first century.

The research literature suggests that many past failures have been caused by such factors as lack of expertise in planning and implementing change, inadequate preparation by the organization and the people affected by the change, and a lack of strategies for sustaining the change after it has been implemented (Liang and Howard 2007). The literature further emphasizes the critical role of effective **leadership**—the ability to implement change, motivate people to accomplish organizational goals, and make decisions and pursue initiatives toward positive outcomes (Bolman and Deal 2003).

Health services leaders, whether they are physicians or trained managers, need to possess specific competencies and skills to manage change and to improve clinical outcomes, patient safety, and quality of care. Spencer and

leadership
The ability to use influence to motivate individuals in an organization to accomplish a particular goal.

Spencer (1993, 9) define *competency* as "an underlying characteristic of an individual that is causally related to criterion-referenced effective and/or superior performance in a job or situation." Others have defined *competency* as behavior that lies behind competent performance, or as a suitable or sufficient skill, knowledge, or ability. This chapter will look extensively at core healthcare leadership competencies, as well as global competencies, which may involve working in different countries, comparing services and systems internationally, and working with individuals and groups from diverse cultures. Cultural engagement, self-directed study, and fieldwork opportunities in university-based education can help individuals elucidate their global competencies.

Understanding Motivation

Leadership can be defined as the ability to use influence to motivate individuals within an organization to accomplish a particular goal. Hence, motivation is central to the concept. The fundamental task of a leader or manager is to ensure that work is completed, and this task is achieved through the motivation of teams and members (Barr and Dowding 2012). Birk (2010) notes that leadership is about relationships and the creation of a vision with which people are able to identify. Leadership titles, therefore, are not as important as the ability to motivate a heterogeneous working population.

Of the various theories related to motivation, one of the most important is by McClelland (1984). In his pioneering work on workplace motivational thinking, McClelland distinguished between three types of motivation: achievement motivation (driven by accomplishment of goals), authority/power motivation (driven by the desire for power and influence), and affiliation motivation (driven by interpersonal relationships). He believed that achievement-motivated leaders were the ones who produced the best results, and they did so by setting goals that are achievable through their own efforts and the efforts of others in the organization. McClelland's work suggested that achievement is more important than material or financial reward, and research tends to support this suggestion. Financial reward may be important in attracting high performers to the job, but recognition, job satisfaction, and the presence of a clear career path are the key elements of organizational retention strategies.

People are intrinsically motivated when they understand why they are doing something. Thus, leaders need to put the correct conditions in place to promote the development of such an understanding. According to Abraham Maslow's (1954) **hierarchy of needs** model, people are motivated by several levels of needs, with physiological needs at the most basic level, safety and security at the next level, followed by love/belonging and esteem, and finally self-actualization at the top level. Applying this model, leaders can achieve staff motivation by taking into consideration individuals' physical, spiritual, and emotional needs and by making staff feel secure, needed, and appreciated.

hierarchy of needs
A model, introduced by Abraham Maslow, stating that people are motivated by several levels of needs, with physiological needs at the most basic level and self-actualization at the top level.

> ### Vignette: St. Elizabeth University of Health and Social Work
>
> St. Elizabeth University of Health and Social Work was founded in 2003 as a private university in Bratislava, Slovakia. With more than 60 study programs in public health, social work, nursing, missionary work, health technology, psychology, and related fields, the university serves as an example for other European educational programs seeking to foster effective leadership in a global health context. At St. Elizabeth, physicians, faculty, social workers, government officials, practitioners, educators, students, managers, and researchers work together in solidarity to share experiences and practices around the theme of "Promoting the Dignity and Worth of Peoples." The team's efforts benefit from effective leadership and support from senior management. The university has more than 50 international programs addressing issues of social justice, human rights, collective responsibility, and respect for diversity (European Network for Social Action 2014).

Motivating leaders are good listeners, communicators, and problem solvers. Most importantly, they rely on integrity, experience, and competence rather than authority or power.

Such an approach to motivation is evident in effective leaders from all walks of life. Consider, for instance, the Irish rock icon Bono, who gained fame with the band U2 and is also a prominent activist. He cofounded One, a global, data-driven organization that influences governments and raises money for people living in poverty and fighting disease. In 2016, *Fortune* magazine listed him as one of the world's 50 greatest leaders. His secret? "An ability to convince others that they are the true leaders of change, not him" (McGirt 2016).

Dimensions of Leadership

Although motivation is a central component, leadership also involves a multitude of other dimensions. Great leaders can initiate ideas, assemble effective teams to bring concepts to life, and, ultimately, execute their ideas. They are collaborators in building partnerships with shared goals and priorities. They demonstrate honesty, communication, confidence, commitment, positive attitude, creativity, humor, and intuition. They have the ability to delegate, inspire others, and adopt flexible approaches depending on situations (Maxwell 1999). They show respect for others, provide appropriate feedback, and engage in mentoring and coaching to build genuine working relationships.

The United Kingdom's National Health Service (NHS) has developed a healthcare leadership model that consists of nine dimensions (NHS Leadership Academy 2016):

- Leading with care
- Sharing the vision
- Engaging the team
- Influencing for results
- Evaluating information
- Inspiring shared purpose
- Connecting our service
- Developing capability
- Holding to account

Dye and Garman (2014) also offer a competency model for exceptional leadership, and the foundation of their model is a healthy self-concept. From that foundation, they identify four cornerstones: (1) a well-cultivated self-awareness, (2) a compelling vision, (3) a real way with people, and (4) masterful execution.

Leaders in healthcare settings must also demonstrate the professional competence expected of health professionals. **Professionalism** can be regarded as a sort of "meta-skill" that allows individuals to draw on the technical and practical skills appropriate for a given scenario in professional practice. It involves maintaining high professional standards and making ethical workplace decisions, while also actively fostering the professional development of others (Morrow et al. 2014). Leaders can contribute to the development of professional behavior and practices among staff by providing supportive environments in which staff feel valued, by providing management support, and by recognizing the diversity of professions in the healthcare environment (Jha et al. 2007).

professionalism
The ability to maintain high professional standards and ethics and to draw on the technical and practical skills appropriate for professional scenarios.

Effective managers demonstrate leadership by sharing organizational vision and goals with staff; by motivating, engaging, and empowering staff and key stakeholders; by obtaining, providing, and acting on feedback; and by providing training, guidance, and support. Most importantly, they lead by example, are innovative and open-minded, and have a willingness to take risk and responsibility. In the corporate world, leadership development has been the largest expense item in organizational development budgets. However, investment in leadership development in small-scale healthcare settings is still relatively new. Undoubtedly, leadership competence should be embedded within management at the individual, team, and organizational levels.

Developing Leadership Competence

How should leadership competence be developed in the organizational context? No single approach can fully address this question. Leadership competence depends on individual and organizational circumstances. Ross, Wenzel, and Mitlyng (2002) distinguish between conceptual skills that are needed to solve complex problems; technical skills that are related to specific work tasks; and interpersonal skills that affect one's ability to communicate and relate with others.

Leadership development efforts can enhance leadership knowledge, skills, and attributes (Collins and Holton 2004), but evidence suggests that multifaceted interventions tend to be more effective than single interventions. Leadership development is not simply a matter of developing a curriculum and teaching lessons in a classroom; rather, it involves a comprehensive set of processes designed to support managers and other health professionals in their continuous growth as leaders. Such efforts may include any or all of the following:

- Formal training to help potential leaders understand leadership theory and to help them translate knowledge and skills into practical leadership competence
- Coaching and mentoring by experienced leaders
- Guidance through examples of best practice
- Networking and participation in continuous professional development opportunities
- Regular assessment of strengths and weaknesses to identify areas for improvement in themselves and colleagues

Leadership capacity requires the development of nontechnical skills that cannot be mastered in the classroom. Communication and listening, emotional intelligence, strategic planning, and the ability to work with others as a team are lifelong skills that are built through application in work and real-life situations. Skill development should not be viewed as a one-time activity; rather, it requires constant practice, appraisal, and reinforcement, along with continued refinement and the addition of new knowledge.

The leadership practices and competencies in healthcare organizations have been strongly influenced by the behavioral sciences, with meaningful contributions from sociology, social psychology, educational psychology, political science, and anthropology (Gibson et al. 2012). According to theories of developmental psychology, leadership development is best viewed as the construction of a positive cycle of development whereby "prior learning sets the foundation for future learning, and future learning builds on and reinforces prior learning" (DeRue and Workman 2012, 10). DeRue and Workman (2012) also emphasize the benefits of learning from positive experiences rather than from stressful and unpleasant experiences. When leadership development occurs in this manner, it not only addresses the individual's leadership deficiencies but also builds on strengths and talent to foster the development of new capacities.

Organizational Culture

Good leadership is not simply about managing; it is about empowering staff to become part of the organization's culture and working together to make a real impact (Linstead 1999). Leaders should aim to establish a culture within the organization that inspires commitment, dedication, passion, and enthusiasm among employees. A strong **organizational culture** makes employees feel worthy and willing to go the extra mile—which, in healthcare, can lead to better health services delivery and patient outcomes. Schein (2010) describes organizational culture in three levels: (1) artifacts, (2) beliefs and values, and (3) basic assumptions.

Organizational culture does not evolve overnight, and it is often resistant to change. However, leaders can have a powerful influence on the culture of the organization through role modeling, coaching, and mentoring; by shaping organizational structure and policy; and by dealing effectively with problems and crises.

Leaders can also contribute to a strong organizational culture by developing effective talent management strategies and establishing fair criteria for worker selection, reward, punishment, and promotion. Leaders should ensure that the organization has a transparent process for getting the right people in the right position at the right time. Leaders should also be aware that, although financial rewards might attract people to the organization, nonfinancial rewards are what make workers feel appreciated, proud of their work, and committed in the long run. An effective reward and recognition program does not have to be complicated or expensive. Public recognition in newsletters, upskill training opportunities, and assignment of higher-level work and responsibilities are all forms of reward that can contribute to career advancement and a positive organizational culture.

> **organizational culture**
> A pattern of beliefs, values, standards, and assumptions that is shared by members of an organization and contributes to a sense of belonging.

Managing Obstacles and Failure

As noted earlier in the chapter, organizational change and the introduction of new projects and initiatives often fail to achieve their planned outcomes, or they achieve outcomes that do not closely align with the organization's strategic goals. Failures in healthcare settings can result from inadequate planning and preparation, a lack of organizational readiness, unrealistic expectations from senior executives and policymakers, or a variety of other factors.

Resistance from clinicians and staff is an extremely common obstacle to change processes in healthcare settings. No significant change in clinical practice can be achieved without the cooperation and support of clinicians, and most clinicians highly value their autonomy. Leaders should therefore anticipate clinicians' resistance, adopt a leadership style that is attentive to their needs, and look for ways to increase their engagement (Kumar and Khiljee 2016). Clinicians are unlikely to be receptive to sudden and drastic change, but they may support change that is clearly explained and well planned in a series of incremental steps (Ham 2003).

Often, leaders fear that failure will reflect poorly on their performance, causing peers and subordinates to view them in a negative light. Despite the prevalence of these concerns, healthcare organizations have made only limited efforts to develop processes to manage failure and accommodate its impact (Porter-O'Grady 2013). When confronted with failure, leaders must be able to take responsibility and actively learn from their experiences to ensure future success.

Leadership and Coordination in Emergency Situations

Disasters, acute situations, and humanitarian emergencies require urgent actions by healthcare professionals and ancillary staff. One of the major problems in dealing with such situations involves the coordination of rescuers, firefighters, healthcare workers, medical personnel, and other humanitarian teams. Often, the various groups involved in a disaster response are well trained in particular skills but do not function as a coordinated, integrated team. Achieving this coordination is a key challenge for today's global health leadership.

Lack of coordination is particularly evident during global emergencies, given the general lack of exercises and experiences in operationalizing international health systems. The North Atlantic Treaty Organization (2017) has conducted exercises that highlight the importance of cooperation and collaboration in disaster response, but thus far there is little evidence that global medical teams are prepared to be mobilized to work in a coordinated fashion across regions.

Outbreaks of disease, such as Ebola and Zika, have demonstrated the need for healthcare teams to act cooperatively to prevent death, minimize the emergence of other diseases, and control healthcare costs. In 2015 and 2016, for example, Brazil's government and healthcare community undertook a major effort to assemble medical teams, army personnel, police, healthcare workers, and government workers to address the Zika outbreak (Pinheiro de Oliveira 2016). Similarly, the migrant crisis in Europe has led to attempts to organize medical teams, mobile clinics, and other services so that migrants can be transported for care and treatment. More than 1,260,000 migrants applied for asylum in the European Union (EU) during 2015 (European Parliament 2017).

Traditionally, physicians serving in leadership capacities have held authority within the hierarchy of organizations in their country. However, healthcare teams that are organized for special reasons, such as emergency response, have a much larger scope and greater diversity, potentially including physicians, nurses, social workers, technicians, managers, volunteers, religious personnel, and others. Most physicians have not been trained to provide the type of leadership necessary to organize heterogeneous healthcare teams on this scale.

Today's global healthcare landscape demands a different style of leadership to achieve its goals of improving quality, increasing access, and controlling costs. This type of leadership requires new behaviors, performance requirements, and competencies, including the ability to coordinate and mobilize large and diverse teams of global health professionals. By aligning behavior and establishing a shared vision, healthcare leaders can build teams that are adaptable to change and able to address complex problems. Development of these skills will be essential for responding to future disasters and emergencies, as well as addressing issues related to malaria, HIV/AIDS, meningitis, cholera, tuberculosis, and mental health.

Change Management

Healthcare managers must be able to respond quickly to change, whether in terms of unexpected emergencies, reorganized systems of care, the adoption of new technology, or implementation of quality improvement initiatives (Campbell 2008). Kotter has developed a change management model that is highly useful for healthcare leaders (Kotter and Cohen 2002). It consists of eight steps:

1. Create a sense of urgency
2. Build a guiding team
3. Develop a clear vision and strategies
4. Communicate for buy-in
5. Enable action
6. Create short-term wins
7. Maintain momentum
8. Make the change stick

With these steps, Kotter's model outlines a way to turn negative events into a positive force for change.

Exhibit 6.1 identifies some of the key stakeholders who contribute to organizational change and with whom senior healthcare leaders continually interact. Campbell (2008), like Kotter, stresses the importance of building teams and communicating a vision to encourage buy-in from various groups and stakeholders. Effective leaders develop special teams and committees to address specific strategic objectives and institutional priorities, and they encourage collaboration across departments and divisions.

International Leadership and Collaboration Initiatives

Healthcare teams must possess the adaptability and flexibility necessary to adjust to situations and make appropriate decisions to drive results, and these needs are magnified during major international health events. The power of collaboration in addressing complex humanitarian emergencies and natural disasters comes not only from respected international bodies such as the World Health Organization (WHO) and the Red Cross, but also from public health

EXHIBIT 6.1
Organizational
Change and
Stakeholders

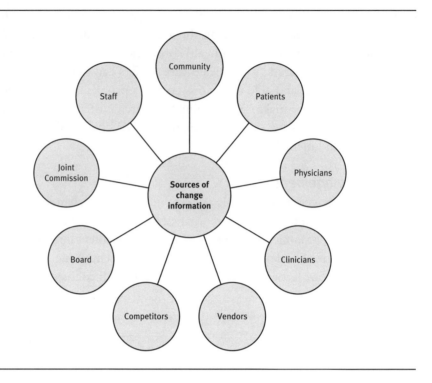

efforts within and between countries. Organizations, countries, and international bodies need to establish a cooperative mechanism to deal with disasters, disease outbreaks, and other emergencies, with plans for providing such services as mobile clinics and field hospitals as needed.

Skolnik (2016) notes that complex humanitarian emergencies are characterized by massive displacement of people; the presence of people in restricted areas; inadequate shelter, food, water, and sanitation; and a need for security to protect the public. Preparations for such scenarios must include plans for addressing such health threats as malnutrition, diarrhea, measles, and malaria; containing potential epidemics; and dealing with long-term concerns related to primary healthcare and mental health.

The WHO, the United Nations (UN), the UN Children's Fund (UNICEF), the UN Population Fund, and the UN Development Programme have worked together to address global health with an emphasis on building international teams. In addition, a number of foundations—such as the Ford, Hewlett, Rockefeller, MacArthur, and Packard foundations—have been active in global health efforts, many of which focus on specific areas such as tuberculosis, pneumonia, malaria, HIV/AIDS, or other infectious diseases. These foundations also support scientific discovery and provide ways of integrating the efforts of multiple global health organizations, programs, and projects. The Bill and Melinda Gates Foundation (2018), for instance, has a major endowment focused on the development of programs to address such issues as HIV/AIDS, malaria, polio, tuberculosis, and other diseases; the development and delivery of vaccines; family planning and maternal health; emergency response efforts; and the translation of scientific discovery into actionable solutions. Funding through the Joint UN Programme on HIV/AIDS (UNAIDS), public–private partnerships for health, WHO-related partnerships, and other international agencies has supported the development of a variety of nongovernmental organizations (NGOs) focused on global health.

All of these international organizations and funding sources stress the importance of leadership. However, they generally do not coherently specify the exact leadership competencies required. In fact, many times the organizations assume that healthcare leaders are physicians who lack formal management training.

The International Hospital Federation (IHF 2015) has developed a platform of key competencies for healthcare leaders and managers, and it has assembled a Global Consortium for Healthcare Management Professionalization to work on implementation of the model throughout the world. The IHF framework stresses the need for effective team building across the spectrum of healthcare delivery systems, across countries, and across regions.

The Institute for Healthcare Improvement (IHI) puts forth the concept of the "**triple aim**," introduced by Berwick, Nolan, and Whittington (2008), as an approach for optimizing healthcare leadership. This approach (discussed in greater detail later in the chapter) centers on the pursuit of three aims: improving the health of populations, improving the patient care experience, and reducing the per capita costs of healthcare. Teamwork, collaboration, and cooperation among healthcare providers are essential for achieving these aims.

triple aim
An approach for optimizing healthcare services by working to (1) improve the health of populations, (2) improve the patient care experience, and (3) reduce the per capita costs of healthcare; advanced by the Institute for Healthcare Improvement.

Strategies for Working with Vulnerable Populations

Working to improve the health of vulnerable populations is a chief concern among global health leaders. The World Bank (2018) categorizes the world's countries into four groups based on income—low income, lower-middle income, upper-middle income, and high income—with the most vulnerable populations falling into the lower-income groups.

Significant gains have been made in global health, yet much remains to be done to address the needs of the most vulnerable. The WHO (2018) reports that 303,000 women died in 2015 during or following pregnancy, with the vast majority of those deaths occurring in low-resource settings. Similarly, of the millions of people who die each year from infectious diseases, lower-income countries are hit especially hard (WHO 2017). Vulnerable populations are at a much greater risk of dying from water-related diseases and diarrheal disease, both of which are preventable and treatable, as well as from noncommunicable diseases (e.g., cardiovascular disease, cancer, diabetes, and chronic lung diseases). A significant maldistribution of the world's healthcare workers—who typically gravitate toward higher-income countries—exacerbates the challenges faced by vulnerable groups.

To develop effective strategies for working with vulnerable populations, global healthcare leaders need to understand health status, determinants of health, risk factors, and the burden of disease, while at the same time taking into account culture, demographics, epidemiologic transitions, and health system organization. They need to be well versed in environmental health, communicable and noncommunicable diseases, nutrition, child health, and reproductive health.

Global efforts to improve health, particularly for vulnerable populations, were a focus of the UN Millennium Summit in 2000, and the meeting produced a set of Millennium Development Goals (MDGs) to guide future work. The eight MDGs, all of which were given time-bound targets, are as follows (UN Development Programme 2018):

1. Eradicate extreme poverty and hunger
2. Achieve universal primary education
3. Promote gender equality and empower women
4. Reduce child mortality
5. Improve maternal health
6. Combat HIV/AIDS, malaria and other diseases
7. Ensure environmental sustainability
8. Develop a global partnership for development

UNICEF (2018) has estimated that 80 percent of all newborn deaths are preventable with the right interventions in the right places at the right time. Effective international cooperation through such organizations as the World Bank, the Global Fund, the UN, and the WHO, therefore, has the potential to save millions of lives in low- and middle-income countries.

Vignette: Charity Education Services and Tropical Medicine

The University of Vienna School of Medicine (Austria), the University of Heidelberg (Germany), and Oxford University (United Kingdom) have launched programs in such areas as charity education services and tropical medicine—areas that are closely tied to the healthcare needs of vulnerable populations. A number of other European universities are developing comparable programs, though the trend has been slower in central and eastern Europe. Countries that were formerly part of the Soviet Union, under communism, historically had been unable to participate in humanitarian efforts.

Diversity and Inclusion

Today's healthcare leaders have a heightened need to embrace diversity and inclusion in their organizations. The US Census Bureau (2015) predicts that, within 30 years, the population in the United States will be mostly nonwhite. As the demographic makeup of society evolves, leaders' abilities to assemble and manage effective teams that are diverse in race, culture, age, and gender become increasingly important. Respect for diversity and inclusion emanates at the top of the organization and filters through every level. It should be reflected in the organization's mission, vision, and core values.

Vignette: A Program in Community Health and Social Work

In 2005, the Catholic University of East Africa, in Nairobi, Kenya, and Trnava University, in Slovakia, developed a joint program in community health and social work, and that program has since been transferred to St. Elizabeth University in Bratislava. The goal of the effort is to develop diverse teams that will work with children in low-income settings and develop cooperative arrangements with NGOs to address issues of poverty and sickness.

Research, Science, and Leadership

Global healthcare management is an emerging field with a unique body of knowledge, and a growing number of writers and researchers have been investigating its specific competencies, practices, and future challenges. Experts have come to recognize that the goals of improving quality of care, increasing access to care, and controlling costs of care can only be achieved through competent leadership.

Global healthcare leaders, whether physicians or nonphysicians, need to possess a broad range of knowledge related to health and wellness, the clinical and business components of care management, and the development of partnerships, network models, and clinical service lines that meet the needs of consumers. They are also expected to have knowledge in the areas of finance and legal and regulatory responsibilities. Zismer (2018) emphasizes the need for leaders to take a strategic approach when dealing with the pressures of cost, quality of care, access, customer satisfaction, and performance. Although his article focuses on the US healthcare system, its concepts are relevant for systems throughout the world. He discusses the importance of strategies and tactics for penetrating new markets, improving financial performance, recruiting and retaining staff, creating market position, and optimizing quality and safety performance.

Vignette: University-Based Partnerships

University-based partnership models tend to be more stable and sustainable than government-funded projects. Whereas government ministers of health or ministers of education (or people in equivalent positions) change office frequently following new elections, Catholic universities have key sustainable elements within their mission and values that remain consistent over long periods. Thus, a commitment to fighting corruption or working with the poor and sick is likely to continue even if the prevailing political parties change.

Researchers are increasingly acknowledging that new delivery models will require expanded roles for nurse practitioners and physician extenders. In assessing the many challenges facing healthcare delivery systems, the Institute of Medicine and the Robert Wood Johnson Foundation have highlighted the ways that strengthening nurse education and training can help organizations address unmet healthcare needs (National Academies of Science, Engineering, and Medicine 2011). Shalala (2014) recommends moving nurses into leadership roles, especially in underserved and hard-to-reach communities. Many regions of the world would be well served to provide better university-based education for nurses, as well as leadership training opportunities focused on patient safety and quality of care.

West, Ramirez, and Filerman (2012) examined the impact of globalization on graduate healthcare management education, based on a pair of studies conducted for the Commission on Accreditation of Health Management Education (CAHME) with funding from Aramark Charitable Fund. The two studies (Phase I and Phase II) collected comprehensive data on international healthcare management education and produced an inventory of 22 countries. The two studies demonstrated that CAHME-accredited programs are globally engaged in a variety of ways and that faculty are interested in research. West, Ramirez, and Filerman (2012, 16) noted that globalization of health management education will continue to grow and mature and that economies and countries need to make sure that there is a "relationship between academia and the production of health professionals who are the profession."

The IHF (2015) and its Global Consortium for Healthcare Management Professionalization have focused on developing and employing a competency model and platform for leadership training. Additional study will be needed for the management of population health, which involves different strategic opportunities and training. Skolnik (2016), in his book *Global Health 101*, highlights the need for trained global health workers especially in dealing with humanitarian services, bilateral organizations, government agencies, consulting firms, foundations, public–private partnerships for health, policy and advocacy organizations, and academia. New designs in public–private partnership models require research to determine efficiency and effectiveness.

Scientific progress has led to new advances and technologies to improve health. The introduction of new diagnostics, drugs, vaccines, and medical devices is especially important in addressing health problems in low- and middle-income countries. Many healthcare systems are looking at ways to target patients across national borders and provide services in other countries. Some such operations are based on the idea of medical tourism, but others actually involve building hospitals and clinics to reach subsets of populations in other countries. Some of the more successful approaches are also looking at establishing multinational health networks.

Today's global health paradigm considers change to be a constant across all organizations and sectors. Goleman (2000), accordingly, suggests that leaders need to be able to react to change and have different styles that can be used depending on the situation. He talks about the styles of coercive leadership, authoritative leadership, affiliative leadership, democratic leadership, pace-setting leadership, and coaching leadership, which effective leaders use in combination. He further emphasizes emotional intelligence, which research has shown to be extremely important in getting good business results. Goleman concludes that effective leaders show flexibility in their leadership styles and are capable of changing to achieve better performance and results.

Marmot (2015), in *The Health Gap*, examines the major health challenges that exist around the globe, with specific attention to the health inequalities and social disadvantages that occur both within and between countries. Confronting these complex global problems will require both significant resources

Vignette: Health Management Education in Slovakia

The BRIDGE (Building Relationships in Developing and Growing Economies) model was developed in the 1990s by the University of Scranton, Pennsylvania, and three Slovakian partners: Trnava University, the Health Management School in Bratislava, and the University of Matej Bel (West et al. 1999). The BRIDGE model is an example of a health management education initiative to train new leaders across several professional disciplines, including economists, physicians, social workers, nurses, government officials, and public health workers. Following the breakup of the Soviet Union, such efforts were particularly important for former communist states that needed healthcare leaders trained in modern management practices. The BRIDGE model is discussed in greater detail later in this chapter.

Vignette: Making Humanitarian Projects Sustainable

Many universities seek relationships with private businesses to secure the necessary funding to make humanitarian projects sustainable. Some teaching, research, and service projects also secure funding through international foundations or public–private university-based partnership models. The Catholic University of East Africa in Nairobi, Kenya, for instance, has successfully worked in partnership with other NGOs to provide comprehensive services for people living in slums.

and competent leadership. Furthermore, Marmot suggests, addressing the societal imbalances related to health equity will require a radical change in the way we think.

Gibson and colleagues (2012) emphasize that organizational leadership occurs within the context of social systems that are shaped by patterns of behaviors. An organization's structure consists of the formalized manner in which people and jobs are grouped and the processes within the organization that affect communication, problem solving, decision making, and socialization of new employees.

Kouzes and Posner (2012, 2) describe the "Leadership Challenge" that centers around the way "leaders mobilize others to make extraordinary things happen in organizations." They propose a framework of "Five Practices of Exemplary Leadership":

1. Model the way.
2. Inspire a shared vision.
3. Challenge the process.
4. Enable others to act.
5. Encourage the heart.

Their approach is based on evidence, with effective practices having been devised from application and research.

Leadership in a healthcare organization requires relationships between senior management, middle management, and lower levels of management. Positive interpersonal skills are a necessity. During turbulent times, effective leaders keep people positive and mobilize their energies toward change (Kouzes and Posner 2012). They create a culture and environment in which people are committed and engaged, performance intensifies, and trust for collaboration grows.

Leadership Traits, Styles, and Approaches

A variety of traits and characteristics have been associated with effective leadership. Effective leaders, typically, demonstrate honesty, vision, competence, intelligence, dependability, ambition, a strong work ethic, and loyalty to the organization and its employees. They understand the mission of the organization and have a clear vision of where they are going and how they will get there. Most leaders exhibit good social and communication skills and an ability to teach others. These leadership traits typically translate into effective decisions with regard to interpersonal relationships, the allocation and management of resources, the design of programs and procedures, and commitment to values and ethics.

Self-Understanding

Leadership has been described as a journey that begins with self-awareness and self-esteem, and effective leaders, over time, come to possess self-efficacy and self-understanding (Gibson et al. 2012). These leaders focus on lifelong learning—a constant process of learning about themselves and improving their knowledge, skills, and competencies—and use this learning to help others within the organization. Exercise 1, at the end of this chapter, provides an opportunity for the reader to engage in the sort of self-examination, reflection, and introspection expected of effective leaders.

Graduate programs in health administration will usually help students to evaluate their leadership style, competencies, values, characteristics, and traits. Some graduate programs require students to engage in comprehensive assessments and evaluations at specific points in their postgraduate studies. The students may be asked to develop a personal mission and vision statement and to complete a personal **SWOT analysis**—an analysis of strengths, weaknesses, opportunities, and threats. Exercise 2 provides an example of a comprehensive student assessment project.

SWOT analysis
An analysis of strengths, weaknesses, opportunities, and threats.

Performance and Effectiveness

Gibson and colleagues (2012), as well as others, stress the importance of assessing leadership in terms of performance and effectiveness, with a focus on evidence and measurable outcomes. Such outcomes can be managerial, financial, or clinical in nature. Gibson and colleagues look at effectiveness using three approaches: the goal approach, the systems approach, and the stakeholder approach.

Under the goal approach, "an organization exists to accomplish goals" (Gibson et al. 2012, 20); thus, the effectiveness of individuals and groups in the organization is reflected in their ability to work together to achieve fundamental outcomes associated with those goals. One tool that can be employed with the goal approach is **management by objectives (MBO)**. In the MBO process, objectives are written in such a way that they are clear, measurable, and useful in assessing outputs and evaluating effectiveness. They are known as **SMART objectives** because they are specific, measurable, attainable, realistic, and time framed. The goal approach has a strong influence on the management and leadership practices in healthcare organizations. Measurement and evaluation are key components.

Under the systems approach to effectiveness, the focus is on the grouping of activities and relationships and on the ways these elements interact in the organization and with the external environment (Gibson et al. 2012). Systems theory enables leaders to understand how people inside the organization perform and to identify common themes to explain behavior and performance within the organization. In systems theory, one element is constantly interacting with a number of other elements, thereby affecting outputs. Systems theory also stresses that organizations are connected to the larger external environment. Managers and leaders must deal with both internal and external aspects of organizational behavior.

The stakeholder approach to effectiveness emphasizes the balance that needs to be achieved across various parts of the system as individuals and groups work together (Gibson et al. 2012). In healthcare, this approach requires attention to customers, shareholders, directors, suppliers, and levels of government and the effects that each of these groups has on the organization. The integration of systems theory and the stakeholder approach differentiates organizations in their ability to manage constant change.

Functions of Management

Healthcare organizations—whether hospitals, long-term care facilities, medical practices, or insurance companies—require managers and leaders who have the appropriate training, competence, and knowledge for the specific entities and sectors of the healthcare environment in which they function.

The concepts of management and leadership are related but distinct. Some leaders may be good managers and some managers may be good leaders, but the two roles differ in terms of responsibility, tasks, and knowledge. Classically speaking, leaders have an appreciation for vision and the ability to assess the external environment. They spend more time communicating and aligning outside groups. Managers, meanwhile, tend to focus more on how the organization is operating. An organization needs both leaders and managers if it is going to move in a forward, functional direction.

Longest and Darr (2008) describe management as a process comprising social and technical functions and activities that occur within organizations to achieve predetermined goals and activities. This definition assumes that people within the organization—more specifically, managers—work through people to carry out desired objectives. Managers implement six key functions:

(1) planning, (2) organizing, (3) staffing, (4) controlling, (5) directing, and (6) decision making.

Styles and Types of Leadership

The types of leadership that an individual leader employs should align with organizational structures, processes, and values. Some leaders tend to be more operational and others more strategic; all leaders, however, need to have a vision and direction for the organization if they want others to follow a course of action.

A variety of leadership styles and approaches have been set forth in the literature and put into practice in healthcare settings. The **situational leadership** approach is based on the idea that the most effective leadership style will depend on the details of the situation and the qualities of the person being influenced (Holsinger and Carlton 2018). Similarly, the **contingency theory** considers the influence of situational variables (relating to leaders, followers, and the situation) on leadership behavior. **Path–goal theory** is a leadership theory that focuses on the use of contingent rewards to influence followers, whereas **transformational leadership** emphasizes efforts to produce positive change in individuals and systems. In looking at contemporary leadership approaches, common themes emerge, including intra- and interpersonal skills, the importance of self-awareness, and the ability to self-regulate. Many approaches also emphasize **servant leadership**—that is, leadership that is sensitive and responsive to followers' needs (White and Griffith 2016). Contemporary leadership models also tend to consider diversity, spirituality, resilience, and the emergence of new leaders.

Models for Learning and Development

The professional development pyramid in exhibit 6.2 provides a way of conceptualizing the relationships between the necessary body of knowledge, skills, and competencies as individuals take on leadership responsibility. In this particular model, people are drawn to management and leadership positions because they have a certain level of interest, desire, or motivation (at the bottom level of the pyramid) rooted in their personal background. To reach the higher levels of the pyramid, they must acquire a body of knowledge through formal education, and they must develop, through training and work experience, the set of skills necessary for specific leadership positions within a particular organization and healthcare setting.

Another basic model of learning, illustrated in exhibit 6.3, suggests that the process begins with people becoming aware of various elements of organizations and leadership positions. Awareness in and of itself is insufficient, but it provides a foundation on which an understanding can be developed through research, undergraduate study, graduate study, and other experiences. In the case of healthcare services, this understanding might encompass healthcare,

situational leadership
An approach based on the idea that the most effective leadership style depends on the situation and the person being influenced.

contingency theory
A leadership theory that focuses on the influence of situational variables (relating to leaders, followers, and the situation) on leadership behavior.

path–goal theory
A leadership theory that focuses on the use of contingent rewards to influence followers.

transformational leadership
Leadership that focuses on efforts to produce positive change in individuals and systems.

servant leadership
Leadership that is sensitive and responsive to followers' needs.

EXHIBIT 6.2
Professional
Development
Model

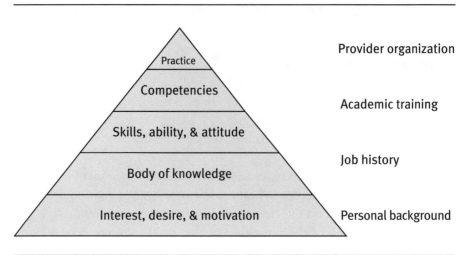

Practice

Competencies

Skills, ability, & attitude

Body of knowledge

Interest, desire, & motivation

Provider organization

Academic training

Job history

Personal background

EXHIBIT 6.3
A Basic Model
of Learning

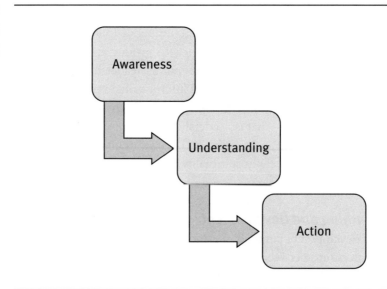

Awareness

Understanding

Action

the various settings and sectors of the healthcare industry, and the organization's internal and external environment. Once that understanding has been achieved, managers and leaders will have the ability to take appropriate action to change services and systems.

Earlier in the chapter, we discussed the IHF's (2015) platform of key competencies for healthcare leaders and managers, which was derived from a Healthcare Leadership Alliance model. In developing the platform, the IHF worked with a variety of organizations and entities across various regions of the world. Over a period of two to three years, the IHF identified five specific domains across which the specific competencies could be categorized: (1) leadership, (2) health and healthcare environment, (3) business skills, (4) communications and relationship management, and (5) professional and social responsibility. Those interconnected domains, which were previously discussed in chapter 4, are shown in exhibit 6.4.

The cascading competency model, shown in exhibit 6.5, considers competencies on a continuum, with individuals progressing from minimal competencies to maximum competencies. The model assumes that people, over

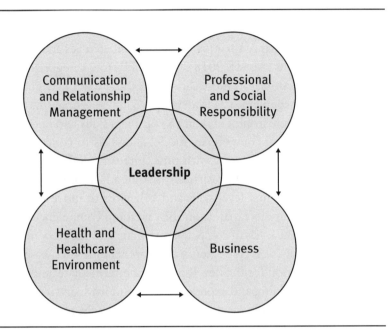

EXHIBIT 6.4
International Hospital Federation Competency Domains

Source: Reprinted with permission from IHF (2015).

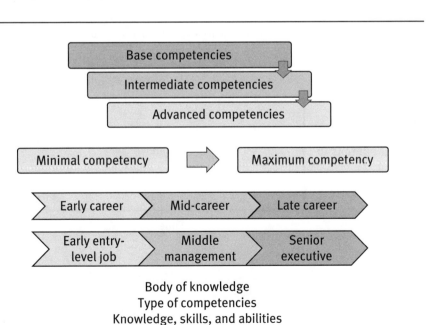

EXHIBIT 6.5
Cascading Competency Model

time, will acquire the body of knowledge, the skills, and the attitudes needed to demonstrate effective and efficient leadership behavior. They develop base competencies upon entering an entry-level position and then proceed to acquire intermediate competencies and, eventually, advanced competencies. These competencies can correspond with the stages of early careerist, mid-careerist, and late careerist. This type of thinking is embedded in the competency assessment tool used by the American College of Healthcare Executives (ACHE), which assumes that individuals develop in their careers and embark on a process of life-long learning to enhance their professional competencies and qualify for future leadership positions (ACHE 2018). The ACHE tool categorizes competencies into five domains similar to those shown in exhibit 6.4: (1) communication and relationship management, (2) leadership, (3) professionalism, (4) knowledge of the healthcare environment, and (5) business skills and knowledge.

The cascading competency model allows us to conceptualize levels of competency training that vary with time, intensity, and career. As individuals are promoted horizontally or vertically within a healthcare organization, they must build on their first-level skills and behaviors to move to the second and third levels. Exhibit 6.6 expands on the cascading competency model to more clearly represent the levels of competency training and the growing intensity from one level to the next. As competency development matures, base competencies serve as a foundation for the development of intermediate and more advanced competencies. Training and experience enable individuals to move from entry-level positions to middle management and, ultimately, to senior management.

The Global Healthcare Management Faculty Forum of the Association of University Programs in Health Administration (AUPHA) has outlined a body of knowledge necessary for the development of competencies for the global healthcare leader. Its key features are shown in exhibit 6.7.

EXHIBIT 6.6
Levels of
Competency
Training

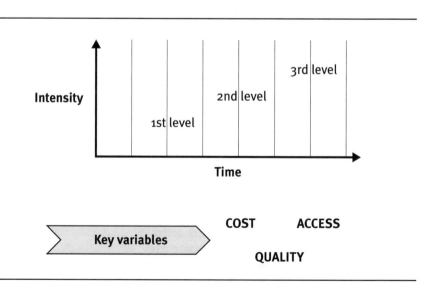

EXHIBIT 6.7
AUPHA Global
Healthcare
Management
Faculty Forum
Body of
Knowledge

The body of knowledge (BOK) takes the following into consideration:

- Relevant and current knowledge on global health issues
- Attitudes and behaviors required for multicultural understanding and effective transcultural communication
- Conceptual and analytical skills required for identifying and effectively applying global managerial best practices
- Competencies necessary for developing community assessment and collaborative partnerships and networks
  - Study abroad
  - Faculty and student collaborative research
  - Service learning
- BOK learning areas
  - Global burden of disease
  - Health systems and services
  - Policy and regulatory environments
  - Cultural influences
  - Communication and marketing
  - Global leadership
  - Data and measurement
  - Medical travel
  - International best practices

Source: Adapted with permission from Dr. Dan Dominguez.

Evidence-Based Management

Physicians and medical education have emphasized the use of evidence-based medicine to develop pathways in clinical protocols, based on research and reliable data, that can lead to improved processes and outcomes. Evidence-based management takes a similar approach to management practices and has led to protocols that are now being applied globally. Kovner, Fine, and D'Aquila (2009), in their important book titled *Evidence-Based Management in Healthcare*, write about the convergence of evidence-based management and evidence-based medicine, highlighting the need for managers and leaders to develop competencies related to the use of research for more efficient and effective decision making. Kovner, Fine, and D'Aquila (2009, 56) explain evidence-based, or EB, management as follows:

> Simply put, EB management is the systematic application of the best available evidence to the evaluation of managerial strategies for improving the performance of health services organizations. What distinguishes EB management from other approaches to decision making is the notion that whenever possible, health service managers should incorporate into their decision making evidence from well-conducted management research.

Kovner and D'Aunno (2017, 17) further discuss why we need evidence-based management. They write:

> Most managers prefer to make decisions solely based on personal experience, but personal judgment alone is not a particularly reliable source of evidence. It is prone to cognitive biases and thinking errors. In addition, managers and consultants are often not aware of the current scientific evidence; in fact, large discrepancies seem to exist between what managers and consultants think is effective and what the current scientific research shows.

Kovner (2014) offers the following steps for evidence-based decision making:

Step 1: Framing the question behind the decision
Step 2: Finding sources of information
Step 3: Assessing the accuracy of the information
Step 4: Assessing the applicability of the information
Step 5: Assessing the actionability of the information
Step 6: Determining whether the information is adequate

The process for applying evidence may also be considered as a series of steps, adapted from the work of Robbins and DeCenzo (2004):

Step 1: Identification of a problem
Step 2: Identification of decision criteria
Step 3: Allocation of weights to criteria
Step 4: Development of alternatives
Step 5: Analysis of alternatives
Step 6: Selection of an alternative
Step 7: Implementation of the alternative
Step 8: Evaluation of decision effectiveness

The abilities to acquire, evaluate, apply, and disseminate knowledge and research data are increasingly important for managers and leaders in healthcare today. Across the countries and regions of the world, healthcare organizations are often required to report data and outcome findings to independent regulatory organizations and to the government, and accountability structures are often extremely formalized.

Organizations need to develop strategic plans and maintain a strategic emphasis on organizational change through the adoption of evidence-based management practices. Shortell and colleagues (2000) emphasize the need for organizational change to be integrated with clinical services and the use of research evidence.

The Triple Aim

The IHI's triple aim, introduced earlier in this chapter, provides an important framework for the development of leadership behaviors in healthcare. As set forth by Berwick, Nolan, and Whittington (2008, 759), the triple aim program has three goals: "improving the experience of care, improving the health of populations, and reducing per capita costs of health care." Across the globe, healthcare systems are striving to improve quality, increase access, and reduce costs, and the triple aim provides valuable guidance for implementing reforms. The effort to curb spending while improving quality and patient safety reflects a meaningful shift toward **value-based healthcare**.

> **value-based healthcare**
> An approach to healthcare that aims to minimize spending while improving quality and patient safety.

Efforts to implement the triple aim program have been linked to improved safety, fewer medical errors, shorter lengths of stay, reduced stroke mortality, better integrated care, improved prevention programs, better pain management, better understanding of genetic disorders, improved cardiac assessment, improved treatment for infectious disease, and significant money savings (Coyne et al. 2014).

Bodenheimer and Sinsky (2014, 573) have suggested an expansion of the triple aim to a "quadruple aim," adding the goal of "improving the work life of health care providers." Positive engagement of healthcare workers is an important aspect of improving the health of populations, particularly as evolving technologies, administrative tasks, and institutional change increase the amount of work-related stress among physicians and other providers. Trained leaders recognize the importance of stress management, ongoing training, and employee-centered leadership.

The BRIDGE Model for Successful Partnerships

In the 1990s, the University of Scranton, Pennsylvania, and three Slovakian partners—Trnava University, the Health Management School in Bratislava, and the University of Matej Bel—developed a partnership framework to assist with the restructuring of health services and systems in central and eastern Europe (West et al. 1999). The framework, known as the BRIDGE (Building Relationships in Developing and Growing Economies) model, stressed the importance of collaboration and cooperation, sustainability, and financial solvency. It also focused on replication—the ability of partnership projects to be repeated in other settings. The project in Slovakia, from 1993 to 2000, was funded through the US Agency for International Development (USAID) in cooperation with the American International Health Alliance (AIHA).

Key features of the BRIDGE model are shown in exhibit 6.8. The model used university-based partnerships with religious affiliations while drawing

EXHIBIT 6.8
The BRIDGE
Framework,
Goals, Design,
Structure, and
Target Audience

The BRIDGE Framework: Building Relationships in Developing and Growing Economies
- Sustainability
- Collaboration and cooperation
- Replication
- Financial solvency
- Assessment and evaluation
- Focus on teaching, research, and service
- Public–private initiatives
- Recognizing local communities

Partnership Design
- Designated project director
- University based
- Religious affiliations
- Health management education
- Points of coordination
- NGO involvement
- Community engagement
- Faculty—rank and tenure

Structural Considerations
- Identified partners
- Critical points of consideration
  - Needs assessment
  - Body of knowledge
  - Levels of education needed
  - Competencies

- Target audiences
- Practical and results oriented
- Adult learning

Structural and Design Considerations
- Application of knowledge, skills, and abilities (KSAs)
- Community health partners
- Organizational stability
- Evaluation and assessment

Model Goals and Objectives
- Needs assessment
- Short courses (5–10 days)
- Continuing education
- University courses
- MHA curriculum
- MBA curriculum
- Concentrations
- Competencies
- Professional development

Target Audiences
- Head doctors
- Nurses
- Economists
- Ministry of Health
- Government managers
- Faculty
- NGO

Note: MBA = master of business administration; MHA = master of health administration; NGO = nongovernmental organization.

upon and recognizing local community healthcare providers as key stakeholders/partners. The focus was on health management education aimed at head doctors, nurses, economists, government employees, public health workers, faculty, and individuals working for NGOs. In addition to specifying key target audiences, the project incorporated principles of adult education, known as **andragogy** (see exhibit 6.9).

andragogy
The principles and practices of adult education.

In implementing the BRIDGE model, a designated project director was appointed in each of the affiliated countries. The identified partners completed a needs assessment and SWOT analysis, reviewed the body of knowledge for health management education, and identified key competencies. The structural design focused on the application of knowledge, skills, and abilities with community health partners. As is true of most grant projects, assessment and

What adult learners look for:	Adult methods of learning:	**EXHIBIT 6.9**
• Competent teachers	• Group interaction	Adult Learning
• Using life experiences	• Simulation	Principles and
• Applying what they learn	• Case analysis	Methods
• Relevancy to their work	• Real projects	
• Group discussion	• Mentoring	
• Working in teams	• Application and integration	
• Sharing ideas	• Support services	
• Current information	• Flexibility	

evaluation were important for monitoring outcomes and making changes to strategic planning. The goals and objectives centered around forms of health management education, including short courses, continuing education, university-based courses, a master of health administration curriculum, and other forms of professional development (e.g., study abroad, fieldwork, mentorship, networking). The BRIDGE model also looked at global health management competencies, public–private sector ventures, and emerging issues in international health.

Partnership-building models such as the BRIDGE framework require that certain conditions be met. For instance, a culture-specific strategic plan needs to be developed in a climate of collaboration and mutual trust. Similarly, measurable goals and objectives must be developed together in a team approach, with shared authority and clear direction (strategic vision). Sustainable partnerships require honesty, trust, and flexibility; respect for cultural differences; willingness to share knowledge, ideas, and information; and the development of positive working relationships.

Professional Identity and Ethics

In general, a profession is distinguished by its professional identity, which is generated through the body of knowledge required for a particular vocation. In the case of health administration, at least in most high-income countries, the professional identity is shaped through the undergraduate and graduate training that individuals receive as they prepare to advance in their careers. This training covers a defined body of knowledge, some of which has been identified through the AUPHA Global Healthcare Management Faculty Network.

In addition to having a defined body of knowledge, professions are also expected to have collegial relationships among professionals, as well as a service orientation. They usually have a social mandate to practice with a community focus. For most professions, coaching and mentoring are important processes associated with professional development.

Professionalism is an important aspect of leadership within an organization. Healthcare leaders and administrators are expected to serve as positive role models for employees, and they must therefore exhibit certain types of behavior. Trust and respect are essential. Other protocols of professionalism include being visible, communicating in a positive manner, motivating others, demonstrating competence, encouraging innovation, and having a strong passion for work.

The American College of Healthcare Executives (ACHE) has a code of ethics that sets forth standards of conduct and ethical behavior for its members across several designated areas of responsibility. The code specifies responsibilities to the profession of healthcare management (e.g., conduct that reflects well on the profession); responsibilities to patients (e.g., confidentiality, quality of care); responsibilities to organizations (e.g., effective management and use of resources); responsibilities to employees (e.g., a safe workplace environment, nondiscrimination policies); and responsibilities to the community and society (e.g., access to health services, advocacy for meaningful reforms) (ACHE 2017). Finally, a professional has a responsibility to report any violations of the code of ethics and employ sanctions where appropriate.

Professionalism requires that leaders and managers have a social awareness, can attend to social disparities and equities, and have a personal plan for lifelong learning and development. Exhibit 6.10 lists forms of education and training that can help with the development of competencies at various stages of a professional career.

cultural proficiency
The ability to relate to and work effectively with members of diverse cultures.

Cultural Proficiency

Effective global healthcare management requires that leaders develop **cultural proficiency** and support its development in others. Cultural proficiency, or

EXHIBIT 6.10
Types of
Education and
Training

- Self-assessment
- On-the-job training
- Residency training
- Career planning
- Case studies
- In-house workshops
- Tutoring
- Grand rounds
- Observation
- Formal education
- Mentoring
- Supervision
- Succession planning
- Professional membership
- Conferences/symposia
- Undergraduate education
- Professional organizations
- Journal clubs
- Study tours
- Community service
- Fellowships
- Fieldwork
- Coaching
- Assigned readings
- Web-based instruction
- Self-study courses
- Graduate programs (MHA/MBA)
- Shadowing
- Audio/video
- Consultants
- Doctoral studies
- Research

cultural competence, is the ability to relate to and work effectively with members of diverse cultures. It requires an understanding of the characteristics and differences that exist across various individuals and groups, as well as the ways those concerns affect the organization, both internally and externally. It also requires awareness of global demographic changes, such as the overall aging of the population. Managers and leaders have a responsibility to understand the implications of cultural change and to institute human resource policies that support diversity in the workforce.

Culture can provide stability and identity for employees and groups of individuals within the organization. Different styles of leadership influence culture differently. Managers and leaders can positively influence the climate of culture in their organizations by serving as role models, clearly establishing values and expectations, involving others in decision making and problem solving, and appropriately delegating authority. Leaders must be aware of the compatibility of subcultures within the larger group. Many mergers and acquisitions fail not because of poor planning but because cultural incompatibility between the two organizations was not properly assessed and addressed.

Values and Spirituality

Effective leadership in healthcare requires not only a wide range of competencies and skills but also a commitment to values that strengthen the profession, provide direction for organizations, and improve interpersonal relationships (Squazzo 2010). Healthcare is about people and the delivery of personalized care, and thus values and ethical behavior must be a top priority. Leadership roles have a powerful influence on institutional values and culture, and leaders should be constantly mindful of the need to establish credibility and respectability with employees and the community.

Wheatley (2002) maintains that conscious spiritual thinking might be needed in management, and Finkelstein (2016) stresses that leaders need

Vignette: Working with Displaced Persons

Rectors (presidents) of a number of European universities have recognized the importance of working with marginalized and displaced persons. St. Elizabeth University in Slovakia, for instance, has a refugee and migrant health task force, and it put together a 50-member rescue team to help during the refugee crisis in Europe, in which large numbers of migrants came to Europe to flee conflict and unsafe conditions in Syria, Afghanistan, Iraq, and elsewhere. Mobile hospitals associated with the task force helped thousands of migrants in 2015 and 2016.

EXHIBIT 6.11
The Jesuit
Paradigm

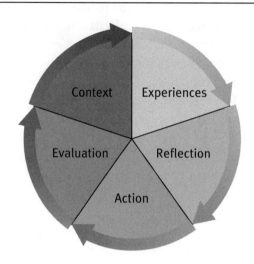

Source: Adapted from Jesuit Institute (1993).

to know their "authentic selves." Both of these authors highlight the need for leaders to thoughtfully reflect about events in their own lives and in the healthcare environment, and to encourage such reflection by others. Exhibit 6.11 illustrates the Jesuit paradigm for growth, development, and change, which includes reflection as a key stage (Jesuit Institute 1993). Reflection can add meaning to the work environment and provide valuable new perspectives about existing conditions and ways to bring about change.

Throughout the world, large numbers of people must navigate chaos and extreme conditions such as warfare, political unrest, ethnic cleansing, and natural disaster. Such situations often necessitate that people maintain a sense of hope and love in the face of adversity. Global healthcare leaders can help foster spiritual health by instilling foundational values and providing positive meaning within their organizations and systems. A framework linking leadership and spirituality can be highly useful for leaders who sit on hospital boards, serve in NGOs, or are members of the medical staff or senior management team.

Work Design

Leaders and managers can address a number of challenges in the work setting by focusing on the ways jobs and groups of jobs are organized. This structure can have a powerful effect on individual and group behavior. Work–life balance is a common concern for employees of many healthcare organizations, and management can respond to such concerns by engaging in work design initiatives. Such initiatives might involve telecommuting; flextime systems, allowing for more flexible work hours; reduced workloads; and per diem employees. Efforts to improve employees' quality of life and work–life balance can help build employee trust, productivity, involvement, and retention.

Leaders and managers can positively influence the organizational culture through job design and analysis. **Job design** is the process of defining the specific tasks, methods, and responsibilities of a given job or position (Dunn 2016). It aims to identify needs that employees have within the organization and to remove obstacles that might interfere with employee performance. Managers may redesign jobs as necessary to attain specific outcomes or to increase employee satisfaction and productivity. The related process of **job analysis** looks at activities of the job, the requirements of the position, and ways the work can best be performed within the organization.

job design
The process of defining the specific tasks, methods, and responsibilities of a given job or position.

job analysis
The process of evaluating the activities of a job, the requirements of the position, and ways the work can best be performed within the organization.

Physician Leadership

In today's healthcare environment, leaders need to have a firm understanding of governance and the physician–administrator team. Physicians play an important role in the leadership of healthcare organizations, and positive relationships between administrators and physicians are vital to organizational success. The key to successfully working with physicians is understanding their interests and values. Physician–administrator relationships are most effective when each side respects the roles and responsibilities of the other and commits to sharing information, solving problems, and making decisions with the other's involvement. Physician leadership must be cultivated within the organization.

Nurse Leadership

Nurses play a critical role in delivering high-quality healthcare services, ensuring patient safety, and generating positive outcomes, and nurse leadership is an important component of organizational success. The countries and regions of the world differ in their standards for nursing education, as well as in the tasks nurses perform and the ways nurses are used in the healthcare system. In most middle- and high-income countries, nursing education consists of four years of university training. In today's healthcare workforce, the use of advanced practice nursing and nurse specialists is imperative.

A 2011 report by the US-based Institute of Medicine (IOM) urged healthcare leaders and healthcare systems to remove outdated practice restrictions for nurse practitioners and to look into new ways of involving nurses in future practice (IOM 2011). Effective use of nurse practitioners can make a meaningful difference to patient education, preventive care, patient satisfaction, and overall wellness. Increasingly, advanced practice nurses are being used for a broad range of responsibilities, including management of chronic disease. Nurse practitioners are an essential part of the team-based medicine approach used for primary care in natural disasters, emerging events, and low-income country projects. In addition, nurse educators are preparing nurses to provide care in such venues as schools, hospices, neighborhood health clinics, and urgent care centers.

Leaders of healthcare organizations need to promote interprofessional collaboration and consider how advanced practice nurses can be used most effectively as part of healthcare teams. They also need to consider how nurses can participate in research to guide the development of health policies and practices.

Strategic Planning

Leaders and managers have a responsibility to ensure proper strategic planning, which requires senior management to work cooperatively with the governing board and medical staff. Healthcare organizations—whether public or private, for profit or nonprofit, governmental or nongovernmental—have mission statements that are rooted in organizational values, and leaders play an important role in translating the organizational mission, vision, and values into decisions and actions affecting the delivery of services. Execution of the organization's strategies requires attention to the needs, wants, and values of strategic partners, key stakeholders, and customers. Within this framework, leaders need to understand clinical ethics, research ethics, and compliance with the applicable rules, regulations, and policies.

The Work of Governing Boards

Oversight of an organization's operations is ultimately the responsibility of the governing board. The board is responsible for monitoring organizational performance; creating a vision for the future; selecting and evaluating senior executives, including the CEO; credentialing the medical staff; and ensuring that the organization meets the healthcare needs of the community. The board must uphold corporate social responsibility as a key part of the organizational culture. It must prioritize the public good and commit resources accordingly.

Executive and physician leaders play an important role in interacting with the board; ensuring that the organization's leadership teams are effective;

Vignette: Functional Networks and Teams for Emergency Response

Effective global healthcare management requires functional networks and teams that can work together to respond quickly and appropriately to natural disasters and other humanitarian emergencies. Such efforts require comprehensive planning and the use of a variety of leadership and management tools, including SWOT analyses. St. Elizabeth University, in Slovakia, has engaged in a number of emergency efforts, including responses to the 2009 earthquake in Pakistan and the 2010 earthquake in Haiti. Another example involved a group of eight staff members and four physicians stationed 25 kilometers from Mosul, Iraq, to help people injured in the battle to liberate Mosul from Islamic State in Iraq and Syria (ISIS) forces.

and helping with the development of skills and expertise at the board level. In today's rapidly changing healthcare environment, boards need to understand the importance of disruptive innovation and be aware of new approaches and opportunities related to population health.

Normally, the governing board of a healthcare organization follows a business model and performs specific organizational functions, with established processes for developing and managing board talent. Governing boards and executive leadership must work in conjunction with the medical staff to ensure that the organization navigates the changes in the healthcare environment. Exhibit 6.12 provides a model for conceptualizing leadership, performance, and clinical outcomes.

Governing boards today are facing increased scrutiny, with new and enhanced standards for transparency, accountability, and conflicts of interest. Many governing bodies are becoming smaller in size and paying closer attention to the composition and educational backgrounds of board members, often seeking members who have a particular expertise. Governing boards are also being asked to engage in self-assessment and succession planning.

Healthcare boards and leaders need to work together to transform their organizations and implement reforms to deliver value-driven care. Doing so will require the development of physician leaders and managers who are effective in the areas of corporate decision making, strategy development, and institutional planning. Dye (2016a, 2016b) stresses the importance of identifying potential physician leaders and providing them with mentoring, executive coaching, and advanced academic training as needed. Kovner (2014) emphasizes that senior decision makers, including the board, need to follow

EXHIBIT 6.12
Leadership and Healthcare Performance

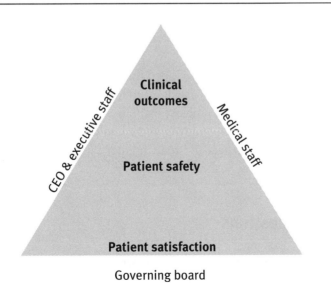

evidence-based management practices, basing their decisions on the best-quality evidence available.

Tsal and colleagues (2015) examined survey data from hospitals in the United States and England to look at the management practices of hospital boards and the relationship between management practices and quality of care. The results of the study suggested that effective governance practices—for instance, attention to quality metrics, use of specific targets, a focus on operations—have a meaningful impact on hospital performance. The study further underscores the importance of strengthening the relationship between board and management performance.

Summary

Today's rapidly changing, increasingly globalized healthcare landscape presents a wide range of challenges for leaders and managers. Leaders must navigate change, motivate others to achieve organizational goals, and ensure the proper use of resources, all while dealing with a wide range of obstacles, limitations, and unexpected events. Success in healthcare leadership requires numerous skills and competencies, as well as a firm understanding of the concept of leadership itself.

Leadership is defined in this chapter as the ability to use influence to motivate individuals within an organization to accomplish a particular goal. Effective leaders are collaborators in relationships based on a shared vision, and they are committed to building an organizational culture with common values, goals, and priorities. They communicate effectively and demonstrate honesty, integrity, confidence, and professionalism in their work. Importantly, effective leaders possess self-awareness and self-understanding, and they are able to adapt their leadership style to particular situations. They practice evidence-based management, applying the best available evidence to the managerial situations at hand.

Leadership skills are best developed through multifaceted interventions that incorporate formal training, coaching and mentoring, regular feedback and assessment, and continuous learning opportunities. The Institute for Healthcare Improvement's "triple aim"—improving the health of populations, improving the patient care experience, and reducing per capita costs—offers a useful framework for optimizing healthcare leadership.

Discussion Questions

1. A diverse workforce includes members with different values and cultural backgrounds. What actions and activities might a healthcare leader or

manager use to increase socialization and productivity within a diverse group?

2. What are the long-term benefits of globalization? How can we enable management teams to develop global healthcare management competencies?

3. Why are communication and interpersonal skills so important to leadership? Identify someone who, in your opinion, exemplifies these skills. What makes that person an effective leader?

4. Discuss the relationship between communication and organizational design. What are some potential barriers to effective communication? How can leaders make sure their messages are heard? What can managers do to improve communication?

5. Many healthcare practitioners deal with significant work–life stress. What can managers do to support employees and help moderate their stress? Discuss the importance of wellness programs and employee assistance programs.

6. What role does team building play in the development of trust among departments or groups? How does a leader diagnose conflict? What can a leader do to resolve differences?

7. Some groups and teams are more productive than others. Describe a team from your own personal experience that performed well on a project. What made that team effective? How did the team evolve? What were the stages of group development?

8. What can a leader do to increase motivation? Discuss positive and negative reinforcement, and give examples. What types of rewards can a leader use to increase productivity?

9. How can evidence-based management practices enhance quality and patient safety? How can leaders foster a culture that promotes safety and continuous learning?

10. Imagine you have been asked to set up a field hospital in Uganda. Where do you begin? What are the major management challenges to be addressed? How would you go about organizing teams? What leadership competencies are needed?

11. Haiti's minister of health has asked for your help in developing primary care services in the town of Jacmel. How would you go about designing the necessary services? What types of teams would you need? How would you evaluate clinical outcomes? What are the major challenges you would expect to face?

12. You have been asked to assemble and develop a new leadership team for a project in Ukraine. What criteria would you use to select people for the team? What type of planning process would you use?

Exercises

Exercise 1: Reflection

Reflection is an important competency that enables us to learn about ourselves and grow as leaders. It helps us think critically about personal and professional decisions, enhance personal achievement and career preparedness, and gain valuable insight into issues of global health and social justice. Dye (2017, 294) points out that "value-driven leaders are self-assessors" who "study their own moves and thought processes" and strive for personal and professional improvement. In addition, reflection is a key aspect of ethical decision making, particularly with regard to issues of fairness and equality. Jesuit colleges and universities have traditionally emphasized reflection, discernment, and engagement.

For this exercise, reflect on yourself and your leadership. Engage in meaningful examination of your behavior, values, thinking processes, and feelings. Ask yourself the following questions:

- What can I change?
- What did I learn?
- How will I change my behavior?
- Are there new ideas I can use at work?
- What competencies do I need to develop?

You may want to develop a one- or two-page document recording your key thoughts, ideas, and future plans. As you reflect, consider the following quotations as they might apply to global healthcare management:

"Of those to whom much is given, much is expected." —Luke 12:48

"We become what we think about." —Earl Nightingale

"You can't escape the responsibility of tomorrow by evading it today." —Abraham Lincoln

"The best way to predict the future is to create it." —Peter Drucker

"When he took time to help the man up the mountain, lo, he scaled it himself." —Tibetan proverb

"I don't know what your destiny will be, but one thing I know: the only ones among you who will be really happy are those who have sought and found how to serve." —Albert Schweitzer

"A positive thinker does not refuse to recognize the negative; he refuses to dwell on it. Positive thinking is a form of thought which habitually looks for the best results from the worst conditions." —Norman Vincent Peale

"You get the best out of others when you give the best of yourself."
—Harry Firestone

"There are no great things, only small things with great love. Happy are
those." —Commonly attributed to Mother Teresa

"Do not go where the path may lead; go instead where there is no path
and leave a trail." —Commonly attributed to Ralph Waldo Emerson

"Between stimulus and response there is a space. In that space is our
power to choose our response. In our response lies our growth and
our freedom." —Viktor E. Frankl

"We must never forget that we may also find meaning in life even when
confronted with a hopeless situation." —Viktor E. Frankl

"Be the change you wish to see in the world." —Commonly attributed
to Mahatma Gandhi

"What counts in life is not the mere fact that we have lived. It is what
difference we have made to the lives of others that will determine
the significance of the life we lead." —Nelson Mandela

Sources: Success (2009); *Forbes* (2018); AZ Quotes (2018a, 2018b, 2018c); IZ Quotes (2018); Albert Schweitzer's Leadership for Life (2018); Quote Investigator (2014, 2017); Quotes.net (2018); Mother Teresa of Calcutta Center (2018); McGregor (2013).

Exercise 2: *Professional Assessment and Development Strategies*

In seeking to achieve meaningful growth, either personally or professionally, individuals must first spend some time assessing where they are at present. Self-awareness and self-understanding are essential for designing an appropriate course of action across the various interrelated areas of our lives. All too often, we fail to recognize how these areas affect our careers.

This Professional Assessment and Development Strategies (PADS) exercise has been designed to help you in your self-assessment. It aims to increase your awareness of specific areas that you might have thought about but have probably never seriously analyzed with the intention of developing a meaningful strategy. This exercise is intended as a starting point around which you can design and implement changes in your life and career. It may also serve as a reference point that you can use to make comparisons over time and to map out future courses of action. Note: PADS is helpful only to the extent that you accurately and honestly assess yourself.

The objectives of this exercise are as follows:

- Complete an assessment of your leadership potential and style.
- Think about areas for change and growth (SWOT analysis).
- Plan your continuing education.
- Develop a realistic action plan for the next two to five years.

- Start changing attitudes, behaviors, thoughts, actions, and perceptions.
- Develop a career plan and road map with benchmarks to measure progress.
- Use the strategic plan to achieve professional goals.
- Prepare a resume.
- Assess leadership competencies.

Complete the PADS exercise via the following steps:

1. Conduct a personal self-assessment and evaluation. Use personal reflection.
2. Use the results of this self-assessment to develop a professional and personal action plan for
   - the next 12 months,
   - 1–2 years, and
   - 3–5 years.
3. Develop a strategic action plan containing the following:
   - Vision
   - Personal mission statement
   - Goals
   - Measurable objectives
   - Time frames
   - Cost projections
   - Responsibility designation
   - SMART criteria (i.e., criteria that are specific, measurable, attainable, realistic, and time framed)
   - Leadership assessment
   - Competency assessment (using the ACHE tool at www.ache.org/pdf/nonsecure/careers/competencies_booklet.pdf)
4. The strategic action plan should address personal and professional areas related to leadership skills and development, career planning, life changes, and so on. Additional requirements:
   - It must be an integrated plan.
   - It must have continuity of thought and action across objectives.
   - It must have quantitative and qualitative forecasting (measurement).
   - It must be a realistic plan.
5. Develop a professional resume containing the following:
   - Personal data
   - Career objective

- Education
- Special training
- Work history
- Professional organizations
- Community experience
- Other sections as needed

6. Consider such areas as physical and mental health, social/interpersonal skills, time management, stress management, family, leisure time, financial goals, plans for future education, areas for spiritual growth, involvement with community and professional organizations, exercise and fitness, nutrition and diet, environmental responsibility, and overall life purpose. Be sure these issues are addressed in your personal/ professional strategic plan.

7. Conduct your own SWOT analysis, develop realistic and measurable objectives (SMART goals), examine mentoring relationships, complete a needs assessment, and think about personal career strategies.

8. Apply a model for strategic thinking to your own career.

9. Develop a written plan.

10. Share your plan with others and get their feedback.

References

Albert Schweitzer's Leadership for Life. 2018. "Who Is Albert Schweitzer?" Accessed May 25. http://aschweitzer.com/abouta.html.

American College of Healthcare Executives (ACHE). 2018. *ACHE Healthcare Executive 2018 Competencies Assessment Tool.* Accessed May 23. www.ache.org/pdf/ nonsecure/careers/competencies_booklet.pdf.

———. 2017. "ACHE Code of Ethics." Accessed May 24, 2018. www.ache.org/ abt_ache/code.cfm.

AZ Quotes. 2018a. "Norman Vincent Peale Quotes." Accessed May 25. www.azquotes. com/author/11448-Norman_Vincent_Peale.

———. 2018b. "Peter Drucker Quotes." Accessed May 25. www.azquotes.com/ author/4147-Peter_Drucker.

———. 2018c. "Victor E. Frankl Quotes." Accessed May 25. www.azquotes.com/ author/5121-Viktor_E_Frankl.

Barr, J., and L. Dowding. 2012. *Leadership in Healthcare*, 2nd ed. Los Angeles: SAGE.

Berwick, D. M., T. W. Nolan, and J. Whittington. 2008. "The Triple Aim: Care, Health, and Cost." *Health Affairs* 27 (3): 759–69.

Bill and Melinda Gates Foundation. 2018. "What We Do." Accessed May 18. www. gatesfoundation.org.

Birk, S. 2010. "The 10 Most Common Myths About Leadership." *Healthcare Executive* 25 (6): 30–38.

Bodenheimer, T., and C. Sinsky. 2014. "From Triple to Quadruple Aim: Care of the Patient Requires Care of the Provider." *Annals of Family Medicine* 12 (6): 573–76.

Bolman, L. G., and T. E. Deal. 2003. "Reframing Leadership." In *Business Leadership: A Jossey-Bass Reader*, edited by J. V. Gallos, 86–110. San Francisco: Jossey-Bass.

Campbell, R. J. 2008. "Change Management in Health Care." *Health Care Manager* 27 (1): 23–29.

Collins, D. B., and E. F. Holton. 2004. "The Effectiveness of Managerial Leadership Development Programs: A Meta-Analysis of Studies from 1982 to 2001." *Human Resource Development Quarterly* 15 (2): 217–48.

Coyne, J. S., P. E. Hilsenrath, B. S. Arbuckle, F. Kureshy, D. Vaughan, D. Grayson, and T. Saygin. 2014. "Triple Aim Program: Assessing Its Effectiveness as a Hospital Management Tool." *Hospital Topics* 92 (4): 88–95.

DeRue, D. S., and K. M. Workman. 2012. "Toward a Positive and Dynamic Theory of Leadership Development." *Oxford Handbook of Positive Organizational Scholarship* (electronic version). Accessed May 14, 2018. https://scholarship.sha.cornell.edu/cgi/viewcontent.cgi?article=1863&context=articles.

Dunn, R. T. 2016. *Dunn & Haimann's Healthcare Management*, 10th ed. Chicago: Health Administration Press.

Dye, C. F. 2017. *Leadership in Healthcare: Essential Values and Skills*, 3rd ed. Chicago: Health Administration Press.

———. 2016a. "Enhancing Physician Engagement." *Healthcare Executive* 31 (1): 70–73.

———. 2016b. "Health Care CEOs Can Build Engagement by Cultivating Physician Leaders." *Trustee*. Published April 4. www.trusteemag.com/articles/1066-health-care-ceos-can-build-engagement-by-cultivating-physician-leaders.

Dye, C. F., and A. N. Garman. 2014. *Exceptional Leadership: 16 Critical Competencies for Healthcare Executives*, 2nd ed. Chicago: Health Administration Press.

European Network for Social Action (ENSACT). 2014. "The Ministry and Scientific Projects of St. Elizabeth University (Bratislava, Slovakia)." Accessed May 17, 2018. www.ensact.com/sites/ensact.com/files/webform/Good%20Practice.docx.

European Parliament. 2017. "EU Migrant Crisis: Facts and Figures." Published June 30. www.europarl.europa.eu/news/en/headlines/society/20170629STO78630/eu-migrant-crisis-facts-and-figures.

Finkelstein, S. 2016. "Managing Yourself: Secrets of the Superbosses." *Harvard Business Review* 94 (1): 104–7.

Forbes. 2018. "Thoughts on the Business of Life." Accessed May 25. www.forbes.com/quotes/82/.

Gibson, J. L., J. M. Ivancevich, J. H. Donnelly Jr., and R. Konopaske. 2012. *Organizations: Behavior, Structure, Processes*, 14th ed. New York: McGraw-Hill.

Goleman, D. 2000. "Leadership That Gets Results." *Harvard Business Review* 78 (3–4): 78–90.

Ham, C. 2003. "Improving the Performance of Health Services: The Role of Clinical Leadership." *Lancet* 361 (9373): 1978–80.

Holsinger, J. W. Jr., and E. L. Carlton. 2018. *Leadership for Public Health: Theory and Practice*. Chicago: Health Administration Press.

Institute of Medicine (IOM). 2011. *The Future of Nursing: Focus on Scope of Practice*. Published January 26. www.nationalacademies.org/hmd/Reports/2010/The-Future-of-Nursing-Leading-Change-Advancing-Health/Report-Brief-Scope-of-Practice.aspx.

International Hospital Federation (IHF). 2015. *Leadership Competencies for Healthcare Services Managers*. Accessed May 14, 2018. www.ihf-fih.org/resources/pdf/Leadership_Competencies_for_Healthcare_Services_Managers.pdf.

IZ Quotes. 2018. "Anonymous Quote." Accessed May 25. https://izquotes.com/quote/354278.

Jesuit Institute. 1993. "Ignatian Pedagogy Document." Accessed May 25. http://jesuitinstitute.org/Pages/IgnatianPedagogy.htm.

Jha, V., H. L. Bekker, S. R. Duffy, and T. E. Roberts. 2007. "A Systematic Review of Studies Assessing and Facilitating Attitudes Towards Professionalism in Medicine." *Medical Education* 41 (8): 822–29.

Kotter, J. P., and D. S. Cohen. 2002. *The Heart of Change: Real-Life Stories of How People Change Their Organizations*. Boston: Harvard Business School Press.

Kouzes, J., and B. Posner. 2012. *The Leadership Challenge: How to Make Extraordinary Things Happen in Organizations*. San Francisco: Wiley.

Kovner, A. R. 2014. "Evidence-Based Management: Implications for Nonprofit Organizations." *Nonprofit Management and Leadership* 24 (3): 417–24.

Kovner, A. R., and T. D'Aunno. 2017. *Evidence-Based Management in Healthcare: Principles, Cases, and Perspectives*, 2nd ed. Chicago: Health Administration Press.

Kovner, A. R., D. J. Fine, and R. D'Aquila. 2009. *Evidence-Based Management in Healthcare*. Chicago: Health Administration Press.

Kumar, R. D. C., and N. Khiljee. 2016. "Leadership in Healthcare." *Anaesthesia & Intensive Care Medicine* 17 (1): 63–65.

Liang, Z., and P. F. Howard. 2007. "Views from the Executive Suite: Lessons from the Introduction of Performance Management." *Australian Health Review* 31 (3): 393–400.

Linstead, S. 1999. "Managing Culture." In *Management: A Critical Text*, edited by L. Fulop and S. Linstead, 82–121. London: Palgrave.

Longest, B. B. Jr., and K. Darr. 2008. *Managing Health Services Organizations and Systems*, 5th ed. Baltimore, MD: Health Professionals Press.

Marmot, M. 2015. *The Health Gap: The Challenge of an Unequal World*. New York: Bloomsbury Press.

Maslow, A. H. 1954. *Motivation and Personality*. New York: Harper & Row.

Maxwell, J. C. 1999. *The 21 Indispensable Qualities of a Leader: Becoming the Person That Other People Will Want to Follow*. Nashville, TN: Thomas Nelson.

McClelland, D. C. 1984. *Motives, Personality and Society: Selected Papers*. New York: Praeger.

McGirt, E. 2016. "Bono: I Will Follow." *Fortune.* Published March 24. http://fortune. com/bono-u2-one/.

McGregor, J. 2013. "What Nelson Mandela Had to Say About Leadership." *Washington Post.* Published June 24. www.washingtonpost.com/news/on-leadership/ wp/2013/06/24/what-nelson-mandela-had-to-say-about-leadership/?utm_ term=.0e1a5292ee15.

Morrow, G., B. Burford, C. Rothwell, M. Carter, J. McLachlan, and J. Illing. 2014. *Professionalism in Healthcare Professionals.* Health and Care Professions Council. Accessed May 14, 2018. www.hpc-uk.org/assets/documents/10003771Prof essionalisminhealthcareprofessionals.pdf.

Mother Teresa of Calcutta Center. 2018. "Quotes Falsely Attributed to Mother Teresa and Significantly Paraphrased Versions or Personal Interpretations of Statements That Are Not Her Authentic Words." Accessed May 25. www.motherteresa. org/08_info/Quotesf.html.

National Academies of Science, Engineering, and Medicine. 2011. "The Future of Nursing: Focus on Education." Published January 26. www.nationalacademies. org/hmd/Reports/2010/The-Future-of-Nursing-Leading-Change-Advancing-Health/Report-Brief-Education.aspx.

NHS Leadership Academy. 2016. "Healthcare Leadership Model." Accessed June 11. www.leadershipacademy.nhs.uk/resources/healthcare-leadership-model/.

North Atlantic Treaty Organization (NATO). 2017. "NATO and Partners Exercise Disaster Response in Bosnia and Herzegovina." Updated September 25. www. nato.int/cps/en/natohq/news_147118.htm.

Pinheiro de Oliveira, A. 2016. "Brazil's Militarized War on Zika." *Global Societies Journal.* Accessed May 18, 2018. www.global.ucsb.edu/gsj/sites/secure.lsit. ucsb.edu.gisp.d7_gs-2/files/sitefiles/Deoliveira.pdf.

Porter-O'Grady, T. 2013. "When It Doesn't Work: Failure Leadership in Healthcare." *Nurse Leader* 11 (2): 42–49.

Quote Investigator. 2017. "Be the Change You Wish to See in the World." Published October 23. https://quoteinvestigator.com/2017/10/23/be-change/.

———. 2014. "I Will Go Where There Is No Path, and I Will Leave a Trail." Published June 19. https://quoteinvestigator.com/2014/06/19/new-path/.

Quotes.net. 2018. "Famous Quotes by Harry Firestone." Accessed May 25. www. quotes.net/quote/881.

Robbins, S. P., and D. A. DeCenzo. 2004. *Fundamentals of Management: Essential Concepts and Applications*, 4th ed. Upper Saddle River, NJ: Pearson Prentice-Hall.

Ross, A., F. J. Wenzel, and J. W. Mitlyng. 2002. *Leadership for the Future: Core Competencies in Healthcare.* Chicago: Health Administration Press.

Schein, E. H. 2010. *Organizational Culture and Leadership*, 4th ed. San Francisco: Jossey-Bass.

Shalala, D. E. 2014. "Nursing Leaders Can Deliver a New Model of Care." *Frontiers of Health Services Management* 31 (2): 3–16.

Shortell, S. M., R. H. Jones, A. W. Rademaker, R. R. Gillies, D. S. Dranove, E. F. X. Hughes, P. P. Budetti, K. S. E. Reynolds, and C. F. Huang. 2000. "Assessing the Impact of Total Quality Management and Organizational Culture on Multiple Outcomes of Care for Coronary Artery Bypass Graft Surgery Patients." *Medical Care* 38 (2): 207–17.

Skolnik, R. 2016. *Global Health 101*, 3rd ed. Burlington, MA: Jones & Bartlett Learning.

Spencer, L. M., and S. M. Spencer. 1993. *Competence at Work: Models for Superior Performance*. New York: John Wiley & Sons.

Squazzo, J. D. 2010. "Today's Leader: Committed to Core Values." *Healthcare Executive* 25 (6): 8–18.

Success. 2009. "Earl Nightingale's Greatest Discovery." Published March 30. www.success.com/article/earl-nightingales-greatest-discovery.

Tsal, T. C., A. K. Jha, A. A. Gawande, R. S. Huckman, N. Bloom, and R. Sadun. 2015. "Hospital Board and Management Practices Are Strongly Related to Hospital Performance on Clinical Quality Metrics." *Health Affairs* 34 (8): 1304–11.

United Nations Children's Fund (UNICEF). 2018. *Every Child Alive: The Urgent Need to End Newborn Deaths*. Accessed May 21. www.unicef.org/publications/files/Every_Child_Alive_The_urgent_need_to_end_newborn_deaths.pdf.

United Nations (UN) Development Programme. 2018. "Millennium Development Goals." Accessed July 16. www.undp.org/content/undp/en/home/sdgoverview/ mdg_goals.html.

US Census Bureau. 2015. "New Census Bureau Report Analyzes US Population Projections." Published March 3. www.census.gov/newsroom/press-releases/2015/cb15-tps16.html.

West, D. J., M. Murgas, V. Rusnáková, and V. Krcmery. 1999. "A Collaborative Health Management Education Partnership in Slovakia: An Analysis of the Model, Outcomes and Sustainable Results After Four Years of Operation." *Journal of Health Sciences Management and Public Health*. Accessed May 21, 2018. www.medportal.ge/journal/n2/11.pdf.

West, D. J., B. Ramirez, and G. Filerman. 2012. "Leadership and Globalization: Research in Health Management Education." *World Hospitals and Health Services* 48 (3): 14–17.

Wheatley, M. J. 2002. "Leadership in Turbulent Times Is Spiritual." *Frontiers of Health Services Management* 18 (4): 19–26.

White, K. R., and J. R. Griffith. 2016. *The Well-Managed Healthcare Organization*, 8th ed. Chicago: Health Administration Press.

World Bank. 2018. "How Does the World Bank Classify Countries?" Accessed May 18. https://datahelpdesk.worldbank.org/knowledgebase/articles/378834-how-does-the-world-bank-classify-countries.

World Health Organization (WHO). 2018. "Maternal Mortality." Published February 16. www.who.int/news-room/fact-sheets/detail/maternal-mortality.

———. 2017. "The Top 10 Causes of Death." Published January 12. www.who.int/en/news-room/fact-sheets/detail/the-top-10-causes-of-death.

Zismer, D. K. 2018. "Managing the Productivity, Enterprise Risk of Strategy (Coach Series, Part 1)." American Association for Physician Leadership. Published January 28. https://news.physicianleaders.org/coach-series-part-1-managing-the-productivity-enterprise-risk-of-strategy-.

STRATEGIC MANAGEMENT AND MARKETING

Steven W. Howard, PhD, Shivani Gupta, PhD, Ana Maria Malik, MD, PhD, and Walter Cintra Ferreira Jr., MD, PhD

Chapter Focus

This chapter introduces the basic process of strategic planning and connects it with the strategic marketing process that enables a healthcare organization to meet its goals and objectives. It addresses the development of an organizational structure, the articulation of an organization's mission and values, establishment of a future vision, and the successful design and implementation of marketing and communications strategies. The chapter encourages systems thinking from diverse perspectives, supported by examples and short cases from multiple countries and from various sectors of the healthcare landscape. After completing this chapter, students should have a basic understanding of the key concepts of strategic management and marketing, and they should be able to draft a strategic plan that incorporates effective communication with desired audiences through targeted channels.

This chapter builds on the leadership concepts of chapter 6 and helps lay the foundation for chapter 8, in which the organization's strategies are operationalized through careful design of processes for day-to-day work and continuous improvement. The concepts of chapters 6, 7, and 8 are all influenced by local and global changes in health policies, health system design, and the external environmental shifts that will be discussed in chapter 14.

Learning Objectives

Upon completion of this chapter, you should be able to

- identify, discuss, and apply key concepts in strategic management;
- understand and explore the role of strategic thought in the healthcare field;
- employ strategic management instruments in organizations and discuss how they have been used;
- explain how marketing relates to an organization's strategic positioning;

- apply the components of marketing and strategic management (assess internal and external environmental trends, analyze target audiences and segments, describe product characteristics, evaluate distribution channels, analyze pricing models, assess types of promotion, evaluate pros and cons of various media, and delineate the methods for evaluating a new product);
- justify various elements of strategy formulation; and
- create and evaluate strategic alternatives, select a strategy, and develop an implementation plan with specific goals.

Competencies

- Articulate and communicate the mission, objectives, and priorities of the organization to internal and external entities.
- Practice and value transparent, shared decision making, and understand its impacts on stakeholders (both internal and external).
- Prepare and deliver business communications, such as meeting agendas, presentations, business reports, and project communication plans.
- Demonstrate an understanding of the function of media and public relations.
- Be aware of one's own assumptions, values, strengths, and limitations.
- Maintain a balance between personal and professional accountability, recognizing that the central focus must be on the needs of the patient/community.
- Balance the interrelationships among access, quality, safety, cost, resource allocation, accountability, care settings, community need, and professional roles.
- Include the perspective of individuals, families, and the community as partners in healthcare decision-making processes, respecting cultural differences and expectations.
- Collate relevant data and information, and analyze and evaluate this information to support or make effective decisions or recommendations.
- Seek information from a variety of sources to support organizational performance, conduct needs analyses, and prioritize requirements.
- Effectively apply knowledge of organizational systems theories and behaviors.
- Manage effectively within the governance structure of the organization.
- Lead the development of key planning documents, including strategic plans, business service plans, and business cases for new services.

- Develop and monitor operating-unit strategic objectives that are aligned with the mission and strategic objectives of the organization.
- Apply marketing principles and tools appropriately for the needs of the community.
- Evaluate whether a proposed action aligns with the organizational business/strategic plan.
- Demonstrate an understanding of the interdependency, integration, and competition among healthcare sectors.

Key Terms

- Continuum of care
- Direct channel
- Directional strategies
- Exclusive distribution
- Intensive distribution
- Marketing
- Marketing integration
- Market research
- Market segmentation
- Market sizing
- Mark-up pricing
- Mission statement
- Parity pricing

- Penetration pricing
- Product portfolio
- Search engine marketing (SEM)
- Search engine optimization (SEO)
- Selective distribution
- Skimming
- Strategy
- Targeting
- Target return pricing
- Triple bottom line
- Value pricing
- Values statement
- Vision

Key Concepts

- Advertising
- Ansoff matrix
- Balanced scorecard
- Buyer behavior
- Competition
- Four *P*s of marketing
- Goals and objectives
- Internal and external environmental analyses
- Marketing plan
- Mission, vision, and values

- Organizational culture
- Perceptual mapping
- Porter's five forces framework
- Pricing methods
- Product life cycle
- Strategic management
- Strategic marketing
- SWOT analysis
- Triple aim
- Utilization of healthcare services

Introduction

Effective leadership in healthcare depends heavily on organizational strategy and effective communication. Strategic management is not simply a matter of designing a good strategy. Rather, it is a process that involves identifying changes in the external environment (e.g., developments in the healthcare landscape, the actions of competitors), understanding the needs of stakeholders, and using and adapting the organization's internal resources accordingly.

Globally, the external environment for healthcare providers is undergoing a dramatic shift with regard to the nature of community needs, the demands of governments and other payers, and the expectations of the population. The demand for healthcare services continues to grow rapidly, yet, at the same time, the demands for improved quality and cost control are also greater than ever before. Although these demands manifest themselves differently in different countries' health systems, the pressures are driving greater competition between healthcare providers. All signs indicate that this dynamic will continue into the future. In this environment, the most successful healthcare organizations will be those with a strong understanding of strategy, as well as the marketing and communications necessary to achieve their strategic goals.

In the nineteenth and twentieth centuries, communicable diseases posed the greatest burden on health systems throughout the world. In the new millennium, however, chronic diseases, such as diabetes and hypertension, and mental health conditions, such as depression, are quickly becoming the most prevalent and costly challenges to public health, even in low-income countries. This trend is the consequence of an aging population, longer life expectancies, advances in medical treatments, and increasingly sedentary lifestyles. Many patients who, just a few decades ago, would have died from their acute or chronic diseases are able to remain alive and productive because of advances in medical technology and improved approaches to care. For these individuals to keep functioning as they grow older, they need multiprofessional and multidimensional care.

These changing conditions suggest the need for a strategic shift, but many elements of past strategic approaches remain in place. Most countries' health systems still place a much stronger emphasis on treating diseases than on preventing them. Most of the indicators used to compare countries are resource-related (e.g., professionals or facilities relative to population) or focused on the negative (e.g., mortality rates). Some argue that, instead, health systems should monitor factors that produce long-term positive or negative health effects, such as healthy diet, regular exercise, or consumption of alcohol, drugs, or sugary beverages. Health systems also must monitor the per capita cost of providing care and the utilization of services that affect cost.

The key is not to simply cut all costs in the short term but rather to understand the evidence-based, appropriate use of goods and services along the whole healthcare continuum in the long term. This approach is reflected in the strong global trend emphasizing payment for value (i.e., results and cost-effectiveness) rather than for volume (i.e., number of services), particularly for high-cost treatments and those lacking a basis in evidence. To help advance this shift, certain services—including vaccinations, disease screenings, maintenance medications for chronic conditions, and other preventive measures—should be actively encouraged. Hence, we see the important interrelationship of strategy and marketing.

Strategy is the art of devising and implementing plans toward the achievement of short-term or long-term goals and objectives. In healthcare, for example, it might include planning for how a provider's organization needs to be structured to flourish under new incentives for evidence-based care and value-based payment mechanisms. **Marketing** is the aspect of strategy that deals with communication, promotion, and distribution of the ideas, products, or services that are key to the strategy (Merriam-Webster 2017). In our healthcare example, marketing might include the communication plans for getting physicians, nurses, and other members of the provider team to understand and commit to the changes needed under the new value-based systems. Marketing might also include communication campaigns to convince members of the public to change their health beliefs and care-seeking behaviors (e.g., not rushing to use antibiotics for every illness, seeing a nurse practitioner first rather than referring oneself to a specialist).

In recent years, the healthcare world has been experiencing a seismic shift toward the empowerment of individuals. Dr. Eric Topol's (2015) *The Patient Will See You Now*, for instance, advocates for the ability of empowered citizens to manage their data (e.g., diets, tests, costs, outcomes) and make their decisions more wisely. At the same time, the world has been marked by growing inequality, both between and within countries and regions. Regional inequities are typical of large developing countries such as India and Brazil (Jayaraman 2014). However, even higher-income countries, such as the United States, have disparities between regions and population segments, with clearly different, though parallel, public and private healthcare sectors. Given that the global healthcare landscape is fragmented by differences in needs, resources, infrastructures, knowledge, and availability of techniques from one country or region to another, pursuit of a new universal goal—such as population health—might seem unachievable.

Countries have developed a variety of approaches for dealing with the complex and ever-changing health needs of their people. Spain, the United Kingdom, Brazil, and Portugal are examples of countries with constitutionally Beveridgean models—meaning that healthcare is provided and funded by the government through tax payments—that have experimented with new

strategy
The art of devising and implementing plans toward the achievement of short-term or long-term goals and objectives.

marketing
The aspect of strategy that deals with communication, promotion, and distribution of the ideas, products, or services that are key to the strategy.

relationships between the public and private sectors. These new public–private partnerships (PPPs) extend beyond traditional nongovernmental organizations and may be either for profit or not for profit in nature. The partnerships have generally been promoted by consulting agencies and large firms but opposed by stakeholders who believe the state should be the main player in the healthcare field. Since 1998, Brazil has used a PPP model called the Social Organization in Health, in which government and private entities work together to finance and deliver healthcare services to populations. The concept of *value* in health-care—defined as outcomes achieved for the money spent—has become one of the most popular topics among healthcare providers, insurers, employers, and government payers, and it represents a central focus for ongoing reform efforts.

Strategic Management

continuum of care
The comprehensive array of health services across all settings, specialties, and levels of intensity.

Since 2010, we have clearly been in an era of networks—not just the ubiquitous social networks but also the networks seeking to integrate the entire **continuum of care** under a single health system (or a few large ones). Such networks may provide services across the continuum under the same ownership or through multiple entities. Corporate mergers and acquisitions have increased as more organizations seek to increase their market power and consolidate links in the value chain. The guiding assumption is that the new, consolidated entities will be able to improve efficiency and efficacy. However, the operations of integrated health networks are extensive, complex, and subject to the social, economic, and political forces of local, national, and global marketplaces, all of which are changing at a rapid pace. Effective management—strategic and otherwise—is a critical part of this scenario. Organizational priorities must be established across multiple dimensions and subsequently managed and monitored.

The Balanced Scorecard

The balanced scorecard (BSC), introduced in chapter 3, is a strategic manage-ment tool that can help drive the pursuit of organizational priorities across multiple dimensions. Presented in a 1992 *Harvard Business Review* article by Kaplan and Norton (1992, 1996), the BSC matrix incorporates at least four dimensions in which strategic results can be monitored: (1) the financial perspective, (2) the learning and growth perspective, (3) the business process perspective, and (4) the customer and stakeholder perspective (see exhibit 7.1).

The BSC can be highly useful in healthcare, though some believe it focuses too heavily on financial results. In a classic article titled "No Mis-sion ↔ No Margin," Meliones and colleagues (2001) highlight the need for healthcare organizations to align the scorecard with the organizational mission and bridge the gap between the financial and clinical aspects of care. Given that organizations need to be concerned with more than one bottom line

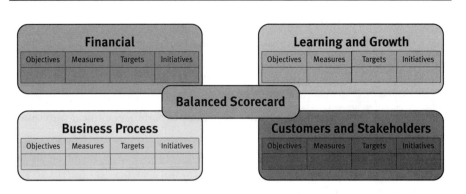

Source: Adapted from Kaplan and Norton (1996).

EXHIBIT 7.1
Balanced
Scorecard
Matrix

simultaneously, the concept of the **triple bottom line** emphasizes results in three areas: (1) profit, (2) people, and (3) planet (sustainability). These areas resemble the parts of the "triple aim" model developed by the Institute for Healthcare Improvement (2017), which strives for the best possible health, the best possible care, and the lowest possible per capita cost. (Some writers have begun recognizing an additional aim, dealing with the workers' engagement, thereby creating a "quadruple aim.")

As a healthcare organization determines its strategic priorities and balances the dimensions of the triple bottom line, the leadership team must ensure that its decisions are consistent with the organization's culture and mission. Like explorers from centuries ago, they must regularly check their navigation to ensure they have their "north star" clearly in sight.

The Organization's Directional Statements

An organization's mission, vision, and values serve as its "north star." They can have both symbolic and practical meaning, depending on how they are designed and communicated throughout the organization. The mission, vision, and values provide the basis for an organization's goals and objectives and guide the organization's strategies to achieve these goals and objectives. Thus, they are often referred to as **directional strategies**.

An organization's mission is, simply put, its reason to exist (Society for Human Resource Management [SHRM] 2012). A **mission statement** is expected to inspire employees and to provide direction for the organization's units based on aligned objectives. Healthcare organizations frequently use such words as *patient*, *health*, *lives*, and *excellence* in their mission statements. For example, Hospital Moinhos de Vento (2018), in Rio Grande do Sul, Brazil, states that its mission is "taking care of lives," with an emphasis on "healthcare excellence and generation of knowledge and innovation" by a "top-performing, humane team." The intent expressed in the mission statement should be lived

triple bottom line
A theory that emphasizes an organization's need to monitor and evaluate results in three areas: profit, people, and planet (sustainability).

directional strategies
The mission, vision, and values that provide the basis for an organization's goals and objectives and guide the organization's strategies.

mission statement
A statement of an organization's reason for existing, intended to inspire employees and provide direction and alignment toward a common goal.

vision
A statement that defines what an organization seeks to become and depicts an ideal future in which the organization has fulfilled its mission and strategic goals.

values statement
A statement that functions as a sort of moral compass and describes how an organization intends to carry out its work.

out in the culture and daily operations of the organization; otherwise, it may come to be seen as little more than hollow words.

The **vision** typically defines what the organization seeks to become and depicts an ideal future in which the organization has fulfilled its mission and achieved its strategic goals (SHRM 2012). For instance, the Cleveland Clinic (2018) has a "Founder's Vision" that applies to all sites and expresses an intention to "be the world's leader in patient experience, clinical outcomes, research and education."

An organization's **values statement** serves as a sort of moral compass, describing how the organization intends to carry out its work. It often expresses the beliefs or ethics of the organization's founders and leaders. Values should be reflected in the decisions of management and in the behavior of employees. Most values statements in healthcare include language about compassion and caring for people in need. At times, however, competitive and financial pressures might cause actions at an organization to become decoupled from stated values. Treating patients differently based on their purchasing power, for instance, would be considered ethically unacceptable and a violation of values.

An organization's mission, vision, and values should guide its strategic planning process. They should facilitate the development of appropriate goals and marketing strategies that allow the organization not only to communicate with stakeholders but also to achieve competitive advantage and superior performance. The relationship between directional strategies, marketing strategies, and goals and objectives is illustrated in exhibit 7.2.

If the directional statements are true and genuine, people throughout the organization will live by them on a daily basis. In many cases, the directional

EXHIBIT 7.2
Directional Strategies, Marketing Strategies, and Goals and Objectives

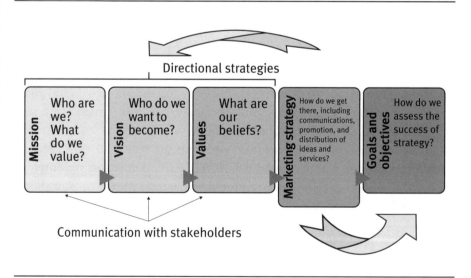

statements are felt deeply by employees of the organization and represent their reason to be working there. Some organizations expect employees to memorize the directional statements, in part because accreditors may ask about them during site visits. Management should enforce the directional statements and review them over time to ensure that they continue to fit the organization's focus and culture and are clearly understood by employees.

Exhibits 7.3 through 7.11 provide examples of directional statements from healthcare organizations in various countries. Note the similarities and differences based on country, culture, type of healthcare organization, and for-profit/not-for-profit status.

Exhibits 7.9 through 7.11, in comparison with exhibits 7.3 through 7.8, highlight some of the ways that countries, cultures, secular/religious nature,

---

EXHIBIT 7.3
The Orthopedics Institute's Mission, Vision, and Values

The Instituto de Ortopedia e Traumatologia—or Orthopedics Institute—at Hospital da Clínicas is part of the Faculty of Medicine of the University of São Paulo, Brazil.

Roughly translated, the institute's mission is as follows: "To deliver specialized healthcare in the area of Orthopedics and Traumatology; to develop teaching and advanced research activities; to acknowledge internal and external clients; and to promote outreach actions."

Its vision is "to be recognized as a Centre of Excellence in knowledge management in Orthopedics and Traumatology."

Its values are "ethics, competency, humanization, promotion of institutional image, pioneering, educational emphasis, value for human beings, heritage defense, and continuous improvement."

Source: Instituto de Ortopedia e Traumatologia (2017).

EXHIBIT 7.4
Austral Hospital's Mission and Values

The Hospital Universitario Austral in Buenos Aires, Argentina, is part of Austral University and is linked to the Catholic organization Opus Dei.

The hospital's mission, roughly translated, is as follows: "To be a university organization aimed at healthcare, teaching, and biomedical research; committed to truth and life, especially emphasizing quality work and patient safety; directing all of its work toward service to individuals and the development of human and Christian values."

The values of Austral University and its hospital derive from the Christian vision of culture and the world. They include the dignity of each and every person and his/her development, freedom of consciousness, spirit of coexistence without discrimination, respect to life, importance of the family, fairness and equity, help to the needy, charity as a main characteristic, freedom, and peace.

Source: Hospital Universitario Austral (2017).

EXHIBIT 7.5
Hospital Infantil
Sabará's
Mission, Vision,
and Values

Hospital Infantil Sabará is a private pediatric hospital in São Paulo, Brazil.

It presents the following, roughly translated, as its mission: "To provide healthcare to children and teenagers, with ethics, high quality, comfort, and safety, in a motivational environment for caregivers and partners, seeking to continuously be in the scientific and technological forefront."

Its vision is "to be recognized as the best pediatric hospital by means of excellence in services, nurturing children, teenagers, their families, physicians, and all other caregivers, in a sustainable way and with social commitment."

Sabará's values are as follows:

- *Care with sustainability.* We respect the health of our foundation by means of a management-driven process, efficiency, and excellence, continuously seeking innovation, quality, and satisfaction of our caregivers, children, and their families.
- *Children and their families.* To take care of children and their families is our reason to exist. We do this with compassion, nurturing, and respect.
- *Ethics.* To behave respectfully and with transparency in our attitudes, with responsibility and integrity in fulfilling our commitments and relationships.
- *Ways of delivering care.* To care requires respect and commitment with the common goals.
- *Our caregivers.* We value our caregivers, acknowledging their competencies and encouraging knowledge and innovation with respect and confidence.

Source: Hospital Infantil Sabará (2017).

EXHIBIT 7.6
The All India
Institute
of Medical
Sciences'
Objectives
Statement

The All India Institute of Medical Sciences (AIIMS) is one of the most respected government-funded academic medical centers in India. In place of statements of mission, vision, and values, AIIMS has an objectives statement:

- To develop a pattern of teaching in undergraduate and postgraduate medical education in all its branches so as to demonstrate high standards of medical education to all medical colleges and other allied institutions in India.
- To bring together in one place educational facilities of the highest order for the training of the personnel in all important branches of the health activity.
- To attain self-sufficiency in postgraduate medical education.

Source: All India Institute of Medical Sciences (2017).

EXHIBIT 7.7
Dr. Lal
PathLabs' Vision
and Mission

Dr. Lal PathLabs is a large, private, for-profit laboratory in India. It presents its directional statements somewhat differently, in some ways combining the attributes of values statements within its vision and mission.

Its vision is as follows: "Dedicated to improve the health of patients through unsurpassed diagnostic insight. Committed to be the undisputed leader in providing world class diagnostic services, maintaining the highest ethical standards and quality."

Its mission begins: "Where Quality, Service, Innovation is a way of life." The mission continues: "We shall achieve excellence in diagnostic testing, information and services to become India's most valued company to patients, customers, colleagues, investors, business partners and the communities where we work and live in."

The website adds: "Leadership in Diagnostics, through Technology & Innovation Excellence in Diagnostics, is our mantra; Quality at your Doorstep Turning Data into Insight."

Source: Dr. Lal PathLabs (2017).

EXHIBIT 7.8
Fortis
Healthcare's
Mission, Vision,
and Values

Fortis Healthcare, a fully integrated healthcare system in India, presents its directional statements in the traditional mission, vision, and values format.

Its vision is "Saving & Enriching Lives."

Its mission is "to be a globally respected healthcare organization known for Clinical Excellence and Distinctive Patient Care."

Fortis lists its values as follows:

Patient Centricity
Commit to "best outcomes and experience" for our patients.
Treat patients and their caregivers with compassion, care and understanding.
Our patients' needs will come first.

Integrity
Be principled, open and honest.
Model and live our "Values."
Demonstrate moral courage to speak up and do the right things.

Teamwork
Proactively support each other and operate as one team.
Respect and value people at all levels with different opinions, experiences and backgrounds.
Put organization needs before department / self interest.

Ownership
Be responsible and take pride in our actions.
Take initiative and go beyond the call of duty.
Deliver commitment and agreement made.

(continued)

EXHIBIT 7.8
Fortis
Healthcare's
Mission, Vision,
and Values
(continued)

Innovation
Continuously improve and innovate to exceed expectations.
Adopt a 'can-do' attitude.
Challenge ourselves to do things differently.

Source: Fortis Healthcare (2018).

EXHIBIT 7.9
Vellore Christian
Medical
College's Vision
Statement

Vellore Christian Medical College (and affiliated health system) in Tamil Nadu, India, presents the following vision statement: "The Christian Medical College, Vellore, seeks to be a witness to the healing ministry of Christ, through excellence in education, service and research."

Source: Christian Medical College, Vellore (2017).

EXHIBIT 7.10
Ascension's
Mission, Vision,
and Values

Ascension, the largest Catholic health system in the United States, has the following mission:

Rooted in the loving ministry of Jesus as healer, we commit ourselves to serving all persons with special attention to those who are poor and vulnerable. Our Catholic health ministry is dedicated to spiritually-centered, holistic care which sustains and improves the health of individuals and communities. We are advocates for a compassionate and just society through our actions and our words.

Its vision is as follows:

We envision a strong, vibrant Catholic health ministry in the United States which will lead to the transformation of healthcare. We will ensure service that is committed to health and well-being for our communities and that responds to the needs of individuals throughout the life cycle. We will expand the role of laity, in both leadership and sponsorship, to ensure a Catholic health ministry in the future.

Ascension lists the following values:

- *Service of the poor:* Generosity of spirit, especially for persons most in need
- *Reverence:* Respect and compassion for the dignity and diversity of life
- *Integrity:* Inspiring trust through personal leadership
- *Wisdom:* Integrating excellence and stewardship
- *Creativity:* Courageous innovation
- *Dedication:* Affirming the hope and joy of our ministry

Source: Ascension (2017).

EXHIBIT 7.11
HCA's Mission
and Values

HCA, headquartered in Nashville, Tennessee, is one of the largest for-profit health systems in the United States. Its website presents the following mission and values statements:

> Above all else, we are committed to the care and improvement of human life.
>
> In pursuit of our mission, we believe the following value statements are essential and timeless:
>
> - We recognize and affirm the unique and intrinsic worth of each individual.
> - We treat all those we serve with compassion and kindness.
> - We trust our colleagues as valuable members of our healthcare team and pledge to treat one another with loyalty, respect, and dignity.
> - We act with absolute honesty, integrity, and fairness in the way we conduct our business and the way we live our lives.

Source: HCA Healthcare (2018).

and not-for-profit/for-profit status lead to different kinds of directional statements. For instance, note the differences between the earlier statements (exhibits 7.3 through 7.8) and that of the Vellore Christian Medical College in India (exhibit 7.9). Furthermore, note the similarities between the Vellore statement and those of Ascension, the largest Catholic health system in the United States (exhibit 7.10). Finally, contrast these statements with the combined mission and values statement of the for-profit US health system HCA (exhibit 7.11).

Internal and External Environmental Analyses

Environmental analysis is key to both strategic management and marketing. Effective analyses need to take into account both internal and external conditions, paying attention to other organizations in the market, what they do, and how they do it. The two most commonly used models for environmental analysis are the SWOT analysis (Andrews 1971) and Porter's five forces model (Porter 1979).

SWOT analysis, as noted in chapter 6, is an analysis of strengths, weaknesses, opportunities, and threats, and the four elements can be placed on a matrix as shown in exhibit 7.12. The first two elements (strengths and weaknesses) reflect features of the internal environment, or attributes of the organization itself, whereas the latter two elements (opportunities and threats) represent features of the external environment. Although the external factors are difficult to control, organizations still need to thoroughly understand and prepare for them. The internal factors are, theoretically, easier to act upon, but certain organizational actors (sometimes called "corporate antibodies") are often present, working behind the scenes to maintain the status quo and thwart the intended strategic changes. When organizations discuss environmental analysis,

EXHIBIT 7.12
SWOT Analysis

	Helpful (to achieving the objective)	**Harmful** (to achieving the objective)
Internal origin (attributes of the organization)	**Strengths**	**Weaknesses**
External origin (attributes of the environment)	**Opportunities**	**Threats**

Source: Adapted from Andrews (1971).

SWOT is often the first approach that comes to mind; however, it is only one of several tools that can be used for this purpose.

Another approach is Michael Porter's framework, shown in exhibit 7.13. Developed around the start of the 1980s, the model identifies five competitive forces, the first of which is the threat of new entrants. At any given time, organizations in a market are competing for similar resources. When new entrants arrive, the existing organizations need to be aware of and prepared for what might happen. For instance, UnitedHealth arrived in the Brazilian market in 2012 after buying a major insurance/HMO company called Amil (Elton

EXHIBIT 7.13
Porter's
Five Forces
Framework

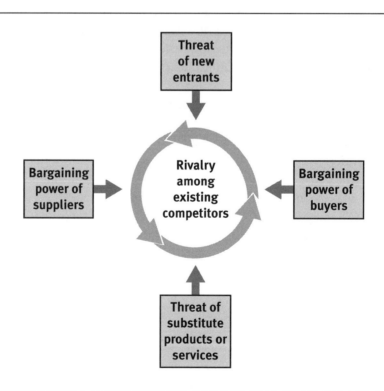

Source: Adapted from Porter (2008).

2017). Since then, United/Amil and all the other insurers in Brazil (i.e., their competitors) have been preparing for what might change as a result of new competitors entering the market. Two other forces in Porter's framework are the bargaining power of suppliers and buyers, respectively. Continuing our example, Amil had to undergo a long process of reorganization to satisfy its buyers, because they are among the company's most important stakeholders. This reorganization had a major influence on the company's purchasing power. The fourth force in Porter's model is the threat of substitute products or services, because substitutes cause changes in the supply of services. Finally, the fifth force is rivalry among existing competitors. The events of the United/Amil example occurred in a market where the rivalry among competitors was not as important as the other forces. However, the rivalry grew in importance as an economic crisis arrived and the number of (potential) clients was reduced.

Once an organization has thoroughly assessed its internal and external environments, consulted its directional statements to ensure strategic alignment, and set its organizational strategies, it can move forward with the implementation and communication of strategic decisions. The operational implementation is discussed elsewhere in this book, particularly in chapter 8, which focuses on operations management, process design, and quality improvement. The remainder of this chapter will discuss the communications strategy, or marketing, which is equally critical for success.

Strategic Marketing

What do you think of when you hear the word *marketing*? The term carries different connotations around the world, and it is most commonly associated with the advertising of consumer goods, such as Coca-Cola, Nike products, or Toyota automobiles. Marketing, however, represents much more than that. According to the American Marketing Association (AMA 2017), marketing is "the activity, set of institutions, and processes for creating, communicating, delivering, and exchanging offerings that have value for customers, clients, partners, and society at large." Marketing is much more comprehensive than simply the advertisement of goods and services. Advertising may be an important part of a marketing plan, but it is only one component.

If a healthcare organization is to have a strong focus on the customer (i.e., the patient, insured, client, resident, or taxpayer), a marketing plan must come first in its overall strategic plan (Hillestad and Berkowitz 2013). However, the field of healthcare has not always acknowledged the critical role of marketing. Traditionally, people have often been uncomfortable associating the concept of marketing with healthcare. Many cultures have felt that healthcare is not supposed to be treated as a "market" and that organizations are not supposed to "compete" against one another when providing such an important public good. Physicians in Latin America have been known to say, "Markets are places where you buy fish—they should have nothing to do with healthcare!" At the highest level, however, marketing is really about communicating key messages and achieving buy-in and behavior change. Marketing in healthcare might include efforts to persuade consumers to choose one clinic over another, but it also includes activities intended to convince policymakers that a hospital is bringing value to its community and to taxpayers. In some areas, marketing includes important efforts to convince tribal leaders to endorse childhood vaccinations. Kotler and Levy (1969) were the first to discuss marketing in the context of nonprofits. After that point, marketing slowly became a more important part of healthcare organizations' strategic plans.

If marketing concepts are to be useful in global healthcare, particularly in the not-for-profit sphere, we need to clearly define the "customer" or "audience." In the world of traditional consumer products, marketers refer to their intended audiences as "target markets" likely to purchase their goods. However, marketers in the healthcare sector have generally not conceptualized their audiences in the same way—in part because the consumer of healthcare services (i.e., the patient) usually differs from the payer (i.e., the insurance company, government agency, or other source of funds). For healthcare marketers, the target audience is a diverse group that consists of patients, physicians, other providers, insurers, policymakers, caregivers, and family members. It includes not just the actual users of healthcare services but also the host of individuals who influence the users' decisions. A comprehensive strategic marketing plan in healthcare will address most, if not all, of these audiences. As we continue our discussion into the areas of buyer behavior, market research, segmentation, and targeting, we will examine the details of these various audiences and the ways their unique needs can be addressed.

Market Strategy and the Ansoff Matrix

The objectives of an organization's marketing plan cascade from the organization's overarching strategic planning objectives, and a variety of approaches and market strategies have sought to help organizations achieve these objectives. One of the earliest approaches is Igor Ansoff's market strategy matrix, first published in 1957 (Ansoff 1957; Bennett 1994).

The appropriateness of a market strategy is heavily influenced by the nature of the product/service and by whether that product/service will be introduced in an existing market or a new one. These two factors affect the responses, psychology, and buyer behavior of consumers (and nonconsumer buyers) and therefore need to be incorporated in the organization's choice of market strategy and resulting promotional plans. Based on these concepts, the Ansoff matrix consists of four quadrants defined by whether the market is new or existing and whether the product/service is new or existing. The various quadrants correspond with market strategies—market penetration, market development, product development, and diversification—that are considered likely to be appropriate. Exhibit 7.14 shows the Ansoff matrix and provides descriptions and examples of the market strategies.

Buyer Beliefs and Behavior

A variety of factors influence audience members' perspectives and beliefs, which in turn influence their attitudes and decisions about healthcare goods and services. Such factors include culture, ethnicity, race, political system (and healthcare system design), socioeconomic status, age/generation, gender, and lifestyle, among other things (Hsairi et al. 2003; Westing et al. 2004; Wong-Kim, Sun, and DeMattos 2003; Kotler, Shalowitz, and Stevens 2008). Audiences' attitudes and beliefs about healthcare services are influenced not only by their individual-level characteristics but also by the characteristics of the countries where they live. In Japan, for example, consumers have traditionally placed a significant value on frequent wellness checks with a primary care physician (Public Broadcasting System 2008). By contrast, consumers in the United States have traditionally sought consultation from a physician only when they experience symptoms of a health problem. Since the passage of the Affordable Care Act of 2010, many health marketers and health promoters in the United States are campaigning to change this behavior and make routine

	Existing Market	New Market
Existing Product	**Market penetration** Providing more of an existing product/service into an existing market Example: St. Louis Children's Hospital launching a new promotional campaign for its pediatric intensive care unit (PICU) services in the greater St. Louis area (emphasizing ambulance services that more commonly choose competitor's PICU)	**Market development** Taking an existing product/service into a new market Example: Hospital Infantil Sabará opening a new hospital in Rio de Janeiro, starting with the service lines that have been most successful in São Paulo
New Product	**Product development** Providing a new product/service in an existing market Example: Austral Hospital introducing a new state-of-the-art diagnostic imaging center to serve the Buenos Aires metro area	**Diversification** Providing a new product/service in a new market Example: Dr. Lal PathLabs developing a new, faster, more economical tuberculosis test for lower-income regions around Palakkad in Kerala State

EXHIBIT 7.14
Market Strategies

Source: Adapted from Ansoff (1957).

Vignette: Cataract Surgery and Buyer Behavior

During the 1990s and early 2000s, the government of India—in partnership with the World Bank, nongovernmental organizations, and other governments—sought to address the widespread problem of blindness caused by cataracts. In addition to increasing the availability of cataract surgery, proponents needed to influence the beliefs of consumers, who commonly believed that nothing could be done about cataracts.

Initially, treatment was delivered using surgery "camps" that would set up in villages for several days, serve the local population, and then pack and move to another village. This practice resulted in a lack of postsurgical follow-up and poor patient outcomes. To address this problem, more permanent surgery clinics were established, meaning that patients would travel to the surgeons. Better intraocular lenses and surgical procedures also developed over time.

Success of this initiative required a concerted marketing campaign to educate consumers about the clinical advancements and to convince them that outcomes were vastly improved and surgical risks diminished. By the end of the seven-year campaign, more than 15 million people had received much-needed cataract surgeries, and the proportion performed with the newer, improved technique rose from 3 percent at the beginning to more than 40 percent at the end (Levine 2007).

---

wellness visits the new norm. For such an effort to be effective, the marketing plan must identify the attitudes and beliefs of the target audience(s) and explain how those will be accounted for when crafting messages and selecting the media with which to deliver those messages.

Market Research

market research
The process of identifying the information needs for successful market planning, identifying sources of data, collecting the data, and then analyzing and acting on the data.

Market research is the process of identifying the information needs for successful market planning, identifying sources of data, collecting the data, and analyzing and acting upon the data. Market research data are important for identifying the market and its needs, segmenting the market into identifiable and logical audiences, targeting the most appropriate segments, and then understanding the perceptions and decision-making processes of members of the targeted segments (including consumer and nonconsumer audiences).

The first step in market research is generally epidemiological—identifying a potential need in a market. In healthcare, disease prevalence is a good starting point. A marketer can begin the research process by identifying the population affected by a disease and then narrowing the focus to the portion with the interest or ability to take action (taking into account such issues as access to care). The marketer should also consider the competitive dynamics of the market, as discussed in the next section. The presence of another competitor nearby will greatly reduce the portion of people with actionable needs that the organization will be able to serve. Exhibit 7.15 lists many of the factors that marketers in healthcare must consider when conducting market research and forecasting demand. All of these factors—whether geographic, demographic, psychographic, or behavioral—have important impacts on healthcare service demand and utilization.

A key early step in market research is **market sizing**—assessing the total potential need of the community. Secondary data sources, including epidemiological data, are extremely important for assessing the prevalence and incidence of disease and other health needs. In the United States, much of this data comes from the Centers for Disease Control and Prevention and from state and county health departments. For example, a health system seeking to

market sizing
A step in the market research process that aims to assess the total potential need of a community.

EXHIBIT 7.15
Factors Affecting Utilization of Healthcare Services

Geographic	Nation or country
	State or region
	City or metro size
	Density
	Climate
Demographic	Age, race, gender
	Income, education
	Family size
	Family life cycle
	Occupation
	Religion, nationality
	Generation
	Social class
Psychographic	Lifestyle
	• Activities
	• Interests
	• Opinions
	Personality
	Core values
Behavioral	Occasions
	Benefits
	User status
	Usage rate
	Loyalty status
	Buyer readiness
	Attitude

Source: Adapted with permission from Kotler, Shalowitz, and Stevens (2008).

establish new diabetes care clinics or dialysis centers needs to first understand the prevalence and incidence of diabetes and kidney failure in various geographic areas. Ideally, these data would help them prioritize which areas to serve.

Once the total market has been sized, the marketer estimates what proportion of the market will act upon its need. For example, not all people with diabetes will seek out the preventive care services offered at the diabetes care clinic. Those who choose to take action will fill their needs in different ways. Some will self-manage their disease with diet and exercise, some will go to competitors, and some will come to the marketer's clinics. Whereas sizing the total market is relatively easy, determining what subset of that market is realistically addressable by the marketer's firm is one of the marketer's greatest challenges. In some markets, government or industry associations may provide valuable market share data to assist with this effort (see the accompanying vignette for one example). Exhibit 7.16 lists several sources of market research data relevant to healthcare in the United States. Similar sources are available in many other countries.

Vignette: Missouri's Hospital Industry Data Institute

The Hospital Industry Data Institute (HIDI), founded by the Missouri Hospital Association, collects a wide array of data about hospitals in Missouri, and it also collaborates with other states' hospital associations to aggregate additional data. HIDI's collection of data includes information about the attributes of hospitals themselves (from the Annual Licensing Survey), utilization data (including hospital discharges and utilization of emergency and specialty services), and compiled analysis for benchmarking hospitals against one another. Secondary market research data available through HIDI can help hospitals with their strategic market planning, including the assessment of demand for specific healthcare services by service line, as well as competitors' market shares. This information is extremely valuable for organizations pursuing market penetration or market development strategies in the areas served by HIDI (Missouri Hospital Association 2017).

Competition

The analysis of competitors is an important component of the market research function. Marketers of healthcare services need to carefully consider how the addressable market is likely to be split between the various competitors. In the context of this chapter, we define *competitor* as any substitute or alternative choice that customers may use to meet the need in question. For example, a

Centers for Disease Control and Prevention—Data and Statistics	www.cdc.gov/datastatistics/	**EXHIBIT 7.16** Market Research Data Sources in the United States
Center for Health Care Strategy—Fact Sheet on Health Literacy	www.chcs.org/media/CHCS_Health_Literacy_Fact_Sheets_2013.pdf	
Central Intelligence Agency—*The World Factbook*	www.cia.gov/library/publications/the-world-factbook/	
Google AdWords	https://support.google.com/adwords/	
National Health Expenditure Data	www.cms.gov/Research-Statistics-Data-and-Systems/Statistics-Trends-and-Reports/NationalHealthExpendData/nhe-fact-sheet.html	
US Census Bureau—Interactive Population Map	www.census.gov/2010census/popmap/	
US Census Bureau—QuickFacts	www.census.gov/quickfacts/	
WebPageFX—Online Marketing Infographics	www.webpagefx.com/data/	
Salary Estimator	www.salary.com/category/salary/	
Psychographics: Weber-Shandwick Report on Millennial Moms	https://www.webershandwick.com/uploads/news/files/MillennialMoms_ExecSummary.pdf	

cardiac surgery center might consider other surgery centers as its main competition. However, some cardiologists and primary care physicians might dissuade patients from pursuing surgery and instead promote drug therapies as a potential substitute. Therefore, the surgery center's marketing plan needs to include drug therapies (and clinicians who prefer them) in its assessment of competition.

Segmentation and Targeting

Market segmentation is the process of using all the information gathered about a market to divide it into identifiable, actionable subgroups. Segmentation may be based on geographic areas (e.g., urban vs. rural, north-metro vs. south-metro) or governmental boundaries (e.g., county, state, or national borders); the latter may be especially appropriate if licensing or other regulatory differences between areas would affect the marketing or delivery of services or products. Demographics are also highly useful in the segmentation process. For instance, research indicates that women make most of the healthcare decisions in modern households (Rappleye 2015), so market segmentation based on gender might help a healthcare organization develop appropriate marketing

market segmentation
The process of using the information gathered about a market to divide it into identifiable, actionable subgroups.

strategies. Other bases for segmentation may include socioeconomic status, culture/ethnicity, age group, psychographics, and purchasing behaviors. For nonconsumer markets, segmentation might involve job type or specialty (e.g., hospital purchasing agent, surgeon, specialist, hospital administrator, national health system policymaker).

When defining segments, marketers should note that a segment is only useful if it is large enough to warrant the additional financial and human capital needed to customize a part of the marketing plan toward it. Pursuit of a particular segment is not worthwhile if it has too few people, if the people have no ability to take action, or if its needs, attitudes, and beliefs are too similar to those of other segments (Kotler, Shalowitz, and Stevens 2008).

targeting
The process of prioritizing market segments and deciding which to pursue first.

Targeting is the subsequent step of prioritizing the segments that have been identified and deciding which to pursue first. Marketers need to systematically decide which segments to pursue, or at least prioritize the segments based on how their characteristics match with the organization and its strategic objectives. At this point, the process is closely tied to the environmental analyses discussed earlier in the chapter (e.g., SWOT analysis) (Kolter, Shalowitz, and Stevens 2008).

The development of a strategic marketing plan is not a simple, linear process. At multiple points, earlier sections need to be revisited as the later sections unfold. In addressing target segments, for instance, the marketer must circle back to market research and buyer behavior and decision making. Using existing data (internal or external) and possibly gathering new data through primary research, the marketer needs to study the targeted segments to understand their needs, how they think, how they feel (especially about the organization), and what they perceive (Fortenberry 2010). The marketer needs to ask: What will the target market's decision-making process be like as individuals decide whether to choose the organization?

Fortenberry's (2010) perceptual map, shown in exhibit 7.17, provides a useful framework for understanding a target audience's perceptions and decision making. The map is based on two product variables, with Variable 1 on the x axis and Variable 2 on the y axis. Variable 1 might be the perceived quality of the good/service, for instance, and Variable 2 might be price (or perceived price). Different audiences will have different decision-making processes, and their purchasing decisions will weigh the two variables differently—thus, the decisions will be at different points on the perceptual map. Using Fortenberry's map to estimate the position of one's own organization (or specific products/ services) relative to competitors can be a useful exercise. The results should influence the marketing strategy and, more specifically, the promotional plan.

Once the market has been segmented, the prioritized segments targeted, and the target audience's perceptions and decision-making processes mapped, the marketer can proceed to the "four *Ps*" section of the strategic marketing plan.

EXHIBIT 7.17
Perceptual Map

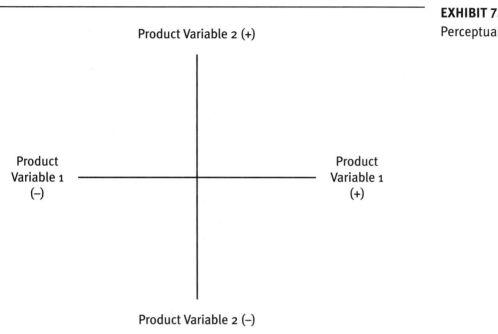

Product Variable 2 (+)

Product Variable 1 (−)

Product Variable 1 (+)

Product Variable 2 (−)

Source: Reprinted with permission from Fortenberry (2010).

The Four *P*s of Marketing

The four *P*s of marketing are product, price, place, and promotion. The concept of the four *P*s developed in traditional consumer goods marketing, but it remains relevant for healthcare products and services. A healthcare marketing plan needs to address all four of the *P*s, though they will not be of equal importance for every plan. For instance, place (or distribution) might be simple for a heart transplant service line but complicated for a wheelchair manufacturer with global markets. Product, price, place, and promotion will be examined in greater detail in the sections ahead.

Product

In the healthcare field, the term *product* refers not only to tangible, physical products but also to intangible services—and even ideas, philosophies, and brands. When planning new products, the market research function is critically important. Products should be developed to meet specific needs of the market, with careful consideration of the organization's and its competitors' strengths and weaknesses. The nature of healthcare, however, introduces significant complexities. Often, we must work with existing products as they are, with little ability to modify them. Consider, for example, an organization that has a well-established and high-quality interventional cardiology service line.

Regardless of whether the product is relatively static or still in formation, the marketer still must analyze and clearly articulate the customer-relevant product attributes. The marketing plan should include a thorough assessment of the strengths and weaknesses of the product relative to customers' needs and expectations, as well as relative to competitors.

The Product Life Cycle

All products, including healthcare services, go through a life cycle. The cycle starts with the introduction stage, then moves into growth and maturity stages, and finally enters the decline stage (see exhibit 7.18). The life cycle stage has a significant impact on the pricing strategy, the place/distribution strategy, and the promotional mix, as well as on other products in the product portfolio.

The strategies and marketing plan for a product in the introduction stage will be significantly different from those for a product in maturity. A product in the introduction stage is not yet widely understood by the target market, so the marketing strategy will need to incorporate education efforts. Consider, for instance, the introduction of the da Vinci surgical robot in 2000 (Mayo Clinic 2018). When the system was first introduced, marketers needed to build awareness, and surgeons and hospital administrators needed to learn the system's technical and clinical advantages, as well as how it could aid in attracting surgeons and patients. Personal selling (which will be discussed in greater detail in the section on promotion) is also an important part of marketing this type

EXHIBIT 7.18
Product Life
Cycle

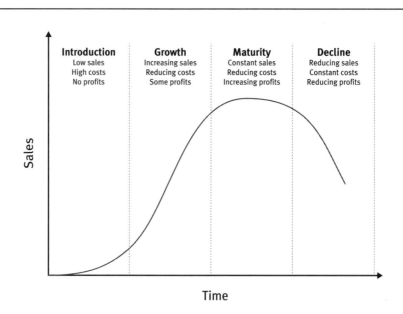

of product. Personal selling is costly, but a product in the introduction stage typically has higher margins and may warrant such an approach.

Now consider a product in the maturity stage, such as hospital linens or socks. At maturity, the market has more competitors, the target audiences are more familiar with the product, and margins are typically lower than they once were. If the product category has little room for further innovation, the marketing is less about educating the audience and more about reminding the audience of its need (or potential future need) and reinforcing the organization's brand as the preferred source for purchasing. Consider the example of aspirin. Everyone knows what aspirin is, but frequent mass-market reminders about the Bayer brand can keep it top-of-mind and support the perception that it is superior to the generic.

The Product Portfolio

As products move through the life cycle, they need to be considered both on their own terms and also in the context of the other products and services offered by the organization. The full line of products offered by an organization is often called the **product portfolio**. A marketing strategy for a single product does not exist in isolation. The marketing plan, therefore, needs to take into account the ways that the pricing, distribution, and promotion of one product might affect the other products in the portfolio. Consider the example of a new natural birthing center. Marketing of the new center might attract women who previously had not been drawn to the hospital's traditional maternity services. However, successful marketing might also have the effect of "cannibalizing" some portion of the organization's existing obstetrics and gynecology business volume.

product portfolio
The full line of products offered by an organization.

Price

Most of the time, when we think about "price," we only consider the amount of money needed to purchase a product. However, price also includes other considerations—other sacrifices that a customer might have to "pay" in addition to the financial price. Such considerations are especially prevalent in healthcare. In most cases, healthcare products are not things that people earnestly wish to consume; with few exceptions, they are products that people consume only if and when they must. (A person would never buy an extra round of chemotherapy just because it was priced at 50 percent off!) Furthermore, in most countries, at least some of the financial prices of healthcare products are fixed by government, often at no cost to the patient. Therefore, we need to look at the other "prices" that consumers pay for healthcare:

- *Time costs.* The time a person spends receiving healthcare represents the loss of time that could be spent doing other things. The loss of time that could be spent working could also mean lost wages.

- *Travel costs.* With relatively few exceptions (e.g., home care services, home-delivered drugs), most healthcare products require the customer to travel. Therefore, the costs associated with private or public transportation, parking, and so on, need to be considered as costs of the product.
- *Discomfort/anxiety/stigma.* Even if patients bear little or no economic cost associated with consuming a healthcare product, they may still be hesitant. Often, patients might not want others in the community to know (or assume) that they have a medical condition. These types of concerns are commonly associated with mental/behavioral health services and sexually transmitted infection testing. This type of cost may vary by segment, as customs and beliefs differ from one group to another.
- *Economic price.* Even if government or private insurance pays most of the economic cost for healthcare services, most countries have at least a nominal price paid by customers at the point of service. Pricing strategies can be an important part of the product portfolio.

When an organization has the latitude to set its prices, the following seven-step process by Kotler, Shalowitz, and Stevens (2008) provides a useful model:

1. Select the pricing objective.
2. Determine demand.
3. Estimate costs.
4. Analyze competitors' costs, prices, and offers.
5. Decide whether to use price as a competitive strategy.
6. Select a pricing method.
7. Select the final price.

penetration pricing
A pricing strategy that involves setting a low price with the goal of quickly gaining market share.

skimming
A pricing strategy that involves setting a high price, often because of intellectual property protections, lack of competitors, or a desire to establish a sense of "prestige" around an organization or product.

Although detailed discussion of the pricing process is beyond the scope of this text, a summary of the seven steps is provided here.

The Pricing Objective
In the first step, the organization needs to decide what it aims to accomplish with its price. **Penetration pricing** involves setting a low price with the goal of quickly gaining market share—in other words, charging a low price to pull volume away from competitors. **Skimming**, on the other hand, involves setting a high price, often because of intellectual property protections, lack of competitors, or a desire to establish a sense of "prestige" around an organization or product. The danger of penetration pricing is that, if a price is unsustainably low, the organization will have to raise it over time, likely causing discontent

among customers and driving some of the customers to competitors. Skimming also has its risks, however. High prices might have the effect of attracting new competitors, failing to gain the desired volume of sales, or setting such high expectations that customers are disappointed. One pricing approach common in healthcare is **parity pricing**—making prices as close as possible to those of competitors.

parity pricing
A pricing strategy that involves setting prices as close as possible to those of competitors.

Determine Demand

In the section of the chapter on market research, we discussed the use of an epidemiological approach to estimate the potential demand in a market. If a firm has experience in a particular product line, it might already have historical data to help determine what demand might be. An organization might also be able to use industry data to gain a better understanding of local or statewide volumes for the product in question (such as the Missouri HIDI data, discussed in an earlier vignette). From these volumes, utilization rates (per 1,000 or 10,000 population) can be calculated and applied to a particular market area.

Estimate Costs

One of the most important parts of the marketing plan is the financial forecast. A crucial point involves whether costs are largely fixed or more variable. The marketer must work with the finance or accounting departments to estimate all the relevant elements of cost that will be related to the product or service line in question. The marketer needs to pay close attention to volume-driven changes in costs. Imagine, for example, that $10 million is to be invested in facilities and staffing and that this amount enables the service line to produce 30,000 patient visits per year (and that most of that cost is fixed, rather than variable), resulting in a modest positive margin. If pricing decisions cause volume to decrease to 15,000 patients, the net effect could be deep financial losses. At the same time, if prices are so low that demand exceeds the 30,000 capacity, the organization will be busy but unable to see more than 30,000 patients—thus, the margin will be lower on a per-patient basis, also resulting in financial losses for the organization.

Analyze Competitors' Costs, Prices, and Offers

Marketers need to consider the positioning of their prices relative to the prices of competitors. If their prices are lower than those of competitors, they may be choosing to lose money on the product/service line, or their cost structure may be lower, thereby enabling lower prices. If the organization believes its product or service is sufficiently superior to that of competitors to justify a higher price, market research is warranted to confirm that the superior features are, in fact, valued by the market. Many a physician—and marketer—has launched a new service line with great faith that its features would command a premium price. Only when it was too late did they learn that the market either did not sufficiently understand the superior features or did not value them enough to justify switching or paying a premium price.

Decide Whether to Use Price as a Competitive Strategy

Generally in healthcare, price is not a highly important aspect of the marketing message, partially because consumer demand tends to be relatively price inelastic. Consumers are often isolated from the true cost of healthcare services. In addition, many organizations—especially large, well-established provider organizations—prefer to avoid price wars and therefore choose not to focus their competitive strategy on price. However, for some organizations, especially start-ups, price can be a primary element of their competitive strategy. For example, independent outpatient imaging centers often focus their messaging on the customer's ability to save money by avoiding traditional, hospital-based imaging departments.

Select a Pricing Method

value pricing
The practice of setting the price for a good or service based on buyers' perceived value.

Theoretically, prices should be set by the market at buyers' perceived value for the good or service—a practice known as **value pricing**. This method also helps resolve questions about the true value of new, unique features. However, all too often, prices give little consideration to the customer. One of the most common legacy pricing methods is **mark-up pricing**. In this method, the cost of producing the good or service is computed and simply grossed up by an amount to allow for any additional fixed costs that must be allocated to it, and to add a margin. A more financially coherent strategy (though still divorced from the customer's concerns) is **target return pricing**. Here, the organization computes costs and projected volumes and then prices the service or good such that the targeted margin or return on investment is achieved. We advocate for value pricing, since it is customer focused and, therefore, should be more sustainable over the long term.

mark-up pricing
A pricing method in which the cost of producing a good or service is computed and grossed up by an amount to allow for additional fixed costs and to add a margin.

target return pricing
A pricing method in which the organization computes costs and projected volumes and then prices the service or good such that a targeted margin or return on investment is achieved.

Select the Final Price

Marketers must carefully consider any concerns and issues raised in the earlier steps and then choose the pricing strategy that best meets the needs of the market and the organization itself (Kotler, Shalowitz, and Stevens 2008). In some cases, the organization will have no control over the price of its products (at least for some customers). For instance, in the United States, federal and state governments, respectively, set the prices they will pay for products covered by the Medicare and Medicaid programs. These prices apply to services rendered to about half the US population, including the elderly and the disabled—two patient groups with the highest utilization rates for healthcare services. In many other countries, including the United Kingdom, national health insurance or national health system structures set the prices for reimbursement to providers. In these cases, the price section of the marketing plan can be simple:

The organization is a price taker, as are its competitors. Differentiation and competitive advantage will need to be found elsewhere.

Place/Distribution

The third of the four *P*s of marketing is place, or the distribution channel that gets most of the goods or services from the point of production to the point of consumption. In healthcare, place is relatively simple and straightforward: Most services are provided directly to consumers (patients) by the producer (clinical staff). This distribution model can be described as a **direct channel**. In these cases, the place section of the marketing plan will likely be quite brief. For example, a family medicine physician might provide her services directly to patients in her medical office. In other cases, however, the distribution model might be more complex. For instance, a cancer patient might receive some consultation services at the physician's office, but other services in a cancer care bundle might be provided at a hospital or surgery center, or at an infusion center. Physical healthcare products generally have more complex paths of distribution. Products such as durable medical equipment (e.g., wheelchairs, crutches, prosthetics) and pharmaceuticals go through complicated, multi-link chains of distribution.

direct channel
A distribution model in which services are provided directly to consumers by the producer.

The three general distribution models are **intensive distribution**, in which the product is available in as many outlets as possible; **selective distribution**, in which the product is available only through select outlets; and **exclusive distribution**, in which the product is only available through one outlet or very few outlets (University of Minnesota Libraries 2015). The marketer's decision about a distribution model is influenced by the customer's decision-making process, and it has significant impacts on capital requirements, brand positioning in the market, and customers' access.

intensive distribution
A distribution model in which a product is available in as many outlets as possible.

Consider aspirin, for instance, a common consumable health product in the mature phase of the product life cycle (or potentially decline). Consumers put little thought or planning into their decision to purchase aspirin, and the analgesic market is highly competitive between brand name drugs and generics. This environment calls for an intensive distribution model, which keeps the product readily available at any corner store or shopping center and requires very little effort on the part of the customer. Contrast this approach with the strategy used for Permobil's high-end motorized wheelchairs. The need to customize products for individual customers and the desire to maintain the image of a premium brand led Permobil to a more exclusive distribution model, in which the product is available only through a small number of select dealers.

selective distribution
A distribution model in which a product is available only through select outlets.

exclusive distribution
A distribution model in which a product is only available through one outlet or very few outlets.

Promotion

The fourth *P* is promotion, the most visible part of the marketing plan. Earlier in the chapter, we emphasized that marketing is not the same as advertising, and many aspects of marketing we have discussed thus far have had little to do with communications to potential customers. The effective communication of messages to targeted market segments or audiences is the primary aim of the promotion mix. This mix includes advertising and a number of other elements in the marketer's tool chest.

Personal Selling

When a product is complex, very costly, high margin, or early in the product life cycle, personal selling is likely to play an important role in its promotion. Consider, again, the example of high-end Permobil wheelchairs, which are represented by a personal sales team at conferences around the world. Personal representation to policymakers and distributors helps ensure that unique individual concerns are addressed and that the product can successfully be made available to consumers and their caregivers in every market. Personal selling is particularly important when the product must be customized to meet the unique needs of individuals (as with the Permobil wheelchairs) or when the message itself must be customized to address individuals' needs and concerns.

Public Relations and Publicity

Public relations (PR) and publicity have historically been the most pervasive elements of the promotional mix in healthcare. PR and publicity efforts include such things as press releases, interviews with media, and sometimes public events (described in the next section). A unique advantage of communication through PR is its credibility, because the audience regards the information somewhat like news, in that it has not been paid for or filtered by the organization. Communication generated through PR is sometimes called "earned media," in contrast to other elements of the promotional mix that might be termed "paid media" or "unearned media." A successful long-term PR strategy involves cultivating strong relationships with members of the media (i.e., media relations) and regularly making spokespersons and experts within the organization (e.g., clinicians, administrators) available for interviews. Marketers should avoid the temptation to reply "no comment" to the media. When something happens in the organization or the community, even if it is bad news, the organization should embrace the opportunity to engage transparently with the media—and, when doing so, it should always be honest.

Sales Promotions and Events

Sales promotions and events are not ongoing activities but rather specific happenings and limited-time offers. For instance, by participating in a community health fair or a fundraising event for a cancer society, a healthcare organization can establish itself as a good corporate citizen of the community while also improving community awareness of the organization in general or certain products or initiatives in particular (e.g., a new cancer center or oncologist).

Sales promotions have long been a staple in the consumer goods industries, and we see it constantly in the advertising around us—buy-one-get-one-free offers, discount coupons, free trial of product X with every purchase of product Y, "rewards points" for every purchase, and so on. Entire companies—Groupon, for instance—have been built on the concept of sales promotions. These tactics are less common in healthcare than in traditional consumer goods, but plenty of opportunities exist. Consider the following possibilities:

- Free mammograms during breast cancer awareness month
- Discounted health insurance premiums when a patient receives a health screening
- An offer where the patient pays for Lasik surgery on one eye and gets surgery on the other eye for free
- A multiple-child visit offer, where a pediatrician sees multiple children together for back-to-school wellness checkups for a single copayment

Direct Marketing

Originally, direct marketing involved the mailing of advertising pieces to consumers' homes. Over time, however, it has evolved to include telephone marketing, emails, text messages, and chat requests. Direct marketing can be used in conjunction with sales promotions, and it is often effective for introducing new products and services (e.g., a newly opened physician office).

Advertising

The most widely recognized element of the marketing mix is advertising. Advertising can take a variety of forms, and the effectiveness of each form depends on the product, the target audience, and the situation. Often, methods will be ideal for certain target audiences but ineffective for others. Exhibit 7.19 presents some of the advantages and disadvantages of advertising, along with those of other promotional tools.

In addition to the traditional forms of advertising, the internet and social media have expanded the variety of media with which to do promotion. Web-based and social media marketing methods offer some significant advantages over older, legacy media, but many of the same concepts apply. **Search engine optimization (SEO)** is an important concept in web-based marketing, and it involves the careful use of words on an organization's website to ensure that the site will appear high on the list of internet search results for a particular product or category. Though it has no direct cost, SEO can be labor intensive. Making sure that the organization remains high in the search results can be an ongoing challenge, given the dynamic nature of internet content and search behaviors. **Search engine marketing (SEM)** is similar to SEO, but it is a paid

search engine optimization (SEO)
The practice of carefully using words on an organization's website to ensure that the site will appear high on the list of search results for a particular product or category.

search engine marketing (SEM)
A form of advertising in which an organization pays for prominent placement on internet search engine pages.

EXHIBIT 7.19
Advertising and Other Promotional Tools: Pros and Cons

Advertising		Personal Selling		Public Relations		Sales Promotion	
Pros	Cons	Pros	Cons	Pros	Cons	Pros	Cons
Attracts new customers	Expensive	Personal service to customers	Expensive	Builds reputation for business	Often non-personal	Usually creates good customer response	When many competitors use similar techniques, advantages are minimized
Draws customers into the store	Information is not always clear or complete	Helps customer satisfy a specific need	Can be too persuasive (high pressure)	Creates goodwill in community	Expensive to sponsor major events	Coupons encourage customers to try new products	
Can be directed toward a specific market		Increases sales through suggestion selling		Can obtain free advertising through publicity	One bad publicity item can be disastrous	Free items usually draw many customers	
				Buyer views publicity as less biased than paid advertising		Creates goodwill	

Source: Developed by Steven W. Howard and Joshua Emerson, incorporating information from Berkowitz (2017).

form of advertising. SEM placements, with the word "Ad" next to them, will often appear at the top or bottom of a list of search results on Google. Google's Keyword Planner can help an organization determine the best terms to use in SEO and SEM; Google's AdWords tool can help with planning the budget and placing orders for Google search ads (Google AdWords 2017).

Marketing integration is the practice of tying together all the various elements of an organization's promotional mix. Just as a composer strives to create harmony among the various instruments in an orchestra, an effective marketer strives to ensure that all the elements of the promotional mix reinforce one another and work toward the same objective. The timing, messaging, and "look and feel" of the various elements should be coordinated to support the aims of the marketing campaign and accomplish the organization's strategic goals.

> **marketing integration**
> The practice of tying together the various elements of an organization's promotional mix.

Crafting the Message

Effective promotion requires not only the selection of appropriate elements in the promotional mix but also the crafting of an appropriate message. Messages should be tailored to each segment being targeted and modified as necessary to suit each element in the promotional campaign. Rossiter and Percy (1997) emphasize four components of an effective message. First, the message needs to establish the category need, helping consumers realize or remember that they have a need for a certain type of product or service (e.g., "Having a baby is one of the most exciting moments in your life. . . ."). Second, the message must establish brand awareness, impressing upon the audience that the organization is an option in the product category. Third, the message should engender a positive brand attitude, making the audience feel that the organization's brand and product could be a positive choice for them (e.g., "Mercy Hospital has been the leading choice of women in the metro area for more than 100 years. . . ."). Fourth, the message, by the time it has been delivered, should inspire the target audience to take action to learn more or to decide in favor of the advertised brand or product (e.g., "Call today to learn more about how Mercy could be the best choice for you and your family during this important time of your life. . . .").

Evaluation

Evaluating the results of a marketing campaign is a critical final step that is too often ignored. The evaluation should link directly back to the goals that were developed in the market strategy section of the plan. Most healthcare organizations, especially nonprofits and governmental entities, have highly constrained resources for marketing. Therefore, marketers need to understand which elements of the promotional mix are most effective and then reallocate resources as appropriate to those elements that yield the best results. A common "gross measure" is to simply monitor changes in sales, admissions, or call volumes during and after a promotional campaign. This approach is imperfect, however, because factors other than the campaign itself might influence the recorded results. Also, this gross measure does not help the marketer understand which of the promotional elements were effective and which were not. A marketer needs approaches that hone in on the effectiveness of each promotional element.

The effectiveness of traditional media campaigns (e.g., direct mail, print, outdoor, broadcast) can be measured by having the audience respond via unique website addresses or telephone numbers. Toll-free numbers can be purchased from vendors, and call volumes can be monitored online. By using different numbers and website addresses for different ad designs, media, and geographic markets, marketers can gain valuable insights about which approaches yield the best results. In general, marketing campaigns should be given a few months to see if they will perform as expected; however, those campaigns that continue to produce paltry results might need to be discontinued so that funds can be reallocated to other approaches that get a better response.

Compared to traditional print formats, electronic media provide significantly greater opportunities for detailed evaluation, often in real time. The technique of "A/B testing" can be used quickly and effectively with online ads and SEM. The marketer can produce "A" and "B" versions of an ad (modifying text, graphics, or whatever is hypothesized to improve the ad's appeal and response rate) and run the versions online simultaneously, with the versions presented to users at random. By tracking the statistics for each, the marketer can quickly determine which version is more appealing to the audience. The low-performing version can then be deleted, and a new "B" version can be put in its place. By iteratively following this process, the marketer can optimize ad designs much more quickly than in the past. Google Analytics can help organizations track the traffic an ad generates (i.e., the click-through rate) and the "stickiness" of website visitors (i.e., how long they remain on the linked web page) (Google AdWords 2017).

Summary

Strategic management in healthcare involves studying the organization's international and external environments (via SWOT and five forces analyses), understanding the needs of customers and other stakeholders, and allocating the available resources in support of the organization's goals and objectives. The organization's directional statements establish the mission, vision, and values upon which the strategic planning process is based. One of the most important aspects of strategic plan implementation is marketing, which encompasses a broad range of activities associated with the creation, communication, delivery, and exchange of products and services. The Ansoff matrix is one of many tools that exist to help organizations develop their market strategies. Once healthcare leaders have identified, researched, and assessed their target audiences, they can implement strategies across the four *P*s of marketing—product, price, place, and promotion—to help achieve their strategic aims. When the principles of marketing are tailored to the unique context of health and healthcare services, they provide an effective model for influencing attitudes, beliefs, and actions in ways that benefit the health of individuals and populations and help the organization achieve its strategic goals.

Discussion Questions

1. How are the SWOT analysis and Porter's five forces framework related to each other?

2. How might Porter's five forces framework help an organization identify opportunities and threats in its external environment?

3. Individually or in groups, review the mission, vision, and values statements from organizations of various countries, profit/nonprofit statuses, and religious affiliations. What are your major observations? In what ways are the statements similar or different? Do you think the differences are deliberate or by chance? Would you propose changing any of them to better suit the organizations or the communities they serve?

4. Individually or in groups, think of a healthcare organization with which you are familiar. Construct mission and vision statements for the organization, taking into account the patient population that the organization serves. What are the most important characteristics you chose to emphasize in your directional statements? Why?

Case Exercise: Environmental Scanning / Internal Analysis
Students should form groups, discuss the following cases, and answer the questions at the end of each.

Case 1
In 2000, hospital and health system managers from the São Paulo, Brazil, and Atlanta, Georgia, metropolitan regions answered questionnaires about strategic management. When the responses were evaluated, the main differences between the two countries were in the following areas: (1) the importance given to strategic planning/management, (2) the amount of health management education the respondents had received, and (3) the use of data systems. Respondents from the two countries had a similar view of future challenges (answers were limited to a horizon of five years). In 2016, Brazilian hospitals were surveyed with the same objective. Use of external databases was still not very popular (even when they belonged to

(continued)

the same network). More hospital managers and planners had taken formal courses in health/hospital management, but strategic management was used more often among the managers of private hospitals than among those of public ones. The balanced scorecard and Lean were the tools most likely to be described as useful, but respondents still had some degree of skepticism about the utility of the BSC in the healthcare field. If you compare the healthcare environment in the year 2000 with that of 2016, what changed?

Case 2

A number of hospitals in Brazil became a network through merger and acquisition. Now, instead of 10 or 12 100-bed hospitals operating independently in different Brazilian states, the group manages approximately 2,000 beds across the entire service area. The fact that it is called a "network" does not mean it is well coordinated: No referral system exists among units, purchasing is independent, logistics are not integrated, professional education is not aligned, and information systems (including medical records) are not connected. If a patient who has been discharged from one hospital shows up at the emergency department of another, his record will not be tracked. What is the rationale for mergers and acquisitions in the hospital field? Is efficiency an important goal? Is it achievable? What steps should a newly merged network like this one take to improve efficiency? What are its next moves?

Case Exercise: Market Segmentation and Buyer Behavior

Students should form groups and discuss the following scenarios. Each group should choose one scenario and submit a written response addressing how the organization in question should segment the market and describing the buying process a member of a prioritized segment would go through.

Scenario 1

A hospital is introducing a new service line in its existing market service area. The hospital has long been a popular choice for maternity services, but the marketing director has heard about a nationwide trend toward all-natural birthing centers (free of epidurals and other pain medications). In the new birthing center, women are primarily aided in labor and delivery by midwives or doulas, and only by physicians when medically necessary.

The labor and delivery rooms are more homelike than traditional patient rooms and are nearly devoid of medical technology.

Scenario 2
A drug manufacturer has developed a new medication to help people with diabetes better manage their HbA1c levels. The drug provides somewhat better results than the standard metformin alone, but it costs approximately double.

Scenario 3
A drug manufacturer is producing a new generic version of ibuprofen that is extended release and will last longer than existing pills.

Scenario 4
An academic medical center with a Level 4 trauma center has added a new trauma surgeon who is a nationally recognized leader in the field. The center has also added new equipment and processes fully in line with evidence-based guidelines.

Case Exercise: Market Strategy

Students should form groups, discuss the following case, and answer the question at the end.

Market development occurs when an organization takes its existing products or services into a new market segment. This strategy is widely used in healthcare, as in the cases of UnitedHealth entering the Brazilian market and the Mayo Clinic opening a new location in Jacksonville, Florida. Market penetration strategies—in which an organization aims to grow its share within an existing market—are also common in healthcare. An example might be a marketing campaign by St. Louis Children's Hospital aiming to attract families who might otherwise take their children for specialty healthcare services at the nearby Cardinal Glennon Children's Hospital.

In their groups, students should choose one or two familiar healthcare organizations and then discuss what strategy or strategies would be most appropriate. What are the advantages and disadvantages of each?

Case Exercise: Product Portfolio Decisions

Students should form groups and discuss the following case in light of what they have learned about strategy and marketing.

Stephanie had just been hired as the new vice president of marketing and strategy at a small, physician-owned Medicare Advantage (MA) health insurance company. One of her first challenges was to revitalize the organization's product portfolio. The portfolio had become stale and was beginning to struggle against large national insurance companies that had recently made aggressive inroads into the local market.

In the MA subsector of the insurance industry, individual beneficiaries have the option to receive their government health insurance benefits through a private health insurer, known as a Medicare Advantage Organization (MAO). When individuals choose this option, the government gives the MAO an amount of funding that approximates the monthly cost of providing care to a beneficiary. In some areas of the country, this monthly capitated payment is more than sufficient to provide a standard health benefits package; in other areas, however, it is insufficient. When the capitated amount is sufficient, the MAO can offer the plan to a beneficiary for no premium (such plans are commonly known as "$0-premium plans"). However, when the capitated amount is short of the cost of providing care, or when the specific benefit plan is more generous (i.e., a "richer benefits plan"), then the MAO must charge a premium to the beneficiary.

When Stephanie arrived on the job, her MAO offered one plan for $59 and another for $85. Just the previous year, however, four different competitors had entered the market with $0-premium plans. Stephanie is conflicted. She would like to win some of the "low end" business in the $0-premium end of the market, but her organization would make less profit on those plans. If she introduces a $0-premium plan next year, she is relatively certain it will cannibalize sales of her organization's two existing plans. Perhaps she should cover the entire pricing continuum—plans at $0, $29, $59, $85, and $115. Or maybe she should stick to the two they already have and simply market them more aggressively.

In approaching this decision, what questions does Stephanie need to answer? What are the advantages and disadvantages of the various options? What would you advise her to do, and why? Consider the external environment and internal issues, as well as the consumers and competition.

Case Exercise: Noneconomic Prices

Students should form groups, discuss this case, and answer the questions posed at the end.

Oregon is a mid-sized, predominantly rural state in the Pacific Northwest region of the United States. The state often struggles economically, and historically it has had higher rates of unemployment and lower rates of insurance coverage than many other states. Under Governor John Kitzhaber, a physician, the government sought to reform its healthcare delivery and payment system to invest in better primary care and prevention, with a long-term goal of improving population health and restraining the ever-increasing cost of care. Although physical, mental/behavioral, and dental health have long been segregated in the US health system, policymakers in Oregon recognized the important interrelationships between them and sought to improve their integration and coordination. A common problem in this area is the stigma that often surrounds mental/behavioral health conditions, which has been known to prevent individuals from seeking care.

The key element of the Oregon health reform model was the coordinated care organization (CCO), which aimed to improve coordination of care by bringing providers of physical, mental/behavioral, dental, and public health together under a shared capitated global budget. Although the design held great promise on paper, the issue of buyer behavior—specifically, care-seeking behavior—remained a challenge, particularly in the area of mental/behavioral health. One of the CCOs served a disproportionately high percentage of Hispanic male blue-collar workers, and research showed that stigma and reluctance to seek mental/behavioral healthcare services were especially high among this demographic.

Two clinics within this CCO piloted a solution. Up to this point, the mental/behavioral health clinic was two blocks away from the main medical clinic, with clear signage on both buildings. Thus, anyone watching could plainly see if a person was going to receive mental/behavioral healthcare. As part of the solution, the clinics colocated their medical doctors and mental/behavioral health professionals in the same office suites, and they trained the medical staff on the symptoms of mental/behavioral health problems. In addition, staff began personally escorting patients to the appropriate professionals within the same building—often just across the hall. As a result of these efforts, the percentage of patients who followed through on referrals for mental/behavioral consultations increased dramatically.

In this case, what role did nonfinancial costs play in individuals' decisions to seek care? How did the CCO's actions influence those costs? Now

(continued)

consider healthcare services from a local organization. Provide an example of a service that seems to have obvious noneconomic costs. Provide another example of a service that appears not to have clear noneconomic costs. Students should discuss their findings in groups.

Case Exercise: Evaluating Effectiveness of Media

Recall Stephanie, the vice president of marketing and strategy at the Medicare Advantage health insurance company from an earlier case exercise. Stephanie revitalized her organization's product portfolio and launched a multifaceted marketing campaign later that year. Because she targets Medicare beneficiaries, who are predominantly elderly, and because older age groups tend to have higher newspaper readership, she chose to make newspapers an important part of the promotional mix.

In her primary market area, Stephanie has two main newspapers to choose from: the local *Hometown Tribune* (which has home delivery in the area) and a newer statewide paper called *The Senior News*. *The Senior News* has the capability to regionalize its paper, so Stephanie can run ads only in the southern region edition, the distribution area of which is closely aligned with her primary service area. Rates for a quarter-page full-color ad are much higher for the *Hometown Tribune* ($1,000) than they are for *The Senior News* ($300). In addition, *The Senior News* is targeted specifically at the older age group, whereas *Hometown Tribune* aims to address all age groups in the primary service area.

Stephanie decided to buy ads for two months in both papers. She put unique toll-free telephone numbers in the two versions of the ad, and both numbers automatically forwarded callers to her organization's main sales and customer service personnel. Each week, Stephanie checked the volume reports on the toll-free number vendor's website. Surprisingly, the number used in the *Hometown Tribune* ad recorded an average of only 3 calls per week (and 1 or 2 of those may have been wrong-number calls, as they were only about 10 seconds in duration). In contrast, *The Senior News* generated 10 to 15 calls per week (again, 1 or 2 were likely wrong numbers). After this pattern persisted for seven weeks during the height of the Medicare Advantage marketing season, Stephanie stopped using the *Hometown Tribune* and reallocated most of the savings to larger and more frequent ads in *The Senior News*.

In groups, students should discuss how Stephanie's actions relate to the marketing concepts described in the chapter. How might Stephanie's promotional mix decisions and ways of evaluating the effectiveness of media have been different if she were targeting a different age group?

Case Exercise: Nuance in Evaluating Effectiveness of Websites

The National Agency for Private Health Insurance and Plans (ANS), a government agency in Brazil, wanted to understand how Brazilians were seeking information about the universal health system and private supplemental plans, so administrators checked the statistics for the ANS website and related web searches. They initially believed their online efforts had failed. The website had only a small number of hits, and search data showed relatively few searches for the ANS name or for supplementary care (the official term used in the Brazilian universal health system for private health plans that supplement the public plan). However, after some discussions with users, the administrators realized the general population did not use the ANS's technical terms when searching; instead, they used more general terms, such as "convênio médico" (the equivalent of "health plan"). Once the administrators gained a better understanding of the public's search habits, the ANS began using the more popular terminology on its websites (thereby improving the agency's position in search results) and in paid advertising (thereby placing the ANS site near the top of the search results pages). These efforts led to a marked improvement in the agency's ability to connect with its intended audience.

What marketing techniques have the ANS administrators used to enhance the agency's online communications? What actions are likely to be necessary in the future?

Additional Resources

ABIM Foundation. 2018. "Choosing Wisely: Promoting Conversations Between Providers and Patients." Accessed June 8. www.choosingwisely.org.

Bisognano, M., and C. Kenney. 2012. *Pursuing the Triple Aim: Seven Innovators Show the Way to Better Care, Better Health, and Lower Costs.* San Francisco: Jossey-Bass.

Elkington, J. 1997. *Cannibals with Forks: The Triple Bottom Line of 21st Century Business.* Oxford, UK: Capstone.

Gawande, A. 2014. *Being Mortal: Medicine and What Matters in the End.* New York: Metropolitan Books.

Kaplan, R. S., and D. P. Norton. 1992. "The Balanced Scorecard: Measures That Drive Performance." *Harvard Business Review* 70 (1): 71–79.

Marmot, M. 2015. *The Health Gap: The Challenge of an Unequal World.* New York: Bloomsbury.

Mintzberg, H., J. Lampel, J. B. Quinn, and S. Ghoshal. 2002. *The Strategy Process: Concepts, Contexts, Cases,* 4th ed. Upper Saddle River, NJ: Prentice Hall.

Moss, M. 2013. *Salt, Sugar, Fat: How the Food Giants Hooked Us.* New York: Random House.

Pena, F. P. M., A. M. Malik, and F. M. Viana. 2016. "Gestão Estratégica em Saúde." In *Gestão em Saúde,* 2nd ed., edited by G. Vecina Neto and A. M. Malik, 113–29. Rio de Janeiro, Brazil: Guanabara Koogan.

Project Management Institute (PMI). 2018. "About Us: What Is Project Management?" Accessed June 8. www.pmi.org/about/learn-about-pmi/what-is-project-management.

Radnor, Z. J., M. Holweg, and J. Waring. 2012. "Lean in Healthcare: The Unfilled Promise?" *Social Science and Medicine* 74 (3) 364–71.

References

All India Institute of Medical Sciences. 2017. "Introduction." Accessed September 5. www.aiims.edu/en/about-us.html?id=91.

American Marketing Association (AMA). 2017. "Definition of Marketing." Accessed September 5. www.ama.org/AboutAMA/Pages/Definition-of-Marketing.aspx.

Andrews, K. R. 1971. *The Concept of Corporate Strategy.* New York: McGraw-Hill.

Ansoff, I. 1957. "Strategies for Diversification." *Harvard Business Review* 35 (5): 113–24.

Ascension. 2017. "Mission, Vision and Values." Accessed September 5. http://ascension.org/living-the-mission/mission-vision-values.

Bennett, A. R. 1994. "Business Planning: Can the Health Service Move from Strategy into Action?" *Journal of Management in Medicine* 8 (2): 24–33.

Berkowitz, E. N. 2017. *Essentials of Health Care Marketing,* 3rd ed. Burlington, MA: Jones & Bartlett Learning.

Christian Medical College, Vellore. 2017. "Vision Statement." Accessed September 5. www.cmch-vellore.edu.

Cleveland Clinic. 2018. "Mission, Vision, Values." Accessed June 14. http://my.clevelandclinic.org/about/overview/who-we-are/mission-vision-values.

Dr. Lal PathLabs. 2017. "About Us." Accessed September 5. www.lalpathlabs.com/about-us.aspx.

Elton, C. 2017. "UnitedHealth Pauses Brazil Acquisition Spree to Strengthen IT." Global Healthcare Insights. Published July 19. https://globalhealthi.com/2017/07/19/unitedhealth-brazil-acquisition-technology/.

Fortenberry, J. L. Jr. 2010. *Health Care Marketing: Tools and Techniques.* Sudbury, MA: Jones & Bartlett.

Fortis Healthcare. 2018. "About Us." Accessed June 8. www.fortishealthcare.com/about-us.

Google AdWords. 2017. "Keyword Planner." Accessed September 5. https://adwords.google.com/home/tools/keyword-planner/.

HCA Healthcare. 2018. "Our Mission and Values." Accessed June 14. http://hcahealth
care.com/about/our-mission-and-values.dot.

Hillestad, S. G., and E. N. Berkowitz. 2013. *Health Care Market Strategy*, 4th ed.
Burlington, MA: Jones & Bartlett Learning.

Hospital Infantil Sabará. 2017. "Missão, Visão e Valores." Accessed September 5. www.
hospitalinfantilsabara.org.br/quem-somos/missao-visao-e-valores/.

Hospital Moinhos de Vento. 2018. "Quem Somos." Accessed June 14. www.hospital
moinhos.org.br/quem-somos/.

Hospital Universitario Austral. 2017. "Institucional." Accessed September 5. www.
hospitalaustral.edu.ar/institucional/.

Hsairi, M., R. Fahfakh, R. Bellaaj, and N. Achour. 2003. "Knowledge, Attitudes and
Behaviours of Women Toward Breast Cancer Screening." *East Mediterranean
Health Journal* 9 (1–2): 87–98.

Institute for Healthcare Improvement (IHI). 2017. "The IHI Triple Aim." Accessed
September 5. www.ihi.org/Engage/Initiatives/TripleAim/Pages/default.aspx.

Instituto de Ortopedia e Traumatologia. 2017. "Missão, Visão e Valores." Accessed September 5. www.iothcfmusp.com.br/pt/institucional/missao-visao-e-valores/.

Jayaraman, V. R. 2014. "5 Things to Know About India's Healthcare System."
Forbes India. Published September 11. www.forbesindia.com/blog/
health/5-things-to-know-about-the-indias-healthcare-system/.

Kaplan, R. S., and D. P. Norton. 1996. *The Balanced Scorecard: Translating Strategy into
Action*. Boston: Harvard Business Review Press.

———. 1992. "The Balanced Scorecard—Measures That Drive Performance." *Harvard
Business Review* 70 (1): 71–79.

Kotler, P., and S. J. Levy. 1969. "Broadening the Concept of Marketing." *Journal of
Marketing* 33 (1): 10–15.

Kotler, P., J. Shalowitz, and R. J. Stevens. 2008. *Strategic Marketing for Health Care
Organizations*. San Francisco: Jossey-Bass.

Levine, R. 2007. *Case Studies in Global Health: Millions Saved*. Sudbury, MA: Jones
& Bartlett Learning.

Mayo Clinic. 2018. "Robotic Surgery." Accessed June 15. www.mayoclinic.org/
tests-procedures/robotic-surgery/about/pac-20394974.

Meliones, J. N., R. Ballard, R. Liekweg, and W. Burton. 2001. "No Mission ↔ No Margin:
It's That Simple." *Journal of Health Care Finance* 27 (3): 21–29.

Merriam-Webster. 2017. "Marketing." Accessed September 5. www.merriam-webster.
com/dictionary/marketing.

Missouri Hospital Association (MHA). 2017. "HIDI Data Collection." Accessed
September 5. http://web.mhanet.com/hidi-data-collection.aspx.

Porter, M. E. 2008. "The Five Competitive Forces That Shape Strategy." *Harvard
Business Review* 86 (1): 78–93.

———. 1979. "How Competitive Forces Shape Strategy." *Harvard Business Review*
57 (2): 137–45.

Public Broadcasting System (PBS). 2008. "Sick Around the World." Accessed September 5, 2017. www.pbs.org/wgbh/pages/frontline/sickaroundtheworld/.

Rappleye, E. 2015. "Women Make 80 Percent of Healthcare Decisions." Published April 13. www.beckershospitalreview.com/hospital-management-administration/women-make-80-percent-of-healthcare-decisions.html.

Rossiter, J. R., and L. Percy. 1997. *Advertising and Promotion Management,* 2nd ed. New York: McGraw-Hill.

Society for Human Resource Management (SHRM). 2012. "Mission & Vision Statements: What Is the Difference Between Mission, Vision and Values Statements?" Accessed September 5. www.shrm.org/resourcesandtools/tools-and-samples/hr-qa/pages/isthereadifferencebetweenacompany%E2%80%99smission,visionandvaluestatements.aspx.

Topol, E. 2015. *The Patient Will See You Now: The Future of Medicine Is in Your Hands.* New York: Basic Books.

University of Minnesota Libraries. 2015. *Principles of Marketing.* Published October 27. http://open.lib.umn.edu/principlesmarketing/.

Westing, M., A. Ahs, K. Bränd Persson, and R. Westerling. 2004. "A Large Proportion of Swedish Citizens Refrain from Seeking Medical Care—Lack of Confidence in the Medical Services a Plausible Explanation?" *Health Policy* 68 (3): 333–44.

Wong-Kim, E., A. Sun, and M. C. DeMattos. 2003. "Assessing Cancer Beliefs in a Chinese Immigrant Community." *Cancer Control* 10 (5 Suppl.): 22–28.

PROCESS DESIGN AND CONTINUOUS QUALITY IMPROVEMENT FOR OPERATIONAL CHANGE IN GLOBAL HEALTH

Eduardo Álvarez-Falcón, MPhil, Mariepi Manolis Cylwik, and Xinliang Liu, PhD

Chapter Focus

This chapter will introduce operations management principles, models, tools, techniques, and methods that are widely used for quality improvement (QI) in global health settings. It will also provide an overview of concepts considered most relevant for students and healthcare managers seeking process improvements that will truly add value for clients, constituents, stakeholders, communities, and the health sector as a whole. Sections of the chapter specifically address the value chain, process and service design, benchmarking, Lean, and Six Sigma. Finally, the chapter will highlight the importance of knowing the level of operational change desired by the organization or system, to aid in the selection of appropriate QI instruments.

Learning Objectives

Upon completion of this chapter, you should be able to

- introduce key operations management concepts to drive operational quality improvements in healthcare processes,
- describe the main operational quality improvement tool kits that have permeated the health sector internationally,
- recognize the value and potential uses of selected quality improvement models in global health settings,
- appraise the mixture of best practices available to face complex healthcare and health system issues, and
- apply effective comprehensive improvement approaches to advances in global health management and policy.

Competencies

- Demonstrate an understanding of the interdependency, integration, and competition that exist among healthcare sectors.
- Demonstrate an understanding of system structure and the organization of healthcare services.
- Understand and balance the interrelationships among access, quality, safety, cost, resource allocation, accountability, care setting, community need, and professional roles.
- Assess the performance of the organization as part of the system of healthcare services.
- Use monitoring systems to ensure that legal, ethical, and quality/safety standards are met in clinical, corporate, and administrative functions.
- Promote the establishment of alliances and the consolidation of networks to expand social and community participation in health networks, both nationally and globally.
- Effectively recognize and promote patients' and their families'/caregivers' perspectives in the delivery of care.
- Include individuals, families, and the community as partners in healthcare decision-making processes, respecting cultural differences and expectations.
- Effectively manage the supply chain to achieve timeliness and efficiency of inputs, materials, warehousing, and distribution so that supplies reach the end user in a cost-effective manner.
- Effectively manage the interdependency and logistics of supply chain services within the organization.
- Develop and implement quality assurance, satisfaction, and patient safety programs according to national initiatives.
- Develop and track indicators to measure quality outcomes, satisfaction, and patient safety, and plan continuous improvement.
- Incorporate management techniques and theories into leadership activities.
- Analyze problems, promote solutions, and encourage decision making.
- Promote ongoing learning and improvement in the organization.
- Respond to the need for change, and lead the change process.

Key Terms

- Benchmarking
- Best in class
- Best practice
- Co-design
- Design thinking
- DMAIC cycle
- Flow
- Inputs
- Jidoka
- Just-in-time (JIT) production
- Kaizen event
- Kanban
- Key success factors (KSFs)
- League table
- Lean
- Lean Six Sigma (LSS)
- Operations management

- Outputs
- Patient journey map
- Plan-do-check-act (PDCA)
- Process design
- Process mapping
- Process redesign
- Pull
- Sensei
- Service blueprint
- Service design
- Six Sigma
- Supply chain management
- Total quality management (TQM)
- Value
- Value chain
- Value system

Key Concepts

- Access to care
- Continuous process improvement
- Continuous quality improvement
- Disruptive improvement
- Effectiveness
- Efficiency
- Incremental improvement
- Innovation

- Operations
- Patient-centered care
- Performance gaps
- Quality
- Statistical process control
- Value-added and non-value-added activities
- Value-based healthcare
- Waste

Introduction

The term *operations*, borrowed from the field of industrial engineering, encompasses all the activities required to create and deliver an organization's products

operations management
The managerial function of creating and delivering an organization's products or services.

or services to its clients. **Operations management**, then, focuses on the function of creating and delivering these products or services.

Products are tangible in nature, whereas services are intangible. Products are produced before they are delivered, whereas services are produced and delivered at the same time. Often in healthcare, products and services do not exist in isolation but rather are combined within a wider array of activities. Given the nature of the healthcare field, this chapter places a greater weight on health services than on health products, though we have aimed to achieve somewhat of a balance.

inputs
The tangible and intangible resources needed to carry out a process or provide a service (e.g., people, expertise, materials, energy, facilities, funds).

The operations management function focuses **inputs**, or resources, being transformed through activities into **outputs**, or outcomes, within the boundaries of closed systems and in relation to opened systems. Thus, operations management is concerned with the design, improvement, and management of the systems that create the organization's products or services, as well as with the ways those systems relate to their environment. The result of an operation's function is measured in terms of the personal, economic, or social value that it produces, depending on whether the organization is in the for-profit or not-for-profit sector.

outputs
The goods, services, or outcomes produced by a system.

Today's global healthcare leaders need to be familiar with—and, over time, master—a repertoire of operational tools if they are to respond effectively to operational challenges and improvement opportunities. This chapter will discuss, in a purposeful order, a number of key tools and concepts to help the reader better understand operations management and its application in the health sector.

The Value Chain and Value System

Michael E. Porter's (1985) value chain model provides a fundamental framework to facilitate better understanding of operations management. A classic management model, it underpins the various operational tools and concepts discussed in this chapter.

value
In competitive terms, the amount that clients (buyers) are willing to pay for what an organization provides them; in not-for-profit terms, the nonmonetary benefit received by clients, constituents, or users.

The Value Chain Model

In competitive terms, **value** is the amount that clients (buyers) are willing to pay for what an organization provides them (Porter 1985). In not-for-profit terms, value is the nonmonetary benefit received by clients, constituents, or users. It may include economic value (e.g., benefits for citizens, government services, prosperity for providers/suppliers, labor) or social value (e.g., community happiness, protection, health, safety). Walters and Lancaster (2000) explain that value represents a preferred combination of benefits compared with acquisition costs. It is the goal for any generic strategy, whether for profit or not for profit.

Two aspects of value are key (Walters and Lancaster 2000):

1. The perceived value, or the utility combination of perceived benefits delivered to the customer through one activity minus the total cost of acquiring the delivered benefits (perceived price). This aspect also takes into account the benefits that would be available through alternative value offers from other sources.
2. The organizational means—primary and support activities, structure, linkages, lines of business, and so on—for maximizing value to customers. Products or services derived from these processes represent the organization's value proposition for its clients.

By matching the means that an organization is able to provide (i.e., its value proposition) with the defined needs and wants of the market or clients and the satisfaction of those needs and wants according to perceived value, we can identify value-driven **key success factors (KSFs)**. These KSFs are sources of competitive advantage and sustainability.

The **value chain** is the sequence of internal organizational activities (e.g., acquiring, producing, selling, delivering, collecting) and external organizational activities (e.g., system relationships) that together create a product or service to meet clients' needs and wants (i.e., demand). By improving inputs, processes, and outputs to satisfy clients, value can be added to the chain of the organization's activities. A simplified representation of the value chain model is shown in exhibit 8.1.

The Value System

An organization rarely undertakes all the activities involved in delivering products or services to the final customer on its own; rather, the organization operates as part of a wider arrangement called the **value system**. The value system is the set of organizational value chain relationships that creates products or services (Johnson and Scholes 2002). It can be viewed as a forward or backward integration of several value chains, with value being added through interrelated products or services to meet a series of client or customer needs.

The management of interface relationships in the value system is called **supply chain management**. It is driven by the need to meet KSFs along the series of chains, and it is facilitated by efficient management of activities and costs to maximize value. In the case of a health system, the supply chain includes activities at various provision levels—such as primary, secondary, and specialized care—as well as other personal and nonpersonal healthcare activities. A simplified supply chain in a healthcare value system is shown in exhibit 8.2. The configurations of the value chain and value system underpin the concepts of process design and process improvement and the way those concepts apply to health organizations and systems.

---

key success factors (KSFs)
A series of factors considered critical for an organization's ability to meet client and customer needs and wants and to achieve sustainability (not for profit) or competitive advantage (for profit).

value chain
The sequence of internal and external organizational activities that together create a product or service to meet clients' needs and wants.

value system
The set of internal and external value chain relationships that work together to create products or services.

supply chain management
The management of interface relationships in the value system.

EXHIBIT 8.1
Simplified Value Chain Model

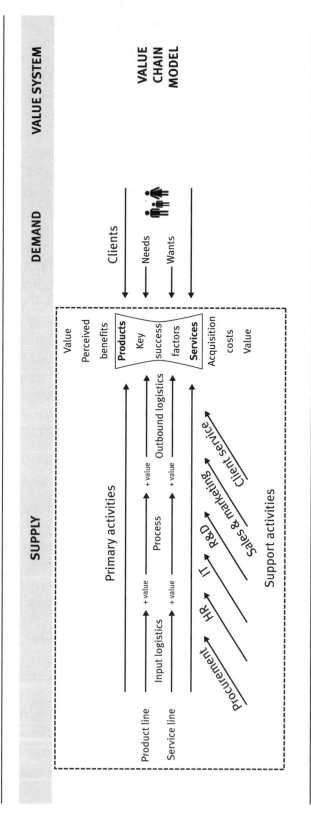

Note: HR = human resources; IT = information technology; R&D = research and development.

Source: Developed by Eduardo Álvarez-Falcón; adapted from Porter (1985).

EXHIBIT 8.2
Simplified Supply Chain in a Value System in Healthcare (primary, hospital, and rehabilitation care)

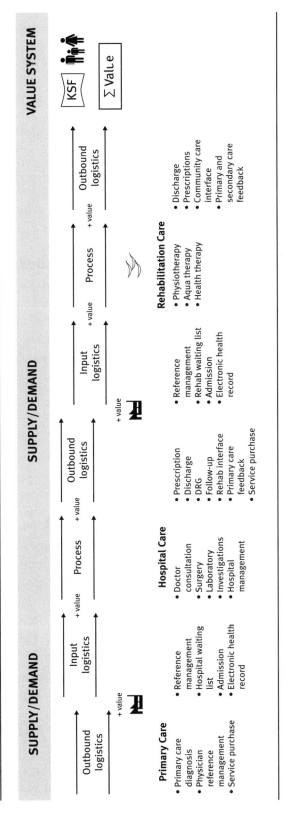

Note: DRG = diagnosis-related group; KSF = key success factor.
Source: Eduardo Álvarez-Falcón.

Process Design in Healthcare

One of the chief concerns of healthcare delivery systems and operations management is the delivery of value, which leads to the question: How do we design services to achieve value-based healthcare? Addressing that question requires familiarity with the disciplines of process design, service design, and design thinking. Those disciplines, their key principles, and the ways they relate to service innovation and improvement are the focus of the upcoming sections.

Value can be an ambiguous term in healthcare, as it may relate to a number of different concerns, such as speed of delivery, technical quality, or cost of care. In this section, we follow Porter's definition of value—patient health outcomes per dollar spent (Porter and Lee 2013).

process design
The discipline focused on the set of processes, actions, and steps to produce a product or service that delivers particular results for the customer.

service design
An emerging field concerned with the design of services and ways to improve and innovate services through the application of established design processes and skills.

process redesign
The task of modifying an existing process to achieve incremental improvement.

The Relationship Between Process Design and Service Design

Process design involves determining the set of processes, actions, and steps to produce a product or service that delivers particular results for a given customer (Davenport 1992). **Service design**, meanwhile, is concerned with planning, developing, and improving the services provided.

Designing the processes that produce a product or service (process design) and designing the product or service (product design or service design) are interrelated activities: Decisions taken during the latter have an impact on the former, and vice versa. In the manufacturing industry, a clear distinction usually exists between product design and process design; in healthcare, however, the two are not as easily separated.

Process Design/Redesign

In industrial engineering, process design is distinguished from the related concept of **process redesign**. The term *process design* is used to describe the design of a new process or set of activities. It suggests setting up activities that are fundamentally new or promoting a disruptive improvement or innovation; thus, it refers to a change process. The term *process redesign* refers mostly to modifying an existing process to achieve incremental improvement. Although this distinction is relatively clear in industrial engineering, it tends to feel arbitrary in healthcare. The main focus of the activities of value-based healthcare is the generation of better patient-reported outcomes. Therefore, whether the aim of the process is disruptive improvement or incremental improvement, the service design methods and principles remain the same.

Value-Based Healthcare: A Paradigm Shift for Designing Services

The healthcare landscape has changed dramatically over time. Health systems that initially developed from a Fordist model of mass production centered around the concept of ill health have had to adapt and transform to keep pace with emerging challenges and an evolving market. Globally, healthcare providers must contend with changing demographics, the increased prevalence of chronic disease, a greater variety of healthcare facilities and resources, and the continuous development of new technologies. Rising costs and uneven quality have come to characterize healthcare systems throughout the world (Porter and Lee 2013). Furthermore, these systems have grown over time, leading to high levels of duplication among providers and the disjointed delivery of services. At the same time, patient demands have evolved, with disease prevention and chronic disease management moving to the forefront.

These and other developments have triggered a shift toward a new approach that focuses more on patient-centered services and systems, with the aim of achieving the best patient-defined outcomes in the most cost-efficient way. Porter and Lee (2013) emphasize that the central goal of healthcare delivery must be maximizing *value* for patients, not *volume*.

This shift has been evident in strategies taken by the National Health Service (NHS) in the United Kingdom. The 2000 NHS Plan, for instance, highlighted the need for the health system to be redesigned around patients' needs (NHS England 2000). Since 2009, NHS England has adopted such tools as Patient Reported Outcome Measures (PROMs) and Patient Reported Experience Measures (PREMs) to assess the quality of care from the patient's perspective (NHS England 2017). In addition, the Francis Inquiry report of 2013 highlighted the importance of the patient experience (Health Foundation 2018), and the Department of Health's (2011, 8) operating framework restated the spirit of the NHS Constitution, with a key theme of "putting patients at the centre of decision making."

Design Thinking in Service Design

This shift to patient-centered, value-driven healthcare service design requires a fundamental departure from past models of healthcare process design. Traditionally, engineering and manufacturing methods have been applied to healthcare operations, and such methods can be highly effective for problems that are well defined. However, these solutions are less applicable for situations with human system constraints (Gruber et al. 2015) and for the rising challenges facing healthcare. Today's healthcare challenges are what Rittel and Webber (1973) described as "wicked problems"—problems whose nature and systems context tend to be unclear or highly complex.

A growing amount of attention has been devoted to applications of **design thinking** to improve public services. Design thinking—essentially, "thinking like a designer"—was popularized as an approach to creative problem solving largely through the work of Tim Brown (2008) and Roger Martin (2009). Brown (2008, 86) describes design thinking as "a discipline that uses the designer's sensibility and methods to match people's needs with what is

design thinking
A problem-solving discipline that takes a human-centric approach to service innovation and improvement, with the customer/ user experience at its core.

technologically feasible and what a viable business strategy can convert into customer value and market opportunity." It reflects a human-centric approach to service innovation and improvement, with the customer/user experience at its core. Design thinking incorporates the concept of **co-design**—the active involvement of all stakeholders (e.g., employees, partners, customers, citizens, end users) in the design process to ensure that the end result meets their needs and is usable. The design thinking process is illustrated in exhibit 8.3.

Stanford Healthcare regards design thinking in the healthcare sector as a way to improve the patient experience. Wykes (2016) describes it as "a step-by-step approach to problem-solving that involves observing and interviewing people as they go through an experience, and then using that information to

co-design
An approach that seeks the active involvement of all stakeholders (e.g., employees, partners, customers, citizens, end users) in the design process.

Vignette: Stanford "D School" Collaboration

During the planning for the new Stanford Hospital, the university worked in conjunction with its Hasso Plattner Institute of Design (commonly known as the "d school") to redesign the emergency department experience (Wykes 2016). The new hospital is scheduled to open to patients in 2019 (Stanford Health Care 2018).

EXHIBIT 8.3
Co-design and the Design Thinking Process

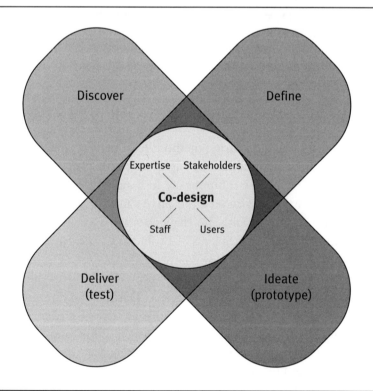

Source: Mariepi Manolis Cylwik.

prototype and test ways of improving the product or process." Other healthcare organizations, including Kaiser Permanente and India's Aravind Eye Care Systems, are also using design thinking to innovate and restructure their services (Brown 2008).

Core Principles of Service Design

Service design departs from traditional models of process design and creates an interdisciplinary platform for service improvement and transformation, with the user at the center of the process. It addresses the design, improvement, and innovation of services and systems through the application of established design processes and skills (Sangiorgi 2009). The Service Design Network (2017) defines it as follows:

> The activity of planning and organizing people, infrastructure, communication and material components of a service in order to improve its quality and the interaction between service provider and customers. The purpose of service design methodologies is to design according to the needs of customers or participants, so that the service is user-friendly, competitive and relevant to the customers.

Service design combines methods from such areas as management, design, engineering, and anthropology.

Service design can be used to improve an existing service or to create a new service from scratch, and it is gaining significant global popularity in healthcare. Health managers, therefore, need to understand its basic principles and know when and how they might be applicable. The core service design principles and benefits are presented in exhibit 8.4.

Vignette: Collaborations in the United Kingdom and the United States

A number of collaborations in the United Kingdom and the United States have brought service design approaches to healthcare concerns. In the United Kingdom, for instance, the Design Council (2011) worked with the government's Department of Health in an effort to reduce violence and aggression in hospitals' accident and emergency departments. Similarly, the Royal College of Physicians of Edinburgh (2018) consulted the Helen Hamlyn Centre of Design as part of an effort to navigate the pressures of the acute medical units across Scotland. In the United States, the Mayo Clinic (2017), following a collaboration with IDEO (a global design company), established a resident service design team to aid in its health services processes.

EXHIBIT 8.4
Principles and
Benefits of
Service Design/
Redesign

PRINCIPLES	
User-centricity	Services should be designed based on patient needs rather than on the internal needs of the organization. Services should be *experienced* through the perspective of the users—both patients and the frontline workforce.
Collaboration	Service design should be based on a genuine comprehension of the purpose of the service, the demand for the service, and the ability of the service provider to deliver. All stakeholders should be included in the service design process.
Holistic focus	Services should be designed to deliver a unified and efficient system rather than component-by-component approach, which can lead to poor overall service performance. The entire environment of the service should be considered. Services should be designed with processes to accommodate events that cause variation in general processes.
Prototype	Services should be prototyped before being developed in full. This step should happen in collaboration with all relevant stakeholders.
Iteration	Services should be developed as a minimum viable service (MVS) and then deployed. They can then be iterated and improved to bring additional value based on patient feedback.

BENEFITS
• Improves understanding of what value means for the patient
• Identifies pain points (real or perceived problems) and inefficiencies on the patient journey
• Improves waste management
• Improves understanding of limitations related to the environment and first-line workers
• Engages stakeholders
• Encourages alignment, problem solving, co-design, and ownership of solutions
• Helps with change management, implementation, and sustainability
• Allows for testing and fine-tuning, while keeping costs down

Source: Mariepi Manolis Cylwik.

The Four Stages of Design Thinking

In applying design thinking to the health services sector, the customer journey, rather than the process workflow, is used as the frame of reference for the design. Problem framing is central to the design thinking approach.

The design thinking / service design process occurs in four stages:

1. Discover
2. Define
3. Ideate
4. Deliver

These stages, which are illustrated in exhibit 8.5, are somewhat similar to those of the DMAIC (define, measure, analyze, improve, control) cycle, which will be discussed in the section of the chapter dealing with Six Sigma. The design process is highly iterative, moving backward and forward between stages, rapidly testing hypotheses through prototyping, and engaging users throughout the process. In this manner, it differs from DMAIC, which is cyclical in nature.

User engagement is essential for problem framing and for scoping opportunities for design interventions. Through prototyping and visualization of alternative potential solutions, the design approach considers how effective and technically robust proposals are and also how well they align with users' lives and needs and the broader context of the system.

The discovery phase is not limited to quantitative data collection; rather, it incorporates acute observation of the users and of the system's context and constraints. A clear understanding of behavioral patterns—which can be achieved through the use of ethnography, visual anthropology, and co-creation workshops (Gruber et al. 2015)—is an important element in designing solutions that will be endorsed.

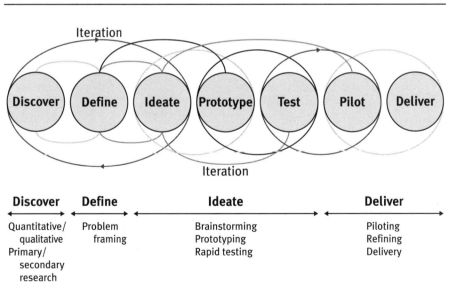

EXHIBIT 8.5
The Four Stages of the Design Thinking / Service Design Process

Source: Mariepi Manolis Cylwik.

process mapping
A tool for examining the activities involved in the delivery of a service and the ways those activities are managed.

patient journey map
A visual representation of a patient's journey through a set of clinical services.

Process Mapping and Patient Journey Maps

Because the customer journey serves as the frame of reference for the application of design thinking to healthcare, **process mapping** and **patient journey maps** are essential. In service design, process mapping involves an examination, from the user's perspective, of the activities involved in the delivery of a service and the ways those activities are managed. It provides a detailed overall picture that helps leaders and teams to

- identify key elements of service,
- understand the links between the various elements over time,
- identify problem areas and opportunities, and
- create empathy with various types of users.

The patient journey map is a process map specific to healthcare. It provides a visual representation of a patient's journey through a set of clinical services, showing the various interactions and touch points. It is useful for understanding healthcare processes from the patient's perspective and identifying problems and potential improvements (Trebble et al. 2010).

Process mapping can help multidisciplinary teams make sense of clinical practices, develop a shared understanding of key issues from the users' perspective, and identify workflow issues such as functional bottlenecks. Data collected from patient journey maps can help organizations redesign the patient pathway, improve the quality and efficiency of clinical management, and shift the focus of care toward activities most valued by the patient.

Exhibit 8.6 provides an example of a patient journey map, with a condensed visual summary of patient actions and experiences linked to the steps

EXHIBIT 8.6
A Generic Example of a Patient Journey Map

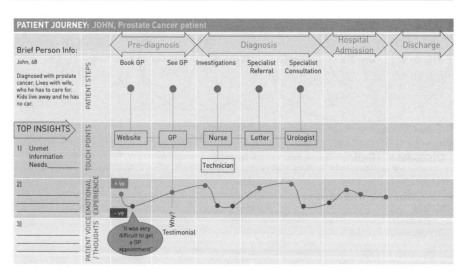

Source: Mariepi Manolis Cylwik.

of a healthcare process. Such maps can be specific to a particular service (e.g., visit to a general practitioner), or they can be more macro in nature, taking into account the coordination of multiple services (e.g., the steps from diagnosis to treatment of prostate cancer).

When process mapping is applied to healthcare, the terms *users* and *patients* are sometimes used interchangeably. However, healthcare systems have other types of users besides patients, and the perspectives of these individuals (e.g., clinicians, nurses, administrators) must also be considered.

Service Blueprint

A **service blueprint** is an operational planning tool that provides guidance for how a service will be provided, specifying the physical environment, staff actions, support systems, and infrastructure needed for delivery of a service across its various channels. The service blueprint was adapted from the flow analysis tool (FAT), a tool widely used in manufacturing. It builds on detailed process mapping to create a visual schematic that incorporates everything from points of patient contact to backstage processes. It provides a way to detail every aspect of a service and more closely examine what is happening at every stage of the process. It allows for the analysis of patient flow across complex processes, the identification of waste and non-value-added activities, and the assessment of roles and responsibilities related to management of patient flows.

> **service blueprint**
> An operational planning tool that provides guidance on how a service will be provided, taking into account physical environment, staff actions, support systems, and infrastructure.

Co-design

The co-design approach (illustrated previously in exhibit 8.3) emphasizes the active involvement of all stakeholders (e.g., employees, partners, customers, citizens, end users) in the design process to ensure that the resulting project is usable and meets their needs. This stakeholder involvement adds value by helping to identify value-added and non-value-added activities from the points of view of the people involved in service consumption and delivery. It can be a useful strategy for change management, as it helps give stakeholders a feeling of ownership toward the solution, thereby making resistance less likely. Changes with broad stakeholder ownership tend to have a higher probability of success and sustainability.

Vignette: International Co-design Efforts

In the United Kingdom, the King's Fund, in cooperation with the Health Foundation, launched a Patient and Family-Centred Care (PFCC) initiative that used a co-design approach to transform healthcare services with patients and staff. The initiative addressed a wide range of areas, from pediatric accident and emergency care to care for older adults. A new organization

(continued)

called the Point of Care Foundation (2018) developed from the King's Fund program and continues with "a mission to humanise healthcare."

A 2005 initiative by the NHS Institute for Innovation and Improvement similarly applied design methods with a focus on patient experiences, leading to an approach called Experience-Based Co-Design (EBCD). The approach was first piloted for head and neck cancer services in England and was later rolled out to other cancer services nationally. An international survey of EBCD projects in healthcare services identified 59 projects that had been implemented in six countries (Australia, Canada, England, the Netherlands, New Zealand, and Sweden) between 2005 and 2013, with another 27 projects in the planning stage (Donetto, Tsianakas, and Robert 2014).

Quality in Healthcare

Quality is a diffuse, multidimensional concept, and little consensus exists over how it is to be measured or operationalized. No single definition of the term is regarded as completely correct and comprehensive.[1] In healthcare, the following definition from the Institute of Medicine (IOM) is often used: Quality is "the degree to which health care services for individuals and populations increase the likelihood of desired outcomes and are consistent with current professional knowledge" (IOM 2001, 44).

One stream of the literature on this topic regards quality as a desired attribute of the outcomes produced by organizations; in this sense, the word *quality* is used to describe some product or service. Another stream of the literature expands the focus of quality to include organizational processes and practices beyond those of prior definitions, so that the term refers to an overall experience and encompasses the culture of the organization (Cole and Scott 2000). We regard these two streams of *quality* definitions as complementary, and both approaches are used in health systems internationally.

Because of its complexity and multidimensionality, quality in healthcare requires systems for measurement and analysis that capture both objective and subjective quality dimensions. One basic framework for analysis and measurement, set forth by Donabedian (1988), distinguishes between quality in structure (inputs), in process, and in outcomes. This classic approach to quality care is reflected in the value chain model discussed earlier in the chapter and shown in exhibit 8.1. Quality in health systems may also be approached through four underlying perspectives:

1. *The outcomes.* This perspective focuses on the benefits or effects in economic or societal terms.

2. *The clients.* This perspective considers the attributes needed or desired by clients, customers, and stakeholders.

3. *The process.* This perspective focuses on the internal activities to meet clients', customers', and stakeholders' needs/desires through delivery of products or services (value chain and value system).

4. *The resources.* The resources perspective deals with the tangible and intangible inputs (e.g., human resources, organizational resources, informational resources, systemic infrastructure) required for process activities.

Exhibit 8.7 presents these perspectives—along with quality domains and dimensions, as well as associated methods and measurements—in a practical and simplified manner. Although the focus of this chapter is primarily on the process perspective of quality, a holistic picture spanning all four perspectives is necessary to cover the various areas linked with process design, redesign, and improvement; therefore, this multidimensional approach is key for healthcare managers wishing to master operations management.

Total Quality Management / Continuous Process Improvement

Total quality management (TQM)—also known as *continuous quality improvement (CQI)* or *continuous process improvement (CPI)*—is a management philosophy and business strategy that seeks to establish continuous, organized quality-improvement activities and to involve everyone in the organization in an integrated effort to improve performance at every level (Iles and Sutherland 2001). A systematic TQM approach uses specific models and techniques to achieve change and improve quality in a continuous and incremental manner. One of the chief techniques is the cycle of **plan-do-check-act (PDCA)**, or plan-do-study-act (PDSA), which is used to develop, implement, test, and refine changes and improvements. Versions of the PDCA/PDSA cycle are sometimes known as the Deming cycle or the Shewhart cycle, after W. Edwards Deming and his mentor, Walter Shewhart, who were pioneers of modern quality control. The cycle was developed through Deming's work in Japan in the years following World War II, and it has come to serve as a "template" for the quality movement. Quality techniques from such authors as Juran, Feigenbaum, Ishikawa, and, more recently, Berwick have followed (Berwick 1998).

Exhibit 8.8 shows a PDSA cycle on the outer edge of the diagram. The concentric circles show how the cycle is related to other improvement models and tools—namely, the design process and process reengineering.

Quality improvement efforts in healthcare typically aim to enhance processes by addressing key success factors. The IOM (2001) report *Crossing the Quality Chasm* identifies six improvement aims, which can be separated into the broader categories of quality, time, and cost:

total quality management (TQM)
A management approach that seeks to establish continuous, organized quality-improvement activities and to involve everyone in the organization in an integrated effort to improve performance at every level; also known as *continuous quality improvement (CQI)* or *continuous process improvement (CPI)*.

plan-do-check-act (PDCA)
A quality-improvement approach in which changes are developed, implemented, tested, and refined in repeated cycles; sometimes written as *plan-do-study-act (PDSA)*.

EXHIBIT 8.7

Perspectives, Domains, Dimensions, and Measurements/Methods of Quality in Health Systems

Perspectives	Domains of Quality	Quality Dimensions	Measurements/Methods in Health
1. The outcomes—economic and societal value (includes benefits and effects in both monetary and nonmonetary terms)	• Overall quality—improving the overall quality of the experience of giving and receiving care	• Effectivity—providing services based on evidence of a clear overall health benefit	• Health status—the health benefit received through personal or nonpersonal care • System efficiency—efficiency as a social good in itself and as a basis for determining value in the healthcare market, with systemwide approaches
	• Equity—ensuring that care provided does not vary based on patients' or users' characteristics	• Access to care—offering personal and nonpersonal access to care or health status attainment, given current technology, clinical practices, public health knowledge, and management practices	• Healthcare coverage—regional status or disparities • Responsiveness—responses from patients and constituencies (though many have difficulty determining whether outputs/outcomes are appropriate and reasonable)
2. The clients—based on the voice of the client, customers, stakeholders, or constituencies	• Patient and population engagement	• Patient satisfaction (acceptability)—requires mapping and surveying the patient's entire experience within the product or service delivery system	• Citizen charter / expected service • Surveys of client satisfaction or willingness to recommend provider or use again
		• Information and emotional support—promoting the involvement of the individual and family, informed choice, encouragement, clarification, and confidentiality	• Amount and clarity of information, time spent listening, and time spent encouraging—better patient information and more effective emotional support can lead to shorter stays, less medication, fewer side effects, better compliance, and higher levels of satisfaction (Delbanco 1992)
	• Person-centered	• Amenities and convenience—services reflect the patient's preference for technology, people, facilities, and behaviors	• Clean, fast, accurate, and timely care; patients treated with respect; service available when needed—service inconveniences have "opportunity cost" implications for patients, though offering greater convenience has cost implications for caregivers

(continued)

EXHIBIT 8.7

Perspectives, Domains, Dimensions, and Measurements/Methods of Quality in Health Systems *(continued)*

3. The processes—dealing with models of both personal care and nonpersonal, population-based care	• Models of care—based on deep understanding of cause-and-effect relationships of processes, where results are replicable on a continuing basis • Process quality—aimed at improving the overall quality of the process of producing a product or service	• Technical dimension of quality • Effectiveness—services provided based on evidence that they produce a clear clinical or public health benefit • Efficiency—relating resources (inputs) with satisfactory process outcomes, avoiding waste • Time—reducing waits or delays in processes • Cost—affordability of care • Safety—avoiding harm from health products or services • Regulation and standards	• Clinical standards or clinical pathways—consistency with clinical guidelines, research on outcomes, and evidence-based medicine • Six Sigma and Lean—avoiding variability of product/service, waste, and rework • Wait times—ensuring quick and accurate diagnosis and treatment, reducing cycle times of care, increasing patients' chances of success and returning to "normal life" • Diagnosis-related groups (DRGs)—comparing processes, costs, and results and coming to a conclusion about the cost/value of activities • Standards, public health accreditation, drug regulation, clinical paths/guidelines, waste management, Joint Commission International accreditation
4. The resources—inputs or assets (both tangible and intangible) needed to activate processes	• Organizational capacity • Leadership	• Quality culture—embedding best practices in the organization's employees and systems and ensuring that they remain in the organizational culture (quality assurance) • Collaboration—building teams or external coalitions • Knowledge and skills—generalizing scientific evidence and best practices • Leadership—the processes of shaping change or assisting with management control	• Accreditation, quality assurance, excellence programs—such as the Malcolm Baldrige National Quality Award (US) or the Business Excellence Model (Europe) • Collective impact—addressing systemwide health issues with quality in the value system • Evidence-based medicine—health services based on evidence • Healthcare management/leadership—the right health management knowledge and skills to address quality dimensions when setting priorities for improvement

Source: Eduardo Álvarez-Falcón.

Quality (of process, product, or service outputs to meet client's needs/wants)

1. *Safety*—avoiding injuries to patients from the care that is intended to help them
2. *Effectiveness*—providing services based on scientific knowledge to all who will benefit; refraining from providing services to those not likely to benefit
3. *Patient-centeredness*—providing care that is respectful of and responsive to individual patient preferences, needs, and values; ensuring that patient values guide all clinical decisions
4. *Equity*—providing care that does not vary in quality because of personal characteristics such as gender, ethnicity, geographic location, and socioeconomic status

Time (for delivery of products or services to meet client's needs/wants)

5. *Timeliness*—reducing wait times and potentially harmful delays (which have the effect of limiting access to care) for those who receive and those who give care

EXHIBIT 8.8
The Plan-Do-Study-Act Cycle, the Design Process, and Process Reengineering

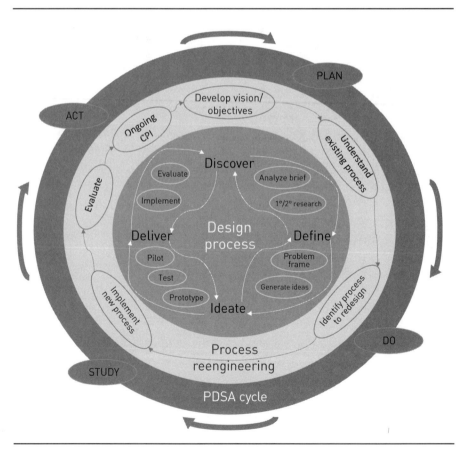

Note: CPI = continuous process improvement.
Source: Mariepi Manolis Cylwik.

Cost (of producing products or services outputs to meet client's needs/wants)

6. *Efficiency*—avoiding rework and waste of equipment, supplies, ideas, and energy

These improvement aims are often in tension with one another, and management decisions typically involve trade-offs. For instance, an option that is fast and inexpensive (satisfying the aims related to time and cost) will often be low in quality. Likewise, an option that is fast and high in quality will likely be expensive, and an option that is low in cost and high in quality will often not be timely.

We encourage the reader to spend time reviewing exhibit 8.7 to develop familiarity with the many facets of quality and the related methods and tools that can be applied in the health systems arena. Many of the quality improvement methods discussed in this chapter—including process design, service blueprints, co-design, PDCA/PDSA, benchmarking, Lean, and Six Sigma—share basic TQM principles.

Benchmarking in Healthcare: Bridging Gaps to Improve Performance

Benchmarking, a practice deeply embedded in the TQM philosophy, involves measuring the performance of an organization against a standard, or benchmark. The standard—which may be absolute or relative to other organizations—is often treated as a goal to be equaled or surpassed, and it is believed to reflect the **best practice**. Many organizations compare their own performance against the performance of their strongest competitor or a benchmark organization renowned as a leader in the field. The highest current performance level in a field is regarded as the **best in class**. The fundamental aim of benchmarking with the best in class is to become the industry leader. This aim is reflected in the Japanese word *dantotsu*, which means "being the best of the best" (*Economist* 2009).

Benchmarking can expose areas where improvement is needed and provide guidance for the adoption of processes or standards that have been associated with superior performance at other organizations (Zairi and Jarrar 2001). Benchmarking is not a measurement itself; rather, it is a process of identifying "gaps" in performance and putting in place action plans to close such gaps. Exhibit 8.9 illustrates the way in which performance gaps can be addressed through benchmarking. Whereas the continuous process improvement approach focuses on incremental increases in effectiveness, benchmarking focuses on competitiveness and best practice.

A variety of benchmarking methodologies have been developed, most notably by Robert Camp of Xerox Corporation (Zairi and Leonard 1994). Three main benchmarking techniques are widely used in health systems: (1) results benchmarking, (2) standards benchmarking, and (3) processes benchmarking.

benchmarking
The process of measuring the performance of an organization against a standard (benchmark).

best practice
A method or activity that has been shown to generate superior results.

best in class
The highest current performance level in a field, often used as a benchmark to be equaled or exceeded.

EXHIBIT 8.9
Bridging
Performance
Gaps with
Benchmarking

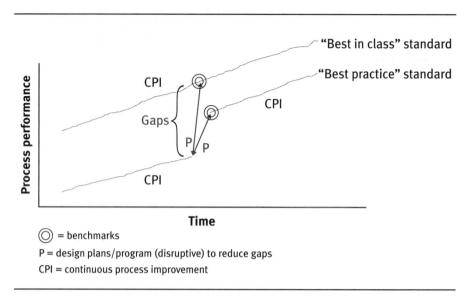

Source: Eduardo Álvarez-Falcón.

Results Benchmarking

Benchmarking based on results (i.e., outputs or outcomes) is perhaps the most noticeable benchmarking technique in the healthcare sector (Zairi and Leonard 1994). It focuses on the systemic effects of personal and nonpersonal care processes on the health status of a population (Donabedian 1988). It considers major clinical benefits achieved, as well as small improvements in patients' clinical results. It also indicates the degree to which a service provider's performance achieves its potential.

Results benchmarking requires a performance standard against which success can be measured. Goals are generally defined in one of two ways:

• Achieving better-than-average outcomes (based on average performance outcomes and variations from mean outcomes—i.e., the standard deviation)
• Achieving the maximum obtainable or best possible outcomes observed in practice (based on proximity to best-in-class providers or an empirical results quality frontier)

league table
A performance table that compares results of similar organizations.

Results benchmarking in healthcare can be seen, for example, when an organization consults published performance tables, or **league tables**, to compare performance across a number of organizations providing a similar service. Such tables are made available to the public to inform judgment concerning care results and effective use of resources (Jee and Or 1999). This technique needs to be used with caution, however, because it only tells the "end of the story," without considering whether value was added or destroyed in the process. It should not be used in isolation for decision making. Results benchmarking is commonly used for accountability purposes and to incentivize quality performance in the presence or absence of competitive pressures.

Vignette: Performance Benchmarking in the *World Health Report*

The WHO's (2000) *World Health Report 2000* was dedicated to performance assessment for health systems, and it focused significant attention on ways to improve quality internationally.

The report presented a new methodology in which a composite indicator of overall performance is used to enable the ranking (via league tables) and comparison (benchmarking) of health status across countries. In this methodology, health system performance was treated as a relative concept, and assessment of performance took into account what could be achieved for a given set of circumstances (Murray and Frenk 2000). The chief aim of the report was to improve the average health status and reduce inequalities. The report also included two intrinsic goals common to all social systems: (1) responsiveness of the system to legitimate expectations of the population (clients' perspective) and (2) fairness in the financing of the system (Murray and Frenk 2000).

Under the report's methodology, health system performance involved not just the organizations' functions but also the way each function related to the others—in other words, the methodology took into account the structural and organizational arrangements of the value system. The report also acknowledged that factors and interrelationships outside the health system could influence or determine the system's performance.

Various aspects of the WHO report attracted criticism. Some critics questioned the validity and reliability of methods for measuring health attainment, responsiveness, and overall performance, or the value judgments involved in the weighting of domains, goals and priorities, preferred distributions, and other elements. Other critics questioned the use of the WHO's league tables in addressing strategic decisions at national levels, as well as the quality of the data used to measure outcomes (Álvarez-Falcón and Heymann 2006).

Standards Benchmarking

Standards benchmarking is based on standards of performance typically determined through one of three approaches:

- A standard that an effective organization could be expected to achieve (for examples at international levels, see WHO [2000] and Joint Commission International [2018]; for examples at national levels, see Public Health Accreditation Board [2018] and United Kingdom Accreditation Service [2017])
- A standard to promote areas for technical improvement for staff (for examples adapted to national levels in evidence-based medicine, see National Institute for Health and Care Excellence [2017] and the Official Mexican Standards for healthcare [Secretaría de Salud 2015])
- A standard to inform customers, citizens, or stakeholders about expected service standards in key areas (see Care Quality Commission [2018])

These forms of benchmarking are used globally for accreditation or certification of health services processes. These benchmarks change over time, and organizations must remain up to date. Use of outdated benchmarks could potentially inhibit improvement or innovation.

Vignette: Official Mexican Standards

In Mexico, some national standards are enforced by a type of government regulation called a Norma Oficial Mexicana (NOM), or Official Mexican Standard. NOMs spell out guidelines for a variety of activities related to health records, family planning services, pregnancies, delivery and postpartum care, obesity treatment, school health, addiction treatment, and epidemiological surveillance. Mexico's General Health Council establishes the standards for hospital certification.

Process Benchmarking

Process benchmarking is probably the most valuable type of benchmarking but also the most complex and costly to perform. It involves the detailed examination of organizations' activities through such methods as efficiency scrutinies and value-for-money studies, with the aim of understanding reasons for variations in performance and incorporating cost-effective best practice. The approach is closely related to economic evaluations (Smee 2001) and activity-based costing (ABC), which provides the basis for the diagnosis-related group (DRG) methodology.

An interesting example involves DRGs in which components incorporate multiple benchmarking techniques focused on statistics (output case mix), technical/medical issues (evidence-based clinical standards), and costs of activities (European Observatory on Health Systems and Policies Series 2011). DRGs are used extensively in the United States, Europe, Latin America, and other parts of the world for planning, payment, and reimbursement in the for-profit and not-for-profit sectors.

Six Sigma and Lean

Over the past several decades, health services organizations have increasingly turned to quality improvement methodologies such as **Six Sigma** and **Lean** as ways to improve patient outcomes. The application of these methodologies in healthcare is driven in large part by the successes of Six Sigma and Lean in the manufacturing industry (Shah, Chandrasekaran, and Linderman 2008). This trend is also influenced by the fact that healthcare payers around the world have placed greater emphasis on quality of care. In the United States, for instance, hospitals can receive additional payments from the Centers for Medicare & Medicaid Services (CMS) if they improve patient satisfaction and lower readmission rates among patients with certain medical conditions (CMS 2017). Healthcare organizations, especially hospitals, are therefore highly motivated to seek new strategies to improve patient outcomes (Amaratunga and Dobranowski 2016; Alessandro, Malcolm, and Jiju 2013; Mason, Nicolay, and Darzi 2015; Roberts and Singh 2009; Tlahuiz 2011). Henke (2009) has estimated that 42 percent of US hospitals use some form of Six Sigma and 54 percent practice some form of Lean.

Six Sigma
A quality improvement methodology, developed at the Motorola corporation in the 1980s, that emphasizes the elimination of variation and error.

Lean
A quality improvement methodology, evolved from the Toyota Production System in Japan, that emphasizes the elimination of waste and unnecessary steps.

Six Sigma

Developed at the Motorola corporation in the mid-1980s, Six Sigma aims to improve quality by identifying and correcting the causes of variations and errors that occur in a process (Harry and Schroeder 2000). The methodology uses sigma levels to reflect the number of defects per million opportunities (DPMO); the higher the sigma level, the lower the number of defects. The goal of Six Sigma is to reduce the rate of defects to a six sigma level, or 3.4 DPMO. To provide an example of DPMO in a healthcare context, a reported incidence of bile duct injury during laparoscopic cholecystectomy of 1 per 1,500 surgeries would translate to 95 DPMO, or a 5.25 sigma level. Sigma is a symbol for standard deviation, and the name *Six Sigma* reflects the goal of having process output within a span of six standard deviations (i.e., the mean plus and minus three standard deviations) (Pyzdek and Keller 2014).

Six Sigma projects in healthcare settings can help reduce waiting time and delays, prevent adverse events, and lower costs (Amaratunga and Dobranowski 2016; Alessandro, Malcolm, and Jiju 2013; Mason, Nicolay, and Darzi 2015; Roberts and Singh 2009; Tlahuiz 2011). Six Sigma represents not only an approach for quality improvement but also a key part of TQM philosophy. Research suggests that successful implementation of Six Sigma requires organizations to undergo a meaningful cultural change (Antony and Banuelas 2002; Banuelas Coronado and Antony 2002).

The DMAIC Cycle

DMAIC cycle
A Six Sigma improvement cycle that consists of five phases: define, measure, analyze, improve, and control.

The cornerstone of Six Sigma is process management through the **DMAIC cycle** of five phases: define, measure, analyze, improve, and control. Each phase of the cycle is built on the prior phases, which helps ensure a scientific design and statistical rigor. The DMAIC cycle provides Six Sigma projects with their conceptual framework, and it distinguishes Six Sigma from other quality improvement approaches. Exhibit 8.10 examines the DMAIC cycle in greater detail.

Lean

flow
A key Lean principle referring to the movement of products or services through the value stream without waits or delays.

pull
A key Lean principle requiring that the production process be triggered only by customer demand.

sensei
A master teacher in the Lean improvement methodology.

The Lean quality improvement approach evolved from the Toyota Production System, which was developed by Taiichi Ohno, Toyota's chief of production, in the years following World War II (Womack, Jones, and Roos 1990). It uses an ongoing cycle of improvement to map out and adapt process steps that generate values from the customer's perspective and to eliminate waste and unnecessary steps. The adoption of Lean in healthcare is driven by the pressure placed on health services organizations to improve efficiency, reduce costs, and streamline the care delivery process.

Five main principles underscore Lean: (1) value, (2) the value stream, (3) flow, (4) pull, and (5) perfection (Cottington and Forst 2010; Ohno 1998). *Value* refers to something that the customer is willing to pay for, or something that changes the finished product in a meaningful way. The *value stream* is defined as the sequence of events involved in producing a product or service. **Flow** is achieved if a product or service travels through the value stream without waits or delays. In supply chain management, flows must be coordinated and integrated both within and among companies. The principle of **pull** requires that the production process be triggered only by customer demand. The final principle, perfection, calls for the complete elimination of waste so that all activities along the value stream are value-added activities. Lean relies on the use of **senseis**, or master teachers, to diffuse new beliefs and promote cultural value shifts.

The following sections will discuss the key Lean tools of waste reduction, *kaizen* improvement events, *jidoka*, and just-in-time production.

EXHIBIT 8.10
The Six Sigma DMAIC Cycle

Phase	Tasks	Tools	Comments
Define	The quality improvement team identifies a project based on the strategic objectives of the organization and the customers' requirements of the process.	A critical to quality (CTQ) analysis can be conducted to identify the needs or requirements of the internal and external customers of the process. A CTQ analysis focuses on quantifiable customer requirements of a product or process that can be used to set performance standards or specification limits. The analysis usually involves focus group discussions, customer surveys, and complaint analysis. A project charter can be used to formally authorize the project. The charter should clearly state the purpose and goals of the project, provide background, identify project stakeholders and team members, authorize responsibilities and resources to the team, and outline project milestones and deliverables.	A "good" Six Sigma project should address an issue that is important to the mission of the organization, focus on a measurable improvement goal, clearly define the project boundaries, and be expected to positively affect the financial performance of the organization (cost savings or revenue gains).
Measure	Team members develop a system to accurately measure how well the target process meets the requirements set by the customers at the baseline or prior to improvement intervention.	Statistical process control (SPC) aims to evaluate the effectiveness of a process in meeting an outcome-related goal. This technique involves identifying a measurable outcome of the process, collecting outcome data over a defined period, determining the statistical distribution of the outcome data, plotting the center and control limits for the process, and assessing whether the process is within or out of control. In a Six Sigma project, it is important to distinguish common cause variation, which is inherent in any process, from special cause variation, which is caused by factors outside the process of interest. Other tools that may be valuable in this phase include process mapping, time value analysis, root cause analysis, Pareto charts, and failure modes and effects analysis.	The team must understand not only how the target process works but also how well it works; thus, it should collect as much information as possible. The baseline performance will be used to evaluate the impact of any intervention in the "improve" phase.

(continued)

EXHIBIT 8.10
The Six Sigma DMAIC Cycle *(continued)*

Phase	Tasks	Tools	Comments
Analyze	The project team analyzes the data and provides information for the development of quality improvement interventions.	In addition to the tools used in the measure phase, statistical analysis, such as analysis of variance and regression, can be used to determine the relationship between various factors and the outcome of interest.	The data collected in the define and measure phases will be used to identify the causes of poor performance.
Improve	The team designs, implements, and evaluates the impact of improvement interventions.	Change management requires identifying and understanding stakeholders, communicating the necessity of change, articulating the proposed changes, and developing a plan to address potential resistance. Pilot testing involves a trial run of process changes on a limited scale prior to deployment throughout the organization. For example, interventions can first be rolled out in a less-busy shift in a single department of the hospital. Results of pilot testing can be used to fine-tune the interventions and eliminate issues that might surface during the full-scale implementation. In this phase, tools from other quality improvement approaches, such as Lean, may be used.	Possible interventions can be identified by reviewing the related literature.
Control	The team works to institutionalize successful process changes to sustain improvement gains.	The new process can be maintained through personnel adjustment, employee training, and process monitoring.	During this phase, the team may also identify opportunities for further improvement as the environment changes, leading to the start of a new DMAIC cycle.

Source: Xinliang Liu.

Waste Reduction

The primary goal of Lean production is to completely eliminate waste from the production process and to produce exactly what the customer wants. In Lean, waste is identified by distinguishing between value-added and non-value-added activities. An activity is considered non-value-added if it does not transform the end product or service in a way that is valuable for a customer, or if it represents rework. Ohno (1998) describes seven types of waste that commonly occur in systems and processes: waste of time, transportation, overproduction, motion, excess inventory, defects, and overprocessing. By some estimates, as much as 95 percent of the work of healthcare practitioners is non-value-added (Hagan 2011)—suggesting that the field has substantial room for efficiency improvement.

Kaizen Improvement Event

A **kaizen event**, which gets its name from the Japanese term for "continuous improvement," is a short-term improvement event, or rapid process improvement workshop, aimed at improving a specific process. Its goal is typically to create a project plan and execute it within one week.

A kaizen event begins with training in the tools of Lean and worker empowerment. Team members then begin to measure and analyze a target process and develop ideas for improvement. A proposal for improvement should be completed by midweek, and, for the remainder of the week, the proposed changes are implemented and their impact assessed. The team reports the results at the end of the week, and a new process should be established the following week. Although the scope of a kaizen project is restricted to allow for completion within one week, rapid cycle improvement can bring quick benefits and create a great sense of accomplishment and pride among team members.

Jidoka

Jidoka is the Japanese term for automation. In Lean production, **jidoka** can be described as "automation with a human touch," referring to the ability to stop a production process immediately when a problem arises so that defects will not be passed on from one step to the next. The word *jidoka* traces its roots to an automatic loom invented by Sakichi Toyoda, founder of the Toyota Group. The loom stopped itself if a thread broke, preventing defective cloth from being produced. One application of jidoka in healthcare involves the use of surgery checklists in operating rooms. The checklists provide members of the surgical team an opportunity to stop the progression of a surgery if protocol has not been properly followed.

Just-in-Time Production

Lean originated from the concept of **just-in-time (JIT) production**, which is based on the delivery of the supplies, equipment, and information needed

---

kaizen event
A short-term improvement event, or rapid process improvement workshop, aimed at improving a specific process; a key tool of Lean.

jidoka
The ability, in Lean production, to stop a production process immediately when a problem arises so that defects will not be passed on from one step to the next.

just-in-time (JIT) production
The delivery of the supplies, equipment, and information needed for a production process at the time they are needed and in the right quantity.

for a production process at the time they are needed and in the right quantity. Generally, JIT is often viewed as an inventory management strategy.

kanban
A Lean production tool that uses signs or signals to automatically control the movement of inventory.

Lean production uses a **kanban** system—named after the Japanese word meaning "sign"—to control the movement of inventory. A kanban system relies on the use of signs that provide information (e.g., item name, code, storage location) related to inventory items in a container. In the production process, when a downstream step consumes all of a certain inventory item, the empty container serves as a signal for the immediate upstream step to fill the container. In this way, the upstream step produces or reorders the inventory only when it is needed and in the amount needed.

The healthcare field consumes a large quantity of medical and surgical supplies, so numerous opportunities exist for applications of JIT and kanban. Italian hospitals, for instance, have effectively used the concepts to reduce or eliminate inventory (Persona, Battini, and Rafele 2008).

Six Sigma and Lean Together

Six Sigma and Lean have distinctive philosophies, tools, and techniques, but they share a number of similar goals and approaches (Andersson, Eriksson, and Torstensson 2006). A comparison of Six Sigma and Lean is provided in exhibit 8.11. Increasingly, the two systems are being implemented concurrently as **Lean Six Sigma (LSS)**. By integrating the two approaches, LSS benefits both from the statistical rigor of Six Sigma and from the cyclical waste reduction of Lean (DelliFraine, Langabeer, and Nembhard 2010).

Lean Six Sigma (LSS)
A combined approach in which elements of Lean and Six Sigma are implemented concurrently.

Six Sigma, Lean, and LSS have been applied in projects to reduce costs, wait time, cycle time, and adverse events, as well as to increase patient volume, patient safety, and patient satisfaction (Amaratunga and Dobranowski 2016; Alessandro, Malcolm, and Jiju 2013; Mason, Nicolay, and Darzi 2015; Roberts and Singh 2009; Tlahuiz 2011).

Implications for Health Policy

Leaders and managers in the healthcare field need to bear in mind that access, efficiency, and quality relate directly to TQM's main dimensions, models, tools, and techniques. Access is related to infrastructure inputs that enable timely care by reducing wait times and harmful delays. Efficiency is related to lowering cost, reducing variability of processes, and avoiding waste. Quality is related to the delivery of good, safe, and evidence-based products and services. Access, efficiency, and quality are instrumental to attaining the WHO's (2000) three primary goals for health systems: health status, responsiveness, and financial fairness and protection.

Operations management approaches are highly relevant for healthcare policy, given that operational activities drive results improvements in interrelated

	Six Sigma	Lean
Goal	To improve the system of interest through continuous improvement cycles	
Approach	Collecting data and using quantitative methods to document quality improvement and progress toward a stated goal	
Theoretical focus	Variation reduction	Waste reduction
Guiding principles	Define Measure Analyze Improve Control	Identify value Identify the value stream Streamline the flow Use pull to drive production Perfection / elimination of waste
Assumptions	Variation reduction will improve system effectiveness.	Waste removal will improve system efficiency.
Improvement cycle	DMAIC (define, measure, analyze, improve, control) cycle	PDSA (plan, do, study, act) cycle
Tools and techniques	Critical to quality (CTQ) analysis, project charter, process mapping, time value analysis, root cause analysis, Pareto charts, failure modes and effects analysis, statistical process control, statistical analysis	Waste reduction, kaizen improvement events, jidoka, just-in-time production
Critical elements	Quantitative analytical techniques and error rates	Use of "*senseis*" (master teachers) to diffuse new beliefs and promote cultural value shifts

EXHIBIT 8.11
Comparison of Six Sigma and Lean

Source: Xinliang Liu.

value chains, thereby producing benefits across the system. Service design thinking, for example, is starting to provide a systemic approach to healthcare strategy, with the service architecture extending from clinical care to community services in a cost-efficient manner, leading to a value-driven care transformation. These operational advances are converging with strategic management in global initiatives—such as Community Balanced Scorecards and the Collective Impact Framework (Results That Matter Team 2018; Collaboration for Impact 2018)—that seek to transform health services while also addressing other complex social issues.

In selecting the best operational change model, or mixture of models, for a policy intervention, decision makers need to consider a variety of organizational and contextual factors and determine the appropriate level of change for a given situation. Exhibit 8.12 provides some guidance on how the models discussed in this chapter correspond with varying levels of operational change.

EXHIBIT 8.12
Improvement
Models and
Levels of
Operational
Change

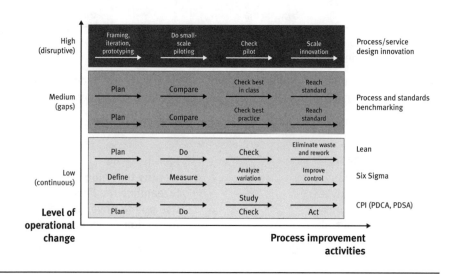

Source: Eduardo Álvarez-Falcón.

Summary

A wide variety of operational change and quality improvement models—process/service design, benchmarking, Six Sigma, and Lean, among others—are being used by health organizations and systems internationally. All of them, either directly or indirectly, apply common principles of TQM in an effort to add value to processes. The relationships and parallels among the various models are shown, in simplified fashion, in exhibit 8.13. Advancements in methodologies in such areas as process/service design are providing platforms with which to explore disruptive innovations, especially when combined with other methods.

In pursuing value-based healthcare, improvement models consider two aspects of value: the value perceived by internal and external clients and the organizational means that add value in the chain of activities. As process improvement advances in global health settings, it emphasizes reconciliation, collaboration, and engagement across all actors involved in a process—an important part of the TQM philosophy.

For purposes of operational change management and decision making, the models presented in exhibit 8.13 operate across four predominant "value added" categories: (1) value added by novel process improvement, or innovation; (2) value added by incremental process improvement; (3) value added by decreasing process variation; and (4) value added by reducing waste, rework, and costs in processes. Examples from each of these categories are presented in exhibit 8.14. Caution needs to be exercised in assigning specific categories to the various models, tools, and techniques, because the methods commonly overlap across multiple categories and are often mixed.

EXHIBIT 8.13

Operational Quality Improvement Models Used in Health Organizations and Systems

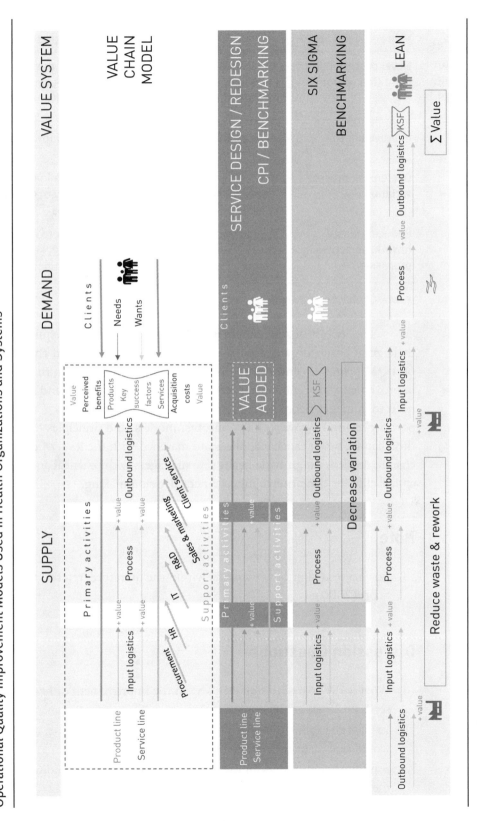

Source: Eduardo Álvarez-Falcón.

EXHIBIT 8.14
Categories
of Value-
Added Quality
Improvement in
Global Health

Value-Added Category	Examples of Models, Methods, Techniques, and Tools
Novel process improvement (innovation)	Innovative or disruptive process/service design/redesign, process mapping, service blueprints, benchmarking (best in class), technological advancements
Incremental process improvement	Process/service design/redesign, process mapping, service blueprints, continuous process improvement, results benchmarking
Decreasing process variation	Six Sigma, standards benchmarking, eliminating defective products, ensuring consistency of evidence-based best practices in clinical processes
Reducing waste, rework, and costs in processes	Lean, jidoka, just-in-time, various efforts to increase process efficiency (e.g., process mapping, service blueprints, standards and process benchmarking)

Source: Eduardo Álvarez-Falcón.

The success of any of these interventions in healthcare requires capable management, an organizational commitment to quality, and the embrace of TQM principles and skills as part of the organization's culture. Process improvements may encounter cultural barriers and resistance, and leaders will need to influence people's mind-sets, encourage openness, and generate support for trying new ways. The concepts, models, and principles discussed in this chapter, when capably applied and matched with the level of operational change desired, can provide healthcare managers with practical and powerful approaches for operational improvement decision making.

Note

1. For major definitions of *quality* within the literature, refer to Cole and Scott (2000).

Discussion Questions

1. What is the role of design thinking in the improvement of healthcare services? What are its limitations?
2. Explain the value of co-design. What challenges might arise, and how would one manage those challenges?
3. A public health agency in the United States has been accredited by the Public Health Accreditation Board, but to be reaccredited in

2020, the agency will need to move to a new set of specifications. The next-generation standards have already been published. Which of the three main benchmarking techniques discussed in the chapter—results, standards, and process benchmarking—is likely to be used? Support your answer by comparing and contrasting the advantages and disadvantages of the three options.

4. A mental health hospital is developing a new partnership scheme with community health centers and private doctors that will require new processes and the redesign of chains of activities. In this scenario, which of the models presented in the chapter is the healthcare manager likely to use? Explain your answer.

5. Think of an organization with which you are familiar, and identify a process that needs to be improved. List the activities you would carry out in each phase of the DMAIC cycle.

6. What are the similarities and differences between Six Sigma and Lean? Provide an example of a specific issue at a healthcare organization that Six Sigma or Lean could help address.

Case Study: Quality Improvement Principles and Methods Adopted by the National Health Service in the United Kingdom

Benchmarking

In 1995, the British government announced its intention to benchmark the performance of central Next Steps executive agencies—that is, the agencies created as part of the Next Steps performance-based reform initiative—against both the private sector and public services in other countries (Panchamia and Thomas 2018). After considering the options for an appropriate methodology, the government determined that the option proposed by the British Quality Foundation would be most advantageous. The British Quality Foundation option involved self-assessment of organizations' performance against standards set out in the Business Excellence Model (BEM) developed by the European Foundation for Quality Management (EFQM), as shown in exhibit 8.15 (EFQM 2006). This methodology was based on the principles and practices of TQM (Dean and Bowen 1999).

Government agencies in the UK also recognized the need to improve the link between their overall strategy and its organization-wide implementation by means of business planning (Cowper and Samuels 2001). Policies directed toward this goal were applied widely in the NHS. The NHS used benchmarking techniques to foster "internal competition," in the absence of true competitive markets. It also encouraged the adoption of best practices

(continued)

EXHIBIT 8.15
The UK/
European
Business
Excellence
Model and
Benchmarking

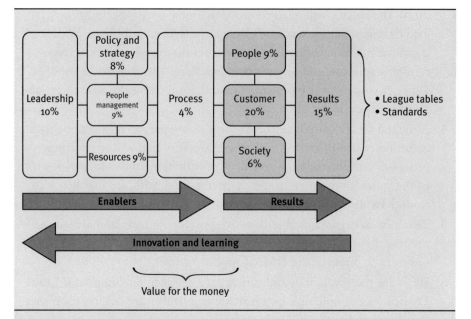

Note: The percentages are weights assigned to the criteria for benchmarking performance.
Source: Adapted from EFQM (2006).

through the use of predetermined standards and comparisons of accomplishments (results). This family of techniques, derived from the BEM, put in place important elements for the development of the NHS Performance Assessment Framework (PAF) (Álvarez-Falcón and Heymann 2006).

The NHS PAF introduced assessment of critical processes through such instruments as standard frameworks (in this case, National Service Frameworks) and value-for-money studies. It also included an outcomes/results measurement dimension in which organizational performance was compared against the best in class (via league tables), as well as performance incentives and rewards, such as budgetary autonomy or access to complementary funds for good performers. In both the process and outcome dimensions, the changes promoted by benchmarking filled in gaps relative to the best in class, thereby making for a balanced approach suitable for strategic or transformational change.

Six Sigma
In the early 2000s, the NHS Modernisation Agency (MA) and its successor, the NHS Institute for Innovation and Improvement (NHSI), began working on the improvement and redesign of NHS processes using improvement

approaches advocated by the Institute for Healthcare Improvement (IHI) in the United States (Young 2005).

From June 2004 to March 2005, the MA initiated a Six Sigma Green Belt initiative, in which more than 50 NHS staff members (mostly from the MA) received formal training and Green Belt certification. The staff worked on 14 projects with the aims of reducing waiting times and variation for patients referred for magnetic resonance imaging (MRI), shortening length of stay for low-risk chest pain patients, avoiding late follow-ups for ophthalmology outpatients, and reducing variability in nurse rostering (Boaden et al. 2005).

The initiative significantly accelerated the adoption of Six Sigma in the complicated environment of the NHS. Although participants in the pilot projects had to deal with chaotic and unstable processes, they began to appreciate the strengths of Six Sigma—particularly, the structured methodology and the well-defined tool set. The Six Sigma pilot projects also inspired growing interest in Lean thinking, with a focus on redesigning a process instead of just improving it (Proudlove, Moxham, and Boaden 2008).

Co-design

In 2005, the NHSI applied design methods with the aim of improving patients' experiences of treatment and care. These efforts led to the Experience Based Co-Design (EBCD) program, first piloted by Glenn Robert and Paul Bate in Luton and Dunstable University Hospital's head and neck cancer service (Bate and Robert 2007; Donetto, Tsianakas, and Robert 2014). The co-design process involved staff, patients, and others involved in the delivery of care, all of whom worked together to identify service improvement priorities and to devise and implement changes (Robert et al. 2015).

The initial pilot led to the development of a tool kit that was subsequently used to enhance touch point experiences for patients in two breast cancer services and two lung cancer services (Tsianakas et al. 2012). The NHS has since used the tool kit to improve a wide range of clinical services related to diabetes, drug and alcohol treatment, emergency care, genetics, and intensive care. Some specific improvements include the following:

- The use of iPad applications to help ventilated patients communicate
- Provision of information for staff and patients on the experience and impact of hallucinations
- Instructions for the correct application of continuous positive airway pressure (CPAP) masks

Additional Resources

Useful Websites
- The Helix Centre, a collaboration between Imperial College London and the Royal College of Art, which houses a multidisciplinary team inside a large London NHS hospital: http://helixcentre.com
- The Open School of the Institute for Healthcare Improvement, an online educational community seeking to help the healthcare workforce to deliver high-quality care: www.ihi.org/education/IHIOpenSchool/Pages/default.aspx
- The Public Health Accreditation Board, which establishes standards for public health departments in the United States: www.phaboard.org/accreditation-process/public-health-department-standards-and-measures/

Recommended Readings
- Brown, T. 2009. *Change by Design: How Design Thinking Transforms Organizations and Inspires Innovation.* New York: HarperCollins.
- Donabedian, A. 2003. *An Introduction to Quality Assurance in Health Care.* New York: Oxford University Press.
- Gladwell, M. 2002. *The Tipping Point: How Little Things Can Make a Big Difference.* New York: Back Bay.
- Heath, C., and D. Heath. 2010. *Switch: How to Change Things When Change Is Hard.* New York: Broadway Books.
- Institute of Medicine (IOM). 2001. *Crossing the Quality Chasm: A New Health System for the 21st Century.* Washington, DC: National Academies Press.
- Kimbell, L. 2014. *The Service Innovation Handbook: Action-Oriented Creative Thinking Toolkit for Service Organizations.* Amsterdam, Netherlands: BIS Publishers.
- McLaughlin, C. P., J. K. Johnson, and W. A. Sollecito. 2012. *Implementing Continuous Quality Improvement in Health Care: A Global Casebook.* Sudbury, MA: Jones & Bartlett Learning.
- McLaughlin, D. B., and J. R. Olson. 2017. *Healthcare Operations Management,* 3rd ed. Chicago: Health Administration Press.
- Porter, M. E., and E. O. Teisberg. 2006. *Redefining Health Care: Creating Value-Based Competition on Results.* Boston: Harvard Business School Press.
- Reason, B., L. Lovlie, and M. B. Flu. 2016. *Service Design for Business: A Practical Guide to Optimizing the Customer Experience.* Hoboken, NJ: John Wiley & Sons.

- Stickdorn, M., and J. Schneider. 2014. *This Is Service Design Thinking.* Amsterdam, Netherlands: BIS Publishers.
- Williams, S. 2017. *Improving Healthcare Operations: The Application of Lean, Agile and Leagility in Care Pathway Design.* New York: Palgrave Macmillan.
- Zidel, T. G. 2017. *Rethinking Lean in Healthcare: A Business Novel on How a Hospital Restored Quality Patient Care and Obtained Financial Stability Using Lean.* Boca Raton, FL: CRC Press.

References

Alessandro, L., B. Malcolm, and A. Jiju. 2013. "Applications of Lean Six Sigma in an Irish Hospital." *Leadership in Health Services* 26 (4): 322–37.

Álvarez-Falcón, E., and T. D. Heymann. 2006. "The United Kingdom's NHS Performance Assessment Framework: A Review of Its Evolution, Present Limitations and Suggestion for Future Direction." Paper presented at the European Academy of Management Conference, Oslo, Norway, May 2006.

Amaratunga, T., and J. Dobranowski. 2016. "Systematic Review of the Application of Lean and Six Sigma Quality Improvement Methodologies in Radiology." *Journal of the American College of Radiology* 13 (9): 1088–95.

Andersson, R., H. Eriksson, and H. Torstensson. 2006. "Similarities and Differences Between TQM, Six Sigma and Lean." *TQM Magazine* 18 (3): 282–96.

Antony, J., and R. Banuelas. 2002. "Key Ingredients for the Effective Implementation of Six Sigma Program." *Measuring Business Excellence* 6 (4): 20–27.

Banuelas Coronado, R., and J. Antony. 2002. "Critical Success Factors for the Successful Implementation of Six Sigma Projects in Organisations." *TQM Magazine* 14 (2): 92–99.

Bate, P., and G. Robert. 2007. "Toward More User-Centric OK: Lessons from a Case Study of Experience-Based Design." *Journal of Applied Behavioral Science* 43 (1): 41–66.

Berwick, D. M. 1998. "Crossing the Boundary: Changing Mental Models in the Service of Improvement." *International Journal for Quality in Health Care* 10 (5): 435–41.

Boaden, R. J., G. Harvey, N. C. Proudlove, R. Greatbanks, A. Shephard, and C. Moxham. 2005. *Quality Improvement: Theory and Practice in the NHS and Evaluation of the NHS Modernisation Agency Six Sigma Initiative.* Manchester, UK: Manchester Business School.

Brown, T. 2008. "Design Thinking." *Harvard Business Review* 86 (6): 84–92.

Care Quality Commission (CQC). 2018. "About Us." Accessed May 30. www.cqc.org.uk/about-us.

Centers for Medicare & Medicaid Services (CMS). 2017. *Hospital Value-Based Purchasing*. Accessed May 30, 2018. www.cms.gov/Outreach-and-Education/Medicare-Learning-Network-MLN/MLNProducts/downloads/Hospital_VBPurchasing_Fact_Sheet_ICN907664.pdf.

Cole, R. E., and W. R. Scott. 2000. *The Quality Movement and Organization Theory*. Thousand Oaks, CA: SAGE.

Collaboration for Impact. 2018. "The Collective Impact Framework." Accessed May 30. www.collaborationforimpact.com/collective-impact/.

Cottington, S., and S. Forst. 2010. *Lean Healthcare: Get Your Facility into Shape*. Marblehead, MA: HCPro.

Cowper, J., and M. Samuels. 2001. "Performance Benchmarking in the Public Sector: The United Kingdom Experience." Organisation for Economic Co-operation and Development. Accessed May 30, 2018. www.oecd.org/unitedkingdom/1902895.pdf.

Davenport, T. H. 1992. *Process Innovation: Reengineering Work Through Information Technology*. Boston: Harvard Business School Press.

Dean, J. Jr., and D. E. Bowen. 1999. "Management Theory and Total Quality: Improving Research and Practice Through Theory Development." *Academy of Management Review* 19 (3): 392–418.

Delbanco, T. 1992. "Enriching the Doctor–Patient Relationship by Inviting the Patient's Perspective." *Annals of Internal Medicine* 116 (5): 414–18.

DelliFraine, J. L., J. R. Langabeer 2nd, and I. M. Nembhard. 2010. "Assessing the Evidence of Six Sigma and Lean in the Health Care Industry." *Quality Management in Health Care* 19 (3): 211–25.

Department of Health, United Kingdom. 2011. *The Operating Framework for the NHS in England 2012/13*. Accessed June 1, 2018. www.gov.uk/government/publications/the-operating-framework-for-the-nhs-in-england-2012-13.

Design Council. 2011. *Reducing Violence and Aggression in A&E Through a Better Experience*. Accessed June 1. www.designcouncil.org.uk/sites/default/files/asset/document/ReducingViolenceAndAggressionInAandE.pdf.

Donabedian, A. 1988. "The Quality of Care. How Can It Be Assessed?" *JAMA* 260 (12): 1743–48.

Donetto, S., V. Tsianakas, and G. Robert. 2014. *Using Experience-Based Co-design (EBCD) to Improve the Quality of Healthcare: Mapping Where We Are Now and Establishing Future Directions*. London: King's College London.

Economist. 2009. "Benchmarking." Published July 27. www.economist.com/node/14116203.

European Foundation for Quality Management (EFQM). 2006. *The EFQM Framework for Managing External Resources*. European Institute of Purchasing Management. Accessed September 5, 2018. http://www.eipm.org/research/EFQM%20EIPM%20Framework%20for%20Exc%20Ext%20Resources.pdf.

European Observatory on Health Systems and Policies Series (EOHSPS). 2011. *Diagnosis-Related Groups in Europe*. Berkshire, UK: Open University Press.

Gruber, M., N. de Leon, G. George, and P. Thompson. 2015. "Managing by Design." *Academy of Management Journal* 58 (1): 1–7.

Hagan, P. 2011. "Waste Not, Want Not: Leading the Lean Health-Care Journey at Seattle Children's Hospital." *Global Business and Organizational Excellence* 30 (3): 25–31.

Harry, M., and R. Schroeder. 2000. *Six Sigma: The Breakthrough Management Strategy Revolutionizing the World's Top Corporation*. New York: Currency.

Health Foundation. 2018. "About the Francis Inquiry." Accessed June 1. www.health.org.uk/about-francis-inquiry.

Henke, C. 2009. "Healthcare Catches on to Lean, Six Sigma." *Quality Progress* 42 (5): 17.

Iles, V., and K. Sutherland. 2001. *Organisational Change: A Review for Health Care Managers, Professionals and Researchers*. London: National Co-ordinating Centre for NHS Service Delivery and Organisation Research and Development.

Institute of Medicine (IOM). 2001. *Crossing the Quality Chasm: A New Health System for the 21st Century*. Washington, DC: National Academies Press.

Jee, M., and Z. Or. 1999. "Health Outcomes in OECD Countries: A Framework of Health Indicators for Outcome-Oriented Policymaking." *OECD Labour Market and Social Policy Occasional Papers*, No. 36. Paris: OECD Publishing.

Johnson, G., and K. Scholes. 2002. *Exploring Corporate Strategy*. Harlow, UK: Pearson Education.

Joint Commission International (JCI). 2018. "About JCI." Accessed May 30. www.jointcommissioninternational.org.

Martin, R. 2009. *The Design of Business: Why Design Thinking Is the Next Competitive Advantage*. Boston: Harvard Business School Publishing.

Mason, S. E., C. R. Nicolay, and A. Darzi. 2015. "The Use of Lean and Six Sigma Methodologies in Surgery: A Systematic Review." *Surgeon* 13 (2): 91–100.

Mayo Clinic. 2017. "Design in Health Care." Accessed June 1, 2018. http://centerforinnovation.mayo.edu/design-in-health-care/.

Murray, C. J. L., and J. Frenk. 2000. "A Framework for Assessing the Performance of Health Systems." *Bulletin of the World Health Organization* 78 (6): 717–31.

National Health Service (NHS) England. 2017. "Patient Reported Outcome Measures (PROMs)." Accessed January 3. www.england.nhs.uk/statistics/statistical-work-areas/proms/.

———. 2000. "The NHS Plan: A Plan for Investment, a Plan for Reform." Published July. https://navigator.health.org.uk/content/nhs-plan-plan-investment-plan-reform-2000.

National Institute for Health and Care Excellence (NICE). 2017. "Evidence Search." Accessed January 31. www.evidence.nhs.uk/Search?q=national+service+frameworks.

Ohno, T. 1998. *Toyota Production System: Beyond Large Scale Production.* Portland, OR: Productivity Press.

Panchamia, N., and P. Thomas. 2018. "The Next Steps Initiative." Institute for Government. Accessed June 7. www.instituteforgovernment.org.uk/sites/default/files/case%20study%20next%20steps.pdf.

Persona, A., D. Battini, and C. Rafele. 2008. "Hospital Efficiency Management: The Just-in-Time and Kanban Technique." *International Journal of Healthcare Technology and Management* 9 (4): 373–91.

Point of Care Foundation. 2018. "About Us." Accessed June 5. www.pointofcare-foundation.org.uk/about-us/.

Porter, M. E. 1985. *Competitive Advantage: Creating and Sustaining Superior Performance.* New York: Free Press.

Porter, M. E., and T. H. Lee. 2013. "The Strategy That Will Fix Health Care." *Harvard Business Review* 91 (10): 50–70.

Proudlove, N., C. Moxham, and R. Boaden. 2008. "Lessons for Lean in Healthcare from Using Six Sigma in the NHS." *Public Money & Management* 28 (1): 27–34.

Public Health Accreditation Board (PHAB). 2018. "About PHAB." Accessed May 31. www.phaboard.org/about-phab/.

Pyzdek, T., and P. Keller. 2014. *The Six Sigma Handbook*, 2nd ed. New York: McGraw-Hill.

Results That Matter Team. 2018. "Community Balanced Scorecards (CBSCs)." Accessed June 7. www.rtmteam.net/page.php?pageName=CBSC.

Rittel, H., and M. M. Webber. 1973. "Dilemmas in a General Theory of Planning." *Policy Sciences* 4 (2): 155–69.

Robert, G., J. Cornwell, L. Locock, A. Purushotham, G. Sturmey, and M. Gager. 2015. "Patients and Staff as Codesigners of Healthcare Services." *BMJ.* Published February 10. www.bmj.com/content/350/bmj.g7714.

Roberts, S., and S. Singh. 2009. "Implementing Lean in Primary Care." *British Journal of Healthcare Management* 15 (8): 380–86.

Royal College of Physicians of Edinburgh. 2018. "Acute Medicine." Accessed June 1. www.rcpe.ac.uk/college/acute-medicine.

Sangiorgi, D. 2009. "Building Up a Framework for Service Design Research." Paper presented at the 8th European Academy of Design Conference, Aberdeen, Scotland, April 1–3.

Secretaría de Salud. 2015. "Official Mexican Standards." Government of Mexico. Published August 20. www.gob.mx/salud/en/documentos/normas-oficiales-mexicanas-9705.

Service Design Network (SDN). 2017. "SDN Manifesto." Accessed January 3. www.service-design-network.org/manifesto.

Shah, R., A. Chandrasekaran, and K. Linderman. 2008. "In Pursuit of Implementation Patterns: The Context of Lean and Six Sigma." *International Journal of Production Research* 46 (23): 6679–99.

Smee, C. 2001. "Improving Value for Money in the UK NHS: Performance Measurement and Improvement in a Centrilised System." Organisation for Economic Co-operation and Development. Published November 5. www.oecd.org/els/health-systems/1960033.pdf.

Stanford Health Care. 2018. "New Stanford Hospital." Accessed June 1. www.sumcrenewal.org/wp-content/files_mf/1510614143NSHFactSheet11.13.17.pdf.

Tlahuiz, M. A. L. 2011. "The Application of Lean Principles and Six Sigma in the Mexican Health Care System." MPhil thesis, University of Leicester.

Trebble, T. M., N. Hansi, T. Hydes, M. A. Smith, and M. Baker. 2010. "Process Mapping the Patient Journey: An Introduction." *BMJ* 341: c4078.

Tsianakas, V., G. Robert, J. Maben, A. Richardson, C. Dale, and T. Wiseman. 2012. "Implementing Patient-Centred Cancer Care: Using Experience-Based Co-design to Improve Patient Experience in Breast and Lung Cancer Services." *Supportive Care in Cancer* 20 (11): 2639–47.

United Kingdom Accreditation Service (UKAS). 2017. "Health & Social Care." Accessed January 15. www.ukas.com/sectors/healthcare/.

Walters, D., and G. Lancaster. 2000. "Implementing Value Strategy Through the Value Chain." *Management Decision* 38 (3): 160–78.

Womack, J. P., D. T. Jones, and D. Roos. 1990. *The Machine That Changed the World.* New York: Free Press.

World Health Organization (WHO). 2000. *The World Health Report 2000.* Geneva, Switzerland: WHO.

Wykes, S. 2016. "Design Thinking as a Way to Improve Patient Experience." Stanford Medicine News Center. Published June 3. https://med.stanford.edu/news/all-news/2016/06/design-thinking-as-a-way-to-improve-patient-experience.html.

Young, T. 2005. "An Agenda for Healthcare and Information Simulation." *Health Care Management Science* 8 (3): 189–96.

Zairi, M., and Y. F. Jarrar. 2001. "Measuring Organizational Effectiveness in the NHS: Management Style and Structure Best Practices." *Total Quality Management* 12 (7–8): 882–89.

Zairi, M., and P. Leonard. 1994. *Practical Benchmarking: A Complete Guide.* Dordrecht, Netherlands: Kluwer Academic Publishers.

MANAGERIAL ETHICS IN GLOBAL HEALTH

Michael M. Costello, JD, and Eva Grey, MD, PhD

Chapter Focus

This chapter examines the topic of managerial ethics in a global health context. It highlights the importance of ethics in managerial decision making, with attention to the additional sensitivity of ethical decision making in situations where two or more cultures come together. The chapter contains a variety of examples of ethical issues that might arise in health settings throughout the world.

Learning Objectives

Upon completion of this chapter, you should be able to

- justify the importance of ethics for global health managers;
- assess the most appropriate ethical theories to be applied in international healthcare settings;
- analyze the shortcomings of certain ethical theories, particularly in working with different cultures and vulnerable populations;
- evaluate situations to support ethical decision making in global health; and
- demonstrate an understanding of ethical sensitivity in global health management.

Competencies

- Analyze problems, promote solutions, and encourage decision making.
- Encourage diversity of thought to support innovation, creativity, and improvement.
- Exercise cultural sensitivity in internal and external communication.
- Demonstrate effective problem-solving skills.

- Advocate for the rights and responsibilities of patients and their families.
- Commit to competence, integrity, altruism, and the promotion of the public good.
- Demonstrate high ethical conduct, a commitment to transparency, and accountability for one's actions.
- Include the perspectives of individuals, families, and the community as partners in healthcare decision-making processes, with respect for cultural differences and expectations.

Key Terms

- Bioethics
- Consequentialism
- Cultural imperialism
- Deontology

- Managerial ethics
- Moral relativism
- Principlism
- Utilitarian ethics

Key Concepts

- Autonomy
- Beneficence
- Character
- Cultural sensitivity
- Ethics
- Global ethics

- Globalization
- Justice
- Morality
- Nonmaleficence
- Responsibility
- Values

Introduction

Being a manager means having to make important decisions that affect an organization and the people the organization serves. Therefore, a central element of managerial development involves instilling in individuals the knowledge and confidence necessary to facilitate effective decision making in difficult situations. An appreciation for the ethical issues that surround specific decisions or sets of decisions is of paramount importance.

managerial ethics The area of study focused on ethical issues and concerns related to managerial responsibilities.

The study of **managerial ethics** seeks to answer questions of what a manager should do when confronted with ethical issues related to managerial responsibilities. Ethical management requires managers to develop an orientation that goes beyond their individual self-interest and leads to a recognition of moral responsibility to the organization and its constituencies. In this chapter, we will examine a number of the key concepts of managerial ethics, with attention to various issues and considerations that are unique to the context of global health.

Ethics in the Context of Global Health

Global health managers have a somewhat more complex set of ethical considerations than would be expected of healthcare managers functioning in a single nation or culture, requiring them to develop a sensitized conscience based on awareness of both the internal and external environments in which the healthcare organization functions. Summarizing the distinctive challenges facing global health managers, Daft (2013, 409) writes: "Organizations operating on a global basis often face particularly tough ethical challenges because of the various cultural and market forces they deal with. The greater complexity of the environment and organizational domain creates a greater potential for ethical problems or misunderstandings." National boundaries and varying cultural traditions are accepted as part of the landscape within which global health managers function, yet globalization is arguably leading to greater uniformity in many dimensions of civilization. Today's health managers must learn to appreciate this dynamic.

The code of ethics of the American College of Healthcare Executives (ACHE 2017) speaks of a manager's responsibilities to four distinct constituencies: (1) the organization, (2) employees, (3) patients or others served, and (4) the community and society. As challenging as these responsibilities are to a manager functioning in a single nation or culture, they become considerably more detailed and nuanced when the manager's scope traverses national boundaries and diverse cultures. Rorty (2014, 9) describes the individual manager's responsibility to the organization: "How the organization acts—the strategies and policies, the choices and decisions that operationalize these values and determine how they affect the day-to-day work of your institution—are to a great extent the responsibility of the leaders, the healthcare administrators."

Global health managers need to possess not only an appreciation of what is traditionally considered managerial ethics but also a working knowledge of professional ethics and **bioethics** as they apply to the supervision of professional individuals in the delivery of healthcare. The concerns of bioethics grow out of the day-to-day issues facing healthcare professionals in the delivery of clinical and research services. Even if the healthcare manager herself does not have a clinical background, her supervisory responsibility for physicians, nurses, and other professional practitioners requires an appreciation for the issues they face in patient care and research. This responsibility becomes more complex in a global context, especially if the manager and professional practitioners have cultural orientations different from one another or from those of the patients.

bioethics
The field of ethical study related to biological or medical practices.

cultural imperialism
The practice of imposing a society's own culture and morality on people of another society.

moral relativism
The tendency to consider morality relative to one's own society, potentially leading to assumptions that the ethical beliefs of people in another society are appropriate for them without question.

A serious consideration of ethics in a global health context requires far more than deference for the moral traditions of the society in which the global health manager is working. In *One World Now: The Ethics of Globalization*, Peter Singer (2016, 163) cautions against the shortcomings of **cultural imperialism** and **moral relativism**. Cultural imperialism occurs when individuals attempt to impose their own society's culture and morality on people of another society, whereas moral relativism occurs when morality is considered relative to one's own society and the ethical beliefs of people in another society are accepted without question as being appropriate for them. Singer (2016, 163) explains:

> Moral relativists imagine they are defending the rights of peoples of non-Western cultures to preserve their own values, but when moral relativism is taken seriously, it undermines all ethical arguments, including those against cultural imperialism. . . . There is, on this view, no way of moving outside the morality of one's own society and expressing a transcultural or objective moral judgement about anything, including respect for the cultures of different peoples.

The discussion of ethical issues tends to generate deep interest from conscientious individuals both inside and outside the organization. Many organizations throughout the world have established ethics committees to help address ethical issues and meet accreditation standards. When such committees are used to aid in the management of a healthcare organization, particular attention must be paid to their makeup. In a healthcare delivery setting, an ethics committee would be expected to comprise both managers and clinical practitioners responsible for delivering patient care, as well as, perhaps, external participants with advanced training in law, ethics, and medicine. The selection of qualified and interested individuals to serve on the committee and present diverse perspectives can have a significant impact on the organization's ethical climate. Particular attention should be paid to the educational preparation that committee members receive prior to initiating their responsibilities to the organization.

Managers play a vital role in shaping the ethical climate of the organization. They need to clarify and communicate organizational values, ethical principles and theories, and decision-making processes, including those specifically for solving ethical dilemmas. They need to ensure not only that ethical principles are being followed but also that people see those principles being followed. In international healthcare settings, people come from various historical, cultural, social, and religious backgrounds, and they often have different goals and priorities. Despite these differences, managers need to help foster the trust necessary for successful cooperation and compliance with group decisions. A sense of "global ethics" needs to exist, based on common values, aims, and principles, with respect for the dignity of every human being without discrimination based on age, sex, ethnicity, religion, or disability. Daft (2013, 406) stresses the importance of managerial commitment to ethical values and the need to communicate those values to members of the organization: "The CEO and other top managers must be committed to specific ethical values and provide constant leadership in tending and renewing the values. Values can be communicated in a number of ways—speeches, company publications, policy statements, and, especially, personal actions. People follow and model what they see managers doing."

Perspectives on Ethical Management

What does it take to be an ethical global health manager? Numerous authors have weighed in on this topic, addressing the ethical development of managers both in general settings and in healthcare specifically.

In his 1988 classic *The Moral Manager*, Walton emphasizes the importance of "character" to a manager's ethical development and ability to lead successfully. In doing so, he addresses one of the oldest questions in moral philosophy: "Can virtue be taught?" Ultimately, Walton (1988, 177) argues that it can: "Example, not exhortation and practice, not principle, take priority: carpenters become carpenters by building houses; pianists become pianists by playing the piano; managers become leaders by leading. The same is true of character: people become virtuous by practicing virtue and by living with moral mentors."

Walton (1988, 219) summarizes many of his thoughts regarding the development of an ethical manager as follows:

- Managers require virtue, an old-fashioned word with ongoing durability.
- Not false pride but a sense of obligation drives executives to demand the best from themselves and, at least, the "better" from subordinates—a point requiring early and frequent statement in the organization's philosophy and through reiteration of its code of ethics.
- As character comes before charisma, so, too, does virtue come before versatility. To understand what virtue is and to live by what virtue demands are two related, but different, things.
- Example is the best teacher, embodying those qualities that constitute virtue—prudence, fairness, fortitude, and temperance—enhances the manager's teaching role.

Walton (1988, 219) also touches on the role of managers in a global economy, stating that "comprehension by executives of their own culture is a necessity, and appreciation of other cultures is a highly desirable auxiliary."

Hartman (2015, 238) suggests that effective ethical decision making involves value judgments that result from the interaction of good character and appreciation of learned principles:

> Your good character does not tell you exactly what to do in most complex situations, and certainly not in situations that, owing to radical changes in the environment, are unlike any you have seen before. It does demand that you make your significant decisions at the right time, in the right way, about the right things, with the right kind of involvement of the right people and for the right purposes. If you have only rules and habits to go by, you will be unable to come to any kind of useful understanding with people who have different rules. If you are not guided by a clear sense of what is important, you will make irrational decisions, and you will be a terrible leader.

The literature of global health management has sought to define *ethics* in the terms of global health. Pinto and Upshur's (2013, 27) *An Introduction to Global Health Ethics*, referencing the work of Benatar, Daar, and Singer (2011), lists seven values to serve as the basis for global health ethics:

- Respect for all human life
- Human rights, responsibilities (duties) and needs—broadly considered
- Equity
- Freedom (freedom from "want," as well as freedom "to do")
- Democracy (in a participatory sense)
- Environmental ethics
- Solidarity

The authors also offer a framework for transformational approaches (Pinto and Upshur 2013, 27):

- Developing a global state of mind
- Promoting long-term self-interest
- Striking a balance between optimism and pessimism
- Developing capacity (to be independent)
- Achieving widespread access to public goods

Global health managers are likely to encounter many of the same ethical issues that more traditional health managers encounter, but additional issues related to global health contexts—and their more diverse employee, community, and patient settings—can be anticipated. For instance, Skolnik (2012) has highlighted human rights concerns as a major issue facing global health managers. Managers in global settings should also be prepared to address such issues as research involving human subjects and the proper management of organizations' financial resources and investments.

Ethical Theories for Global Health

A wide variety of ethical theories can be applied to healthcare provision, but three of the most commonly applied are consequentialism (including utilitarian ethics), deontology, and principlism.

Consequentialism

Consequentialism represents a group of ethical theories that seek to evaluate an action as ethical or unethical based on the action's consequences. One of the most prominent of consequentialist theories is **utilitarian ethics**, which is based on the following principles in combination (Prikasky 2000; Anzenbacher 1994):

1. *The principle of consequences.* No action is morally right or morally wrong in itself. The moral quality is based solely on the consequences of the action.
2. *The principle of utility.* The more good consequences an act produces, the better or more right that act is.
3. *The principle of hedonism.* Good consequences are those that maximize pleasure and minimize pain. Jeremy Bentham is a representative of *quantitative hedonism*—the idea that pleasure is individual and only the amount (quantity) of pleasure matters. John Stuart Mill, meanwhile, represents *qualitative hedonism*—the idea that some pleasures ("spiritual pleasures," for instance) are superior to other pleasures (quality).
4. *The social principle.* The best action is the one that will lead to the highest level of happiness for the largest possible number of people.

consequentialism
An ethical theory in which an action is determined to be ethical or unethical based on its consequences.

utilitarian ethics
A theory based on the idea that the most ethical action is the one that produces the maximum good for the greatest number.

Consequentialism in global health can be counterproductive. Most people are uncomfortable with the idea that "the end justifies the means," and they feel that some actions must be considered inherently wrong regardless of any possible good outcome. In healthcare, some actions might offer the perception of positive outcomes but still be ethically problematic. For instance, a provider might refrain from certain diagnostic or therapeutic interventions to minimize patient pain or discomfort in the short term, but the patient would then lose out on the benefits of those interventions in the long term. Alternatively, an action supported by consequentialist thinking might sacrifice the individual rights of a person or small group to justify positive outcomes for a larger group of patients. For instance, consider the disproportionate suffering of patients receiving the first heart transplants or other experimental operations (Vacha, Konigova, and Mauer 2012).

With utilitarian ethics, similar decisions might be regarded as more or less ethical based on outcomes that are tied to particular circumstances, leading to perceptions of inconsistency with regard to decision making. In global health settings, even more so than in traditional health settings, this type of inconsistency can undermine trust or even be perceived as discriminatory against certain racial or ethnic groups, women, older adults, or other groups.

Deontology

Immanuel Kant refuted utilitarian ethics and instead emphasized that the difference between humans and other animals is human reason—the ability to make rational decisions. He believed that human beings have wisdom and rationality, which help them understand what is good and bad in specific situations, as well as the free will to choose the right decision for themselves. Thus, they should make decisions based on their conscience. According to Kant, general human moral principles exist in everyone's conscience and are binding for every rational being—this obligation is a categorical imperative. A general guiding principle can be formulated: Act always in such ways that the maxims of your actions could become general legislation. We have a moral obligation to do what our conscience perceives as right (Anzenbacher 1994), and our conscience should be cultivated to recognize as right such actions that could be proclaimed as a general law. This approach to ethics based on moral reasoning, rules, and obligation is known as **deontology**. Another important principle of deontology states: Act in such ways that you treat yourself or any other human not as a mere tool, but as a purpose of its own (Vacha, Konigova, and Mauer 2012). In other words, human beings should never be used as tools or as products for sale or exchange.

In global health contexts, deontology has the advantage of treating every human being with respect and protecting individuals' dignity. However, different people's consciences—which reflect personal opinions, as well as cultural and religious backgrounds—may lead people to different decisions in specific situations. In addition, people are often at least partially motivated by passions, as opposed to reason based on ethical imperatives. Therefore, a deontological approach may be difficult to require in all instances.

Principlism

Because ethicists in healthcare have not reached general agreement on either consequentialism or deontology, a third approach, known as **principlism**, has gained prominence. Advanced by Beauchamp and Childress in 1979, principlism is based on four basic principles of bioethics (Beauchamp and Childress 2013):

deontology
An approach to ethics based on moral reasoning, rules, and obligation.

principlism
An ethical approach based on four basic principles of bioethics: (1) beneficence, (2) nonmaleficence, (3) autonomy, and (4) justice.

1. *Beneficence.* Do good; do the best for the patient.
2. *Nonmaleficence.* Do no harm; try to prevent negative consequences.
3. *Autonomy.* Respect the free will of the patient; ensure informed consent.
4. *Justice.* Treat all patients in similar situations equally, in the best possible way, without discrimination.

These principles provide basic guidelines to help solve ethical issues in health-care provision, and they are general enough to be accepted by most scholars. Beneficence and nonmaleficence require the ability to analyze and understand problems and their solutions, weighing potentially positive and negative conse-quences to improve professional competencies. They also push healthcare pro-fessionals to look for what is best for the patients and what should be avoided, so that the rights of the patients can be protected. Autonomy requires that the perspectives of individual patients be included in the healthcare decision-making process, with respect for cultural and religious differences—a major concern in global health management. Finally, a sense of justice prevents global health managers from accepting substandard healthcare for vulnerable communities.

Principlism has become the most commonly accepted ethical approach in bioethics, and specifically in global health ethics. It provides an understandable framework for the decision-making processes of healthcare practitioners, and it can be adapted to various cultural and religious backgrounds. In practical medicine, however, the four principles may sometimes come into conflict with one another. Various authors have stressed one principle over another; other authors have added new principles, such as confidentiality or mutuality, to the original four (DeMarco 2005).

Ethical Issues in Global Health Management

The provision of healthcare in global settings presents many of the same ethical issues that arise in healthcare provision within one's home country, along with several additional concerns. The following sections describe ethical issues of specific relevance to global health management.

Cultural Ignorance of Providers
Cultural sensitivity is essential for global health management. Often, foreign aid is delivered by people who do not understand the local culture and ways of life. They might not speak the local language, and they might lack knowledge about local customs, communication patterns, and prejudices. Healthcare managers who lack cultural understanding will have difficulty not only in cooperating

with local providers and colleagues but also in working with programs' intended beneficiaries. Misunderstanding and poor communication can jeopardize the success of any project. Global health managers need to demonstrate respect for local people, their innate dignity, and their human rights; furthermore, managers must require that the people they manage show that respect as well.

Inflexibility in Promoting Medical Interventions

Global health managers working with a local population might be encouraged to promote certain medical interventions to get the most out of their development aid budget. During their stay, however, they might find out that other activities, whether medical or nonmedical, would actually be more useful for improving the population's health status. Improving nutrition, building wells to secure clean water, constructing toilets and sewage systems, and providing shelter can all help reduce health problems such as malaria or diarrheal diseases. In fact, these types of nonmedical activities can sometimes reduce mortality more than medical interventions, such as early testing or drug therapy, can (Easterly 2006).

Healthcare managers need to observe what works and accept the reality that, in some instances, providing a piece of meat once a week or a glass of milk every day might improve children's health more than medication will (Schavel et al. 2012; Jančovičová and Ondrušová 2012). Achieving this mindset might not be easy, but health managers should nonetheless try it. For example, a program to control parasitic infections could shift from provision of antiparasitic drugs to the building of wells. Similarly, a program to reduce complications related to malaria in babies could shift its focus to improving the nutrition of pregnant women.

"Leftover Medicine"

Global health managers are often tempted to promote medical exports from their own country of origin when working with a recipient country. Such exports might include medical equipment for diagnosis and therapy, as well as medications and other supplies. Bringing such products to a country can have benefits in certain circumstances, but it may also come to be a problem. The continued import of products over the long term can hurt local efforts to manufacture or sell similar products, thereby hampering efforts for self-sufficiency. In such cases, the situation might be worse after the health program ends than it was before the program started. The effect can be especially negative if the imports are based not on the needs of the local population but rather on domestic surplus in the country of origin—in other words, if the products amount to "leftover medicine." For example, a small health clinic in a developing country might receive an extra mammography machine when it would really benefit more from other equipment. Sometimes, surplus just takes up space in the shipping container that could have been used for something more useful.

Global health managers should be able to understand what is useful and what is not, and they should have the courage to politely refuse useless gifts. Managers should pay particular attention to the expiration dates on drugs that are collected for distribution in a foreign country. By the time of arrival, the drugs might be expired or close to expired, causing local authorities to reject them at border crossings.

Tension Between Local/Traditional Medicine and Evidence-Based Medicine

Small health clinics often lack equipment for certain tests, and the equipment favored in highly developed countries is not always appropriate for local conditions. In many cases, the import of complex machines that need "feeding" with specialized diagnostic sets is impractical, and the normal supply or repair costs of such machines might be out of budget in the local community.

Consider this example: A charity health clinic in Kenya received, as a gift from a developed country, a complex analyzer that could measure numerous biochemical substances from a blood sample (e.g., different fractions of cholesterol). However, shipping to Kenya was difficult, and the machine started having problems soon after it was in use. An investigation revealed several possible causes of the problems. For instance, electric current in the local network was inconsistent, and environmental conditions were hotter, more humid, and dusty. These conditions were too much for the sensitive machine to handle, and no repair service for the product was available. Ultimately, the clinic was advised to buy a local machine that was better adapted to the local conditions and had a specific built-in voltage balancer.

In many cases, relatively simple local methods may be available and inexpensive. For instance, a simple test for malaria can be completed by looking at a thick blood smear under a microscope. Managers need to know about such possibilities and provide training for practitioners when necessary.

Another issue is that the guidelines applicable in developed countries are sometimes not feasible in underdeveloped areas. Global health managers should strive to bring state-of-the-art care to even the most vulnerable populations, but such care is not always possible. Developed countries, for instance, use a number of interventions to prevent transmission of HIV from pregnant mothers to their children: They provide anti-HIV drugs to the pregnant mothers with HIV and to their children after birth; they plan the mothers' deliveries via cesarean section; and they advocate formula feeding of the babies rather than breastfeeding (US Department of Health and Human Services 2018). In many rural areas of developing countries, however, such an approach would be counterproductive. In such settings, cesarean sections might not be readily available, and a decision not to breastfeed could introduce health risks for the baby that are greater than the small risk of HIV transmission through breast milk. That said, antiretroviral drugs for expectant mothers and newborns have been made available in many developing countries and should be used according to adjusted guidelines to significantly decrease HIV transmission from mother to child (Suvada, Tumbu, et al. 2010).

"Guinea Pig" Healthcare

Sometimes, the people who wish to participate in global health programs are not sufficiently qualified for the job. In many instances, medical students and even nonmedical personnel might be highly enthusiastic but lacking in the necessary skills, especially with regard to the particular health situation of the recipient country. A related concern involves the harm that can result from the form of "medical tourism" that occurs when doctors travel to exotic locations for a brief opportunity to practice medicine on local residents (Bishop and Litch 2000).

Global health managers need to be aware of their own values, strengths, and limitations, as well as those of their personnel. If managers do not state clear conditions for staff selection, they may end up with healthcare personnel performing procedures for which they have no training or procedures that they would not be able to do in their home country. Such a breach of competency would be regarded as unprofessional and discriminatory toward local patients. This breach should be distinguished, however, from instances where healthcare personnel perform procedures for which they are qualified but that they have little opportunity to perform in their home country. A practitioner might not have performed a certain procedure before but still be qualified to do it after proper training. Such a situation might arise with treatment of diseases that are uncommon in the practitioner's home country (e.g., testing for malaria, treatment for leprosy).

Additional concerns about "guinea pig" healthcare surround the use of local people for research. Research involving local populations must conform to the *International Ethical Guidelines for Biomedical Research Involving Human Subjects*, from the Council for International Organizations of Medical Sciences (CIOMS 2002), as well as the Nuffield Council's (2002) *The Ethics of Research Related to Healthcare in Developing Countries* (Williams 2015).

The testing of medications and vaccines in foreign settings can be challenging and time consuming because of the need to comply with the appropriate ethics or review committees. Furthermore, gaining informed consent from patients can be difficult if language barriers and literacy issues interfere with the sharing of information and the signing of legal papers. However, failure to comply with these requirements can lead to unethical behavior, legal issues, and harm to both the research and the patients. In light of these concerns, the testing of new drugs, vaccines, and procedures should ideally not be performed in a foreign country—especially a developing one.

Nevertheless, in some cases, research might be necessary to prevent, diagnose, or cure diseases (e.g., malaria) that are specific to certain developing countries (Suvada, Bartosova, et al. 2010). Such study should be encouraged, given the fact that, proportionately, fewer resources are invested in the research of diseases specific to developing countries than in the research of diseases common in developed countries (Williams 2015). This kind of research is also beneficial given that, with increasing globalization, some diseases that were previously limited to developing countries might spread around the world.

In a global program, a health manager's work begins with good planning before travel and the selection of qualified team members. Minimal and optimal qualification criteria for the program can help with the evaluation of the individuals who are interested. Some training can be provided before travel, and additional training and supervision can be provided after arrival. Cooperation with local medical specialists and local hospitals should always be encouraged, especially in the management of difficult cases.

Mobility of Physicians

Often, physicians from less-rich countries wish to practice medicine in a richer country, whether motivated by better salary, the ability to practice with better technical equipment, or participation on a specific research project. This movement of physicians can be advantageous for the individuals themselves and for the countries they go to, but it can have a negative impact—in the form of a "brain drain" on the physicians' countries of origin. The World Medical Association, in its "Statement on Ethical Guidelines for the International Recruitment of Physicians," does not recommend that doctors be forbidden to work abroad, but it requests that countries, instead of relying on immigration, work to train a sufficient number of physicians to cover their own needs (Williams 2015).

Physician mobility can also have positive effects, particularly in the case of physicians and other health workers who practice medicine abroad for a limited period and then return to their home countries with new professional knowledge and skills. Healthcare managers should support those solutions that are best for global health provision.

Problematic Motivation of Healthcare Personnel

Physicians, nurses, and other healthcare workers may have a variety of motivations for traveling to a different country and practicing medicine there. In cases where professionals from developed countries travel to help in underdeveloped areas, the most common motivations are positive, such as altruism and solidarity with the less privileged, promotion of good solutions for the vulnerable, desire to learn something new, and willingness to accept the challenge of working with limited resources and living in less comfortable conditions. However, some motivations, whether conscious or unconscious, can lead to problems and potentially endanger a project. Potentially problematic motivations include pride, adventure seeking, and the desire to escape from problems at home or to solve personal problems that could not be solved at home.

Pride becomes problematic when proud individuals think of themselves as "saviors" of the poor and treat the locals as inferior. They might feel that they operate "above" the rules and therefore not comply—even when the rules are important or useful. They might think that any kind of help is good for the underprivileged and perform procedures that would not be acceptable in their home country. Such actions can hurt patients and compromise an entire project.

Young people often seek adventure, and participation in a project in an unfamiliar country can be exciting and requires a certain amount of courage. However, practitioners whose main motivation is adventure might neglect the more mundane aspects of their work, and they may put themselves in disproportionate risk, especially in areas of conflict. Healthcare managers are responsible for safety of the staff, but they cannot be the staff's bodyguard.

Some people may choose to join a foreign mission to escape from problems at home. Consider this example: A young doctor from Europe decided to undertake a six-month project in Sudan, where she had served two years previously. Her brother was in treatment for cancer at the time, and she felt great frustration that she could not help him, even though she was a physician. She justified her decision to go to Sudan based on the need of the local people and the responsibility she felt toward the locals she already knew and had served before. During her stay in Sudan, however, her brother's disease progressed rapidly, to the point that it appeared he had only a short time to live. The doctor then decided that, even though she could not help her brother as a doctor, she needed to be with him as a sister. However, no flight home was available, and the project management in Sudan had no replacement for her. The doctor became distressed and conflicted over her decisions, and her focus and commitment for the work in Sudan suffered.

Similar issues may occur in cases where people feel that traveling away from home will help them solve problems that they were unable to solve at home. For instance, an alcoholic physician might think that practicing medicine in a remote area without the possibility to buy alcohol and without the company of his drinking friends will help him cure his alcoholism. However, the difficult conditions and loneliness of life in the foreign country might trigger his addiction, causing him to seek out forms of alcohol that are not safe. A poisoning from technical alcohol could endanger the doctor's life and also compromise the entire project.

For all of the aforementioned reasons, global health managers should be extremely careful in selecting healthcare personnel based not only on their professional skills and competencies but also on their personality and motivation.

Managers should note that a person's real motivation might not be obvious even to the person concerned (Benca 2016).

Imposition of Foreign Values and Disputed Rights

In recent decades, one of the great problems of global health policy has involved the imposition of programs based on philosophies that are foreign to the cultures being served (Birdsall 2008). Such philosophies are rarely welcomed by local populations and may be regarded as forms of "health neocolonialism." These concerns have affected programs at all levels—even those from major international organizations such as the United Nations (UN), the World Health Organization (WHO), and the UN Children's Fund (UNICEF).

One such philosophy is based on the fear of overpopulation, a concern that was highlighted through the work of the Club of Rome. A number of population-control measures have been implemented based on the hope that a slower population increase in a country will lead to better health and less poverty, and some such measures have become a precondition for countries receiving foreign aid and investment. Measures with a potential impact on population control have included the decriminalization of, and subsequent support for, the practice of abortion; the promotion of affordable contraceptives and other means of preventing or terminating early pregnancy; and support for same-sex partnerships or nontraditional relationships that cannot produce offspring. Such practices can be unfamiliar, or even offensive, to recipients of healthcare services in many areas. For instance, if a remote clinic in a developing country needs antibiotics, antimalarial drugs, and safe birth kits, it may be taken aback by a medical aid delivery of condoms, contraceptives, and abortifacient drugs. Such a delivery might be perceived as suggesting eugenics based on race or ethnicity or implying inferiority of the locals. When aid is perceived in such a manner, trust and cooperation erode, posing a significant threat to global health provision.

The following example demonstrates the damage that can stem from loss of trust and perceived imposition of foreign values. In October 2014, the WHO and UNICEF sponsored a tetanus vaccination campaign in Kenya. However, a Catholic physician group in the country claimed that some vials of the vaccine were laced with HCG (human choriogonadotropin), which could trigger production of anti-HCG antibodies and cause miscarriage in the future pregnancies of women vaccinated in the program (Muchangi 2015). The medical community expected that the WHO and UNICEF would ask several independent laboratories to test the vaccines to prove they were not contaminated, but the organizations responded only with a statement denying the accusation (UNICEF 2015). Because of the lack of proof from independent laboratories, Kenyans were not convinced that the vaccines were safe (England 2015). Ultimately, such instances can lead to reduced compliance with vaccination programs and spur the growth of antivaccination movements worldwide (Grey and Mrazova 2016).

Global health managers need to respect the people receiving health services, treat them on an equal basis, and recognize their cultural and religious beliefs. When healthcare professionals understand the local people well, they can serve as mediators between locals and international authorities, helping to improve communication and cooperation.

Cooperation with Locally Based Providers

Effective global health design and provision require knowledge of local laws, social systems, cultures, traditions, beliefs, and other aspects of life (Easterly 2006). This kind of cultural understanding is best developed through cooperation with locally based providers (e.g., physicians, pharmacies, clinics, large hospitals) and with charity, government, and nongovernment organizations. Health provision should be based on listening and supporting the priorities of locals. Providers' manner of communication should reflect local customs, and newer providers should try to learn from other foreigners who have been based in the area for a while and know the local setting.

People in many parts of the world use traditional local remedies for treatment of diseases, and health managers might question whether such remedies are effective. Health managers should always promote whatever practice works best, but if people believe that a certain local practice helps and the practice does no harm, they do not have to fight against it. Local customs should be discouraged only in cases where they are harmful—as in the case of female genital mutilation, for instance.

Learning to Be Ethical Global Health Managers

Given the complexities of ethical analysis and the need to incorporate moral considerations from diverse cultures, how do global health managers develop the sensitivities necessary to carry out their responsibilities in an ethical manner? The preparation for global health leadership involves information from multiple sources.

In the late 1600s, the British philosopher John Locke wrote of the need for reasoning in ethical analysis. As summarized by Gottlieb (2016), Locke believed that "there is no universal agreement about morals, so morals cannot be innate in any straightforward sense." Thus, people cannot simply memorize a list of ethical principles that can be applied universally. Gottlieb explains: "In matters of morality . . . Locke argued that men must think for themselves. They should not blindly accept the practices and standards of the day, because 'moral Principles require Reasoning and Discourse, and some Exercise of the Mind, to discover the certainty of their Truth.'"

Professional preparation in ethics for global health management would appear, at a minimum, to require an approach from two levels: the preparation of the individual and the application of ethical behavior in an external context. In his *Nicomachean Ethics*, Aristotle wrote of two "complete" virtues: "greatness of soul, or virtue in relation to oneself, and justice, or virtue in relation to another" (Bartlett and Collins 2011, 270). Serious preparation for a global health manager arguably begins with development of the individual's character, as noted by Walton and others earlier in this chapter. This area of development is sometimes known as *virtue ethics*, or ethics based on character. Munson and Lague (2016, 53) define this aspect of ethics as the fundamental idea that "a person who has acquired the proper set of dispositions will do what is right when faced with a situation involving a moral choice." Justice, the second of Aristotle's "complete" virtues, is based on the demonstration of character in addressing an ethical issue with another person or group. It would seem that the exercise of justice becomes significantly more complex when global health managers confront moral issues in cultures other than their own.

Singer (2016) writes that globalization has, in certain respects, resulted in a world community in which members share common moral obligations. This sense of community has developed in large part through geopolitical and technological developments that have broken down barriers between nations and cultures. Singer (2016, 15) writes that "how well we come through the era of globalization . . . will depend on how we respond ethically to the idea that we live in one world. For the rich countries not to take a global ethical viewpoint has long been seriously morally wrong. Now it is also, in the long term, a danger to their security."

Serious students of managerial ethics in a global health context can further their study in several ways, described in the paragraphs that follow. Rather than addressing these elements sequentially, students should look to integrate them into a comprehensive approach that recognizes the contributions of each.

Social and Cultural Observation

In the effort toward ethical and moral development, students can learn much by observing and studying. How do respected individuals in society deal with a certain issue? What seem to be the fundamental beliefs that shape their reactions? Does the legal system address the issues of importance, and does the legal approach seem to lead to just resolution? In more developed nations, popular media may reflect societal beliefs about morality and the corresponding ethical behavior. Likewise, national institutions, including the government itself, might make announcements or publish materials that provide guidance on moral issues.

Religious Influence

For many people, ethical and moral beliefs are developed through the course of their religious upbringing. Religious traditions influence the way adherents think, and in many instances they provide an individual's first exposure to ethics and morality. Religious traditions are commonly reflected in medical practice, often in a person's willingness to serve the underprivileged (Curlin et al. 2007).

The ethical and moral beliefs that are developed through organized religion may continue to influence people's thinking even if religion itself takes a smaller role in the individuals' lives. Indeed, many scholars today refer to "secular bioethics" as a branch of study that has evolved without attributed religious influence.

Individual Reading and Study

Philosophers have written about the human condition since the time of the ancient Greeks, and the published literature on ethics and morality is almost boundless. Ethics is considered one of the main branches of philosophy, and much can be gained by studying the great ethicists of the past. A familiarity with the writings of Plato, Aristotle, Immanuel Kant, René Descartes, Thomas Hobbes, Baruch Spinoza, John Locke, and David Hume, among others, can lay an excellent foundation for ethical reasoning and analysis. Writings from the present day can also enhance a manager's appreciation of ethics and morality. Modern periodical literature can demonstrate the endurance of ethical concepts and reaffirm a manager's ethical commitment.

Formal Education

Graduate and professional education can be a valuable adjunct for managerial preparation, but hopefully not to the exclusion of the other elements described. The study of ethics and morality is a lifelong endeavor. Formal academic course-work in graduate or professional studies should reflect the distinctions between managerial ethics, professional ethics, and bioethics. Professional codes of ethics should be included as part of this study, along with cases that analyze ethical reasoning from a practical standpoint.

Summary

The field of managerial ethics deals with questions of what managers should do when confronted with ethical issues related to their managerial responsibilities. Ethical management requires managers to develop an orientation that goes beyond their individual self-interest and encompasses their moral responsibility to the organization and its constituencies. Global health managers face a uniquely complex set of ethical considerations. They need to possess a firm understanding of not only managerial ethics but also professional ethics and bioethics, while operating in an ever-changing healthcare context spanning multiple diverse cultures. Numerous scholars, from ancient times to the present day, have written about ethics and morality and provided guidance for individuals' ethical development. Of the various ethical theories that can be applied to global healthcare provision, three of the most notable are consequentialism, which focuses on an action's consequences; deontology, which emphasizes reasoning, rules, and obligation; and principlism, which combines the principles of beneficence, nonmaleficence, autonomy, and justice. In applying these principles and carrying out their responsibilities, global healthcare managers must always demonstrate cultural sensitivity toward the populations they serve. A sense of "global ethics" needs to be based on common values, aims, and principles, and it needs to respect the dignity of every human being without discrimination based on age, sex, ethnicity, religion, or disability.

Discussion Questions

1. How do managerial ethics in a global context differ from ethics in a single nation or culture?
2. What is the role of character in the development of a healthcare manager's ethical sensitivity?
3. What is consequentialism? What might be some problems with using utilitarian ethics while providing healthcare services in a foreign country?
4. What are some of the ways in which global health managers might improve their understanding of ethics?
5. What specific ethical issues are likely to arise when providing healthcare services in a developing country?
6. What ethical concerns might need to be considered when conducting biomedical research in a developing country?

Vignette: Healthcare Services for Undocumented Immigrants

The increasing migration of people throughout the world has serious implications for ethical decision making in global health contexts (*Economist* 2016). The arrival of immigrants in a new nation raises difficult questions about responsibility for the provision of healthcare services.

In the United States, the Emergency Medical Treatment and Active Labor Act (EMTALA), a federal statute dating back to 1986, aims to ensure access to care for any citizen experiencing a medical emergency. It requires that hospitals with emergency treatment capacity screen and stabilize all patients who present themselves seeking medical care and who believe they are facing an emergency situation. The Affordable Care Act of 2010,

(continued)

however, prohibits the use of government-subsidized health insurance to finance care for individuals who cannot prove legal immigration status. About a quarter of the approximately 30 million uninsured people in the United States are believed to be undocumented immigrants, according to the US Congressional Budget Office (Radnofsky 2016).

Investigating the situation in the United States, *The Wall Street Journal* found that, of the 25 counties in the United States with the largest undocumented immigrant populations, 20 of them have developed programs using local resources to pay for healthcare services for low-income uninsured immigrants (Radnofsky 2016). Such programs pay for doctors' visits, shots, prescription drugs, lab tests, and surgeries at local providers, with little or no charge to immigrants receiving them. The patients are told that they must prove they live in the county providing the services, but they are not required to demonstrate immigration status. These services are provided to an estimated 750,000 undocumented immigrants at an approximate annual cost of $1 billion.

Critics of the programs maintain that tax revenues provided by US citizens should not be used to provide care for undocumented immigrants. However, proponents of the county-based services argue that federal tax monies are already being used to subsidize the cost of care provided under EMTALA. A local official in Montgomery County, Maryland, states, "If federal programs exclude people who live here and get sick here, then someone has to care for them" (Radnofsky 2016). Another county official suggests that, by providing these basic health services, the county is saving money: "If we don't pay now when it is easy money, we are going to pay later on" (Radnofsky 2016).

References

American College of Healthcare Executives (ACHE). 2017. "ACHE Code of Ethics." Revised November 13. www.ache.org/abt_ache/code.cfm.

Anzenbacher, A. 1994. *Uvod do etiky*. Prague, Czech Republic: Academia.

Bartlett, R. C., and S. D. Collins. 2011. *Aristotle's Nicomachean Ethics: A New Translation*. Chicago: University of Chicago Press.

Beauchamp, T. L., and J. F. Childress. 2013. *Principles of Biomedical Ethics*, 7th ed. New York: Oxford University Press.

Benatar, S. R., A. S. Daar, and P. A. Singer. 2011. "Global Health Ethics: The Rationale for Mutual Caring." In *Global Health and Global Health Ethics*, edited by S. R. Benatar and G. Brock, 129–40. Cambridge, UK: Cambridge University Press.

Benca, J., J. Šuvada, E. Grey, L. Bučko, and M. Nová. 2016. *Globálna rozvojová pomoc*. Příbram, Czech Republic: Dvojfarebný svet and J. N. Neumann Publishing House.

Birdsall, N. 2008. "Seven Deadly Sins: Reflections on Donor Failings." In *Reinventing Foreign Aid*, edited by W. Easterly, 515–52. Cambridge, MA: MIT Press.

Bishop, R., and J. A. Litch. 2000. "Medical Tourism Can Do Harm." *BMJ* 320 (7240): 1017.

Council for International Organizations of Medical Sciences (CIOMS). 2002. *International Ethical Guidelines for Biomedical Research Involving Human Subjects*. Geneva, Switzerland: CIOMS.

Curlin, F. A., L. S. Dugdale, J. D. Lantos, and M. H. Chin. 2007. "Do Religious Physicians Disproportionately Care for the Underserved?" *Annals of Family Medicine* 5 (4): 353–60.

Daft, R. L. 2013. *Organization Theory & Design*, 11th ed. Boston: Cengage Learning.

DeMarco, J. P. 2005. "Principlism and Moral Dilemmas: A New Principle." *Journal of Medical Ethics* 31: 101–5.

Easterly, W. 2006. *The White Man's Burden: Why the West's Efforts to Aid the Rest Have Done So Much Ill and So Little Good*. New York: Oxford University Press.

Economist. 2016. "Looking for a Home." Published May 28. www.economist.com/special-report/2016/05/28/looking-for-a-home.

England, C. 2015. "WHO Puts Kenyan Tetanus Vaccine Under Police Guard to Avoid Testing." *Green Med Info*. Published March 9. www.greenmedinfo.com/blog/who-puts-kenyan-tetanus-vaccine-under-police-guard-avoid-testing.

Gottlieb, A. 2016. *The Dream of Enlightenment: The Rise of Modern Philosophy*. New York: Liveright Publishing Corporation.

Grey, E., and M. Mrazova. 2016. "Did We Fail the Public? Social, Medical and Ethical Reasons for the Anti-vaccination Movement." In *Business and Health Administration Proceedings*, edited by A. Mukherjee, CD-ROM. Chicago: Business and Health Administration Association.

Hartman, E. M. 2015. *Virtue in Business: An Aristotelian Approach*. Cambridge, UK: Cambridge University Press.

Jančovičová, L., and A. Ondrušová. 2012. *Riešenia detskej podvýživy v Keni*. Bratislava, Slovakia: Nadácia Pontis.

Muchangi, J. 2015. "Kenya: 500,000 Women Sterilized—Catholics." *All Africa*. Published February 14. http://allafrica.com/stories/201502150078.html.

Munson, R., and I. Lague. 2016. *Intervention and Reflection: Basic Issues in Bioethics*, 10th ed. Boston: Cengage Learning.

Nuffield Council on Bioethics. 2002. *The Ethics of Research Related to Healthcare in Developing Countries*. Accessed June 20, 2018. http://nuffieldbioethics.org/wp-content/uploads/2014/07/Ethics-of-research-related-to-healthcare-in-developing-countries-I.pdf.

Pinto, A. D., and R. E. G. Upshur (eds.). 2013. *An Introduction to Global Health Ethics*. London: Routledge.

Prikasky, J. V. 2000. *Ucebnice zakladu etiky*. Kostelni Vydri, Czech Republic: Karmelitanske nakladatelstvi.

Radnofsky, L. 2016. "Illegal Immigrants Get Public Health Care, Despite Federal Policy." *Wall Street Journal.* Published March 24. www.wsj.com/articles/illegal-immigrants-get-public-health-care-despite-federal-policy-1458850082.

Rorty, M. V. 2014. "Introduction to Ethics." In *Managerial Ethics in Healthcare: A New Perspective,* edited by G. L. Filerman, A. E. Mills, and P. M. Schyve, 1–17. Chicago: Health Administration Press.

Schavel, M., L. Paskova, E. Misikova, M. Krcmery, A. Mamova, M. Kacanyova, P. Mikulasova, R. Machalkova, I. Duraj, A. Bajcarova, J. Benca, J. Sokolova, N. Kulkova, V. Krcmery, J. Mutuku-Muli, A. Matel, and I. Bartosovic. 2012. "Community Based Interventions Against Protein Calorie Malnutrition: Examples from Programme 'Goat' in Sudan, Rwanda and Burundi." In *Proceedings of the Business and Health Administration Association,* edited by S. J. Saccomano, 174–76. Chicago: Business and Health Administration Association.

Singer, P. 2016. *One World Now: The Ethics of Globalization,* 3rd ed. New Haven, CT: Yale University Press.

Skolnik, R. 2012. *Global Health 101,* 2nd ed. Burlington, MA: Jones & Bartlett Learning.

Suvada, J., M. Bartosova, H. I. Nkonwa, and C. Vertus. 2010. *PMTCT Guidelines for Rural Areas in Uganda.* Nakasero Hill, Uganda: Ministry of Health.

Suvada, J., P. Tumbu, J. Kyiamba, and V. Krcmery. 2010. *Neglected Diseases: Prevention and Treatment in HIV-Infected Children and Adolescents.* Nakasero Hill, Uganda: Baylor College Training Center Uganda/Kampala.

United Nations Children's Fund (UNICEF). 2015. "Statement from WHO and UNICEF on the Tetanus Vaccine in Kenya." Accessed June 20, 2018. www.unicef.org/kenya/media_15665.html.

US Department of Health and Human Services. 2018. "Preventing Mother-to-Child Transmission of HIV." Reviewed May 24. https://aidsinfo.nih.gov/education-materials/fact-sheets/20/50/preventing-mother-to-child-transmission-of-hiv.

Vacha, M., R. Konigova, and M. Mauer. 2012. *Zaklady moderní lékařské etiky.* Prague, Czech Republic: Portal.

Walton, C. C. 1988. *The Moral Manager.* Grand Rapids, MI: Harper Business.

Williams, J. R. 2015. *Medical Ethics Manual,* 3rd ed. Ferney-Voltaire, France: World Medical Association.

BOARDS AND GOOD GOVERNANCE

James A. Rice, PhD, FACHE, Egbe Osifo-Dawodu, MD, Godfrey
Gwaze Sikipa, MD, and Gilbert Kokwaro, PhD

Chapter Focus

In global health, boards of directors, or boards of trustees, are groups of community, business, and health sector leaders who play a crucial role in creating
the conditions within which people who deliver and manage health services are
more likely to succeed. This chapter covers a wide range of concepts related
to boards and good governance, with the intention of helping health system
leaders, especially those in low-resourced countries, explore the power of the
board to improve their systems and health outcomes. In particular, the chapter
describes 5 key practices and 11 essential elements of a good infrastructure for
effective board work.

Learning Objectives

Upon completion of this chapter, you should be able to

- define three practical benefits of an effective board for a healthcare
  organization,
- understand the typology of the governing bodies used within the health
  sectors of low- and middle-income countries,
- define five common risks of poor governance,
- describe five essential governance practices that drive board
  effectiveness, and
- identify five competencies of great board members.

Competencies

- Articulate and communicate the mission, objectives, and priorities of
  the organization to internal and external entities.

- Create an organizational climate built on mutual trust and transparency, with a focus on service improvement that encourages teamwork and supports diversity.
- Demonstrate effective interpersonal relationships and the ability to develop and maintain positive stakeholder relationships.
- Demonstrate reflective leadership by using self-assessment and feedback from others in decision making.
- Demonstrate high ethical conduct, a commitment to transparency, and accountability for one's actions.
- Evaluate whether a proposed action aligns with the organizational business/strategic plan.
- Connect the interrelationships among access, quality, cost, resource allocation, accountability, and community need.

Key Terms and Concepts

- Board of directors
- Board of trustees
- Competency-based governance
- Conflicts of interest
- Continuous improvement
- Culture of accountability
- Decision making
- Diversity
- Education
- Effective meetings
- Ethics
- Good governance
- Governing bodies
- Groupthink
- Health systems strengthening
- Information technology
- Infrastructure for governance
- Member orientation
- Performance dashboard
- Performance indicators
- Policies and regulations
- Resource management
- Self-assessment
- SMART governance
- Stakeholder engagement
- Strategic direction
- Terms of reference (TOR)
- Web portal

A Scenario to Stimulate Strategic Thinking About Good Governance for Health

Imagine you are a senior staff member in a middle-income country's Ministry of Health. The Parliament has asked each community health center to form its own governing body from community leaders and health workers. The terms of reference (TOR)[1] for these new bodies must be drafted within one month for consideration as a regulatory act in Parliament. What considerations should you weave into this proposed new policy? What should be the essential roles and responsibilities of the new community health center governing councils? How should you help the members of these governing bodies become educated about good board work? Consider these questions as you begin your journey into the realm of good board work as presented in this chapter.

terms of reference (TOR)
Documents used to define the scope of responsibilities for leaders, boards, and organizations.

Introduction

Do you want a stronger health system and better health outcomes? Then invest in smarter governance of the programs and organizations of your system.

Whether working in nongovernmental organizations (NGOs), civil society organizations (CSOs)[2], for-profit private sectors, or facilities run under public–private partnership (PPP) arrangements or decentralized/autonomous organizations of ministries of health, the people who lead, manage, or deliver health services benefit when governing bodies and governance decision-making processes are wise and ethical.[3] This point is true particularly for low-resourced health systems in low- and middle-income countries, which are the focus of this chapter.[4]

Governing bodies make decisions about policy, plans, and rules for collective action. When good governance is evident, the members of governing bodies wield power and resources to define, promote, protect, and achieve the health mission of an organization, system, program, district, province, state, country, or institution. For health services organizations, the focus of this collective action is to strengthen health systems to expand access to health services, which in turn leads to better and more sustained health outcomes.

A health system consists of all the people, institutions, resources, and activities that have the primary purpose of promoting, restoring, and maintaining health (World Health Organization 2000). Health systems strengthening (HSS) involves activities in six internationally accepted core functions: (1) human resources for health; (2) health finance; (3) health governance; (4) health information; (5) medical products, vaccines, and technologies; and (6) service delivery (US Agency for International Development 2015).[5] A well-performing health system is one that achieves sustained health outcomes through continuous improvement of these six interrelated HSS functions.

The principles and practices in this chapter apply to most types of organizations, regardless of wealth, and they have relevance both in healthcare and in sectors beyond health. They can also be used in organizations that purchase, finance, or regulate health services. Our focus in this chapter, however, is to support better healthcare and make a greater health impact in health organizations in low-resourced communities around the world.

What Is Governance for Health?

Why do nations and communities need good governing bodies and community engagement? What is good governance? What are the essential practices for high-performing governing bodies? What are the benefits of these governing bodies? This chapter seeks to answer these strategic questions for leaders and managers working in the health sectors of low- and middle-income countries. It also highlights 11 infrastructure factors of good governing bodies that contribute to health system improvement.

Good governance for health is a mission-driven and people-centered decision-making process to achieve optimal health for the populations served. It is carried out by a group of leaders who are organized and entrusted by a government, civil society, private organization, or distinct population of stakeholders. Their job is to protect, promote, and restore the health of the people the entity serves. These leaders may handle one or more high-priority health concerns, such as control of a communicable disease, case management for a noncommunicable disease, or emergency obstetric and newborn care. They can also serve people in rural or urban areas through governmental, nongovernmental, or private-sector organizations. A study for the African Union estimated that more than one million people are serving in more than 170,000 governing bodies in the health sectors of the union's 55 member states.[6]

We believe that good governance advances the mission of an organization or agency to deliver high-impact health services to individuals and communities, especially the most vulnerable populations. Good governing bodies can also engage local community leaders in ways that contribute to political stability and economic development.

Essential Practices and Characteristics

A governing body sets strategic direction and objectives; makes policies, laws, rules, regulations, and decisions; raises and deploys resources; and oversees the work of the organization. It seeks the best ways to achieve its strategic goals and objectives and enhance the long-term vitality of the organization to pursue its mission. To foster good governance for health, the people who govern, the governing bodies themselves, health sector leaders, and managers at all levels must become knowledgeable about good board work. This knowledge should include new organizational forms and practices of governing for health.

Good governance is based on five essential practices, which will provide a key framework for this chapter (*eManager* 2013):

1. Creating a culture of accountability
2. Engaging stakeholders
3. Setting a shared strategic direction
4. Stewarding resources responsibly
5. Continuous improvement of the four practices above

If robust infrastructure is in place for good board work, then continuous governance enhancement—the fifth practice—is easier to apply. Transparency policies will achieve little if the political system does not include the sanctioning of public officials when government corruption is exposed; penalties for service providers when poor performance or absenteeism is revealed; and safeguards or structural reforms in response to evidence of systemic governance problems. In recent years, much attention has been placed on the capacity of citizens to use information, the role of media and civil society groups as intermediaries to make information more accessible, and the extent to which the political space exists for citizens to exert influence and effect change; all of these concerns may be considered when determining the efficacy of governance (Savedoff 2011).

The United Nations (UN) Economic and Social Commission for Asia and the Pacific (2018) asserts that good governance has eight major characteristics. It is

1. participatory,
2. consensus oriented,
3. accountable,
4. transparent,
5. responsive,
6. effective and efficient,
7. equitable and inclusive, and
8. in accordance with the rule of law.

Good government ensures that corruption is minimized, that the views of minorities are taken into account, and that the voices of the most vulnerable in society are heard. It is responsive to both the present and future needs of society.

The various types of organizations that make up a nation's health sector are all likely to have "boards." These boards may go by such names as a *board of directors*, a *governing body*, a *governing council*, a *board of trustees*, a *board of commissioners*, a *board of governors*, a *board of overseers*, or a *health committee*, and their roles and scope of authority may vary widely. The engagement of these groups with multiple stakeholders from their communities can represent a positive force for popular capitalism, democracy, and economic well-being. Health sector managers, therefore, must master a variety of concepts, strategies, and processes for effective health system board work. This mastery can be challenging, however, because of the many obstacles that exist to good governance.

Obstacles to Good Governance

The promise and benefits of good board work can only be achieved when common obstacles are removed, reduced, or worked around. The most common obstacles are as follows:

1. The board is not given adequate authority to govern.
2. The board is unable to recruit talented and ethical people to serve on the board and its committees.
3. Board members do not understand their roles and responsibilities.
4. The board does not receive support (e.g., information, orientation, education, staff help) from managers to successfully engage in wise decision making.
5. The board does not commit to continuously evaluating and refining its governance processes and practices.

This chapter provides information to help board and administrative leaders overcome these obstacles by (a) being ever vigilant to identify and commit to removing each obstacle and (b) understanding and applying positive activities and practices to ensure success.

Leaders Must Take Action for Good Governance

SMART governance Governance that is stakeholder (S) engaged, is mission (M) driven, is accountable (A) to beneficiaries and resource providers, mobilizes resources (R) to support the mission, and demonstrates transparency (T) in all plans and decision making aimed at accomplishing the mission.

If you are a good manager or healthcare provider, you should care about defining and supporting the infrastructure for good health sector governance. What actions should you take to encourage, enable, and empower good governance? What factors are known to facilitate or frustrate good governance? What are the benefits of good governance, and how can various stakeholders help maximize these benefits?

Your answers to these questions will vary somewhat depending on your organization, country, and community context. Your unique approach to good governance will also be shaped by your personal wisdom and influence, as well as by your commitment to ensuring the conditions necessary to continuously improve health services for those most likely to face illness, injury, and disability in your region, district, or catchment area.

Great leaders come in all shapes, sizes, ages, and genders. They represent a variety of backgrounds, experiences, nationalities, languages, cultures, and attitudes, and they come to work with diverse knowledge, skills, and competencies. The practice of **SMART governance** enables leaders and organizations to fully maximize these characteristics. SMART governance is stakeholder (S) engaged, is mission (M) driven, is accountable (A) to beneficiaries and resource providers, mobilizes resources (R) to support the mission, and demonstrates transparency (T) in all plans and decision making aimed at accomplishing the mission.

Leaders can take five key actions to build good governance:

Action 1: Establish, champion, and publicize a clear strategic purpose or mission for the organization and its governing body.

Action 2: Engage and empower competent people to work successfully in the organization's governing processes and decision-making structures.

Action 3: Provide a consistent moral and ethical compass and conscience for the enterprise—whether it is an organization, program, facility, agency, department, council, or ministry—as it strives to achieve its mission.

Action 4: Work with the chairperson of the governing body to define and continuously improve the first four key practices for SMART governance:
1. Cultivating accountability
2. Engaging stakeholders
3. Setting a shared strategic direction
4. Stewarding resources responsibly

Action 5: Support the availability of good information and infrastructure for decision-making processes that are consistent with SMART governance.

Good Governance Benefits Health Sector Leaders

We believe that, if you invest your time, talents, and funds in these five key actions for better governance, you will reap the following five important benefits:

Benefit 1: You will be more effective and efficient at building and operating health systems that save more lives and reduce more sickness.

Benefit 2: You will waste less of your and your colleagues' time when planning, developing, and operating programs and institutions designed to promote, protect, and restore health for all people—especially the most vulnerable and disadvantaged.

Benefit 3: Your career will likely be more satisfying, stable, secure, and economically attractive.

Benefit 4: You, your family, and your community will be prouder of your work and the results you achieve.

Benefit 5: The results you achieve will be more significant and more sustainable.

Why do we believe these bold assertions? We believe in the benefits of good governance because we have seen them in countries throughout Asia, Africa, Latin America, Europe, and North America. We also believe in them because we have forged a clear theory of change that focuses on SMART governance for health and the actions leaders can take to support better systems and better governance.

The work of effective leaders has been previously described in the Management Sciences for Health (2005) book *Managers Who Lead: A Handbook for Improving Health Services.*[7] That book generally describes leaders and managers as the men and women who develop, lead, and manage not only health sector–related organizations but also boards, councils, and commissions dedicated to sustainable health systems strengthening. Roles may also include regional/provincial medical/health directors/officers; regional/provincial nursing officers; and district medical/nursing officers. Such individuals must realize that they have a role to play in health sector governance and that facilitating the work of governance boards/structures is part of their responsibility.

Good governance enables those who lead, manage, and deliver health services to be more effective and efficient by

1. establishing policies, plans, and procedures that remove obstacles affecting leaders and their work;
2. encouraging leaders to be more successful in supporting the governing body to accomplish the essential governing practices of
   - cultivating accountability,
   - engaging stakeholders,
   - setting a shared strategic direction,
   - stewarding resources responsibly, and
   - continuously improving the four practices above;
3. making available the resources—political, human, technological, and financial—that leaders and healthcare professionals need to do their work;
4. expecting, encouraging, and empowering leaders and managers to strive for service delivery that meets or exceeds standards of excellence; and
5. celebrating the organization's journey toward stronger health systems and better health outcomes.

Good Governance Benefits Health Systems

Good board work not only helps health sector leaders better accomplish their work; it also has benefits for health systems and the populations they serve. Good governance creates the conditions in which the "eight rights" improve health systems to achieve better outcomes:

1. The right number of health workers
2. The right quality of health workers
3. The right mix of health workers
4. The right facilities in which to work
5. The right budgets/financing
6. The right medicines, equipment, and supplies
7. The right clinical care protocols
8. The right cultural appropriateness of care

The idea of good governance can be a shallow, false promise—one that is often broken—if it is not understood and demanded by all those who lead, manage, and deliver health services. Good governance does not happen just because you hope it will. Hope is not a strategy. Good governance is more likely to be achieved if one makes a personal commitment to explore the many facets of good and poor governance, then takes action to embrace the good and combat the poor.

Good governing bodies offer the following ten major health system benefits:

1. They improve rapport and engagement with the community, generate support from the community, and enhance understanding of the health needs of people and communities for business planning and market planning.
2. They expand political influence with local and regional politicians to strengthen access to needed resources (whether human, financial, technical, or regulatory).
3. They leverage their members' experience and ideas to help develop better plans to expand equitable access to health services.
4. They encourage leaders to improve accountability to implement plans and improve performance for various constituencies and stakeholders.
5. They help support oversight, accountability, and professional growth for the CEO, the senior management team, and leaders in numerous areas (e.g., medicine and nursing, health promotion, business expertise, finance, legal matters, marketing, process improvement, total quality improvement, public health, epidemiology). They also incorporate the thinking and tools of Six Sigma[8], supply chain management concepts, and expertise in change management in turbulent times and with scarce resources.
6. They shield the CEO from pressures from politicians, health workers, staff, vendors, and unions.

7. They foster an objective view of strategic plans and tactical initiatives by posing challenging questions about meaning and importance.

8. They bring new and objective perspectives to problem definitions and problem resolutions.

9. They support the pursuit of philanthropy, grants, funding, or government backing to achieve the mission.

10. They serve as a sounding board to ensure clarity and to make plans, strategies, and resource investments more effective.

This results-oriented theory rests on five assumptions:

Assumption 1: Governance interventions (e.g., consulting, training, supportive resources, materials) should contribute to group decision making that has the following seven characteristics:
- Mission driven
- Practice based
- People centered
- Open and transparent
- Ethical and honest
- Evidence informed
- Results oriented

Assumption 2: This style of decision making should enable decisions in six spheres that are essential for protecting and strengthening the pursuit of the organization's mission:
- Strategic planning focused on the needs of populations and communities
- Financial planning and budgeting
- Resource mobilization or increased revenues
- Design and delivery of services, and design and implementation of programs
- Quality assurance and service excellence for beneficiaries
- Development and management of human resources

Assumption 3: Decisions in these spheres are more likely to ensure the availability of services that cost-effectively protect, promote, and restore health in all segments of the population because they are delivered
- with the right quality;
- in the right place and time;

- with cultural sensitivity and appropriateness;
- affordably, as measured in terms of a beneficiary's money, comfort, and convenience; and
- with the right numbers and types of health workers who have the right knowledge, skills, attitudes, and competencies and are provided the right compensation, support, and incentives for service excellence.

Assumption 4: The availability of these types of services expands the likelihood that beneficiaries will use the services and that the services will be sustainable.

Assumption 5: The people using the services are more likely to achieve gains in health outcomes that are significant and sustainable.

Master Good Governance Practices

The five essential practices for good governance, as noted earlier, are (1) creating a culture of accountability, (2) engaging stakeholders, (3) setting a shared strategic direction, (4) stewarding resources responsibly, and (5) ensuring continuous governance improvement (*eManager* 2013). These practices have been distilled from principles that evolved over many years through the experiences of frontline health sector leaders and managers. They are also based on several decades of study of governance across a spectrum of organization types in health and other social sectors, including business, government, education, and the arts.

A good set of seven principles for a governing body, as enumerated by the International Planned Parenthood Federation (2007), is as follows:

Principle 1: The governing body ensures member integrity and collective responsibility.

Principle 2: The governing body determines the organization's strategic direction and policies.

Principle 3: The governing body appoints and supports the executive director/CEO.

Principle 4: The governing body monitors and reviews the organization's performance.

Principle 5: The governing body provides effective oversight of the organization's financial health.

Principle 6: The governing body is open, responsive, and accountable.

Principle 7: The governing body ensures its own review and renewal.

Principles for good governance have also been set forth by a variety of organizations, including the Global Fund, the World Health Organization (WHO), the World Bank, the Organisation for Economic Co-operation and Development

Effective Governing Practice	Enabler
Cultivate accountability	Openness and transparency
Engage stakeholders	Inclusion and participation Gender-responsiveness Intersectoral collaboration
Set shared direction	Effective leadership and management
Steward resources	Ethical and moral integrity Pursuit of efficiency and sustainability Measurement of performance Use of information, evidence, and technology in governance

Source: Reprinted with permission from *eManager* (2013).

(OECD), and the Center for Healthcare Governance of the American Hospital Association.[9] Good governance is also taken to be key to the achievement of the UN's Sustainable Development Goal 3, which is to "ensure healthy lives and promote well-being for all at all ages" (UN 2018).

Exhibit 10.1 shows the first four key governance practices that effective boards strive to continuously improve. Improvement can be achieved through annual self-assessments and open conversations among governing body leaders, healthcare workers, and the organization's management team.

Five Imperatives

By designing and institutionalizing SMART governance practices, an organization can improve its performance and become more likely to deliver better health outcomes that can be sustained.[10] The degree to which successful outcomes result from good governance is a function of how well the organization accomplishes five imperatives:

Imperative 1: *Process.* Your governance processes must be inclusive, transparent, and accountable to all key stakeholders (Ciccone et al. 2014).

Imperative 2: *People.* The governing body should include a reasonable number of competent people who reflect the demographic characteristics of the system's beneficiaries and who have influence among those who control power and access to needed resources in the local context (Kickbusch and Gleicher 2012).

Imperative 3: *Practices.* The governing body's leaders must continuously discuss and implement actions that support the five essential practices of governance (*eManager* 2013).

Imperative 4: *Infrastructure.* SMART governance decision making requires a good infrastructure of support staff and information that is accurate and timely (National Leadership Council 2012).

Imperative 5: *Performance.* Health organizations must be dedicated to achieving meaningful results, as measured in service utilization and sustained gains in health status. This imperative requires the commitment to continuously design interventions in a way that enables measurement and study of the factors that maximize the impact of good governance (USAID 2014).[11]

Infrastructure for SMART Board Decision Making

Good governance for health is about the art and science of good decision making relative to the policies, plans, and performance of the governing bodies that are charged with overseeing the work and results of health organizations. High-performing governing bodies have systems and people that develop and manage sound decision-making processes. These processes have numerous elements that must work together in a well-organized and coordinated manner in challenging environments in low-resourced health systems and country contexts.

The decision-making processes for governing bodies should address ten questions:

1. Who makes the decisions?
2. How are parties informed and educated to participate in the decision making?
3. Who advises the decision makers in their process for decision making?
4. What criteria are used in the decisions?
5. How organized, ethical, effective, efficient, and transparent is the process of making decisions?
6. How are the decisions reported to stakeholders and beneficiaries in a way that is understandable and accessible?
7. How can beneficiaries and stakeholders best monitor the implementation of the decisions?
8. Who reports the progress and results of the decisions, and how?

9. How are the decision-making processes continuously improved?

10. How do stakeholders and beneficiaries best ensure improved accountability of the plans and investments based on these decisions and their decision-making processes?

The answers to these questions are informed by a theory of change, illustrated in exhibit 10.2, that shows how good board work leads to stronger health systems and better health outcomes.

Managers seeking to enable good board work need to address key questions about the structures, practices, and infrastructure for governance decision making:

1. *Structures to house good governance.* What are the various types of settings and organizations in which governance decision making is to occur? What characteristics of the governing bodies are best suited for the unique country contexts and organizational settings in which these bodies find themselves? What characteristics will help them to succeed? What types of people are engaged in governance decision making for

EXHIBIT 10.2
Context, Drivers, and Enablers for Good Governance

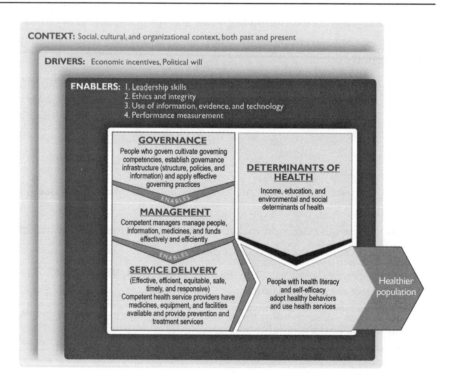

Source: Reprinted from Global Health Learning Center (2018).

health? What are their roles, responsibilities, and relationships? What competencies do they need to ensure that their time and talents are well used to accomplish good governance for stronger health systems and better health outcomes? Each of the challenges in this cluster is addressed below.

2. *Practices.* People engaged in governing bodies should master the five essential practices[12]:

- *Culture of accountability.* Good boards must establish and sustain a culture of accountability through the following activities:
  - Cultivate your personal accountability.
  - Nurture the accountability of your organization to its stakeholders.
  - Foster internal accountability in your organization.
  - Support the accountability of health providers and health workers.
  - Measure performance.
  - Share information.
  - Develop social accountability.
  - Use technology to support accountability.
  - Provide smart oversight.
- *Stakeholder engagement.* Engagement must be optimized to ensure a willingness to help implement decisions of the board. Seven activities help ensure good stakeholder engagement:
  - Extend sincere stakeholder invitations.
  - Achieve sincere stakeholder engagement.
  - Build trust.
  - Engage with patients.
  - Engage with doctors, other clinicians, and health workers.
  - Collaborate with other sectors.
  - Practice gender-responsive governance.
- *Strategy development.* Six activities are key to accomplishing wise and successful strategic plans:
  - Define the target population health goals.
  - Establish a shared vision among key stakeholders.
  - Enable leadership in the organization.
  - Create a successful strategic plan.
  - Implement the strategic plan.
  - Report progress to the key stakeholders.

- *Stewardship of resources.* Resources (e.g., labor, equipment, supplies, money) are often in scarce supply. The six key activities for the efficient use of these resources are as follows:
  - Wisely raise and use resources.
  - Practice ethical and moral integrity.
  - Build management and effective purchasing capacity.
  - Measure performance.
  - Use information, evidence, and technology in governance.
  - Eradicate corruption.
- *Continuous improvement.* Improvement of the above practices helps sustain an effective and high-performing board. Seven activities support the continuous improvement of the board's decision-making processes:
  - Cultivate governance competencies.
  - Build diversity in the governing body.
  - Organize governance orientation and continuous governance education.
  - Perform regular governance assessments.
  - Run effective governing body meetings.
  - Make governance policies.
  - Use governance technologies.

3. *Infrastructure to enable practices.* Exhibit 10.3 shows 11 key systems and infrastructure elements that affect people's ability to participate effectively in governance decision-making processes and practices to maximize the vitality of organizations and their governing bodies. These 11 elements will be discussed at length in the upcoming sections.

Element 1: Types of Governing Bodies

Various types of governing bodies exist, and they have different degrees of control over the affairs of the health sector organizations they govern. These organizational structures can be established in different ways for both governmental and nongovernmental initiatives.

What problems arise from poor governance in health organizations? A survey of public health sector managers across 20 countries identified the following five major risks associated with poor health system governance (International Federation of Public Health Associations 2012):

1. The organization's plans do not reflect the needs of the populations they exist to serve.
2. The organization is not successful in mobilizing resources to implement their plans.

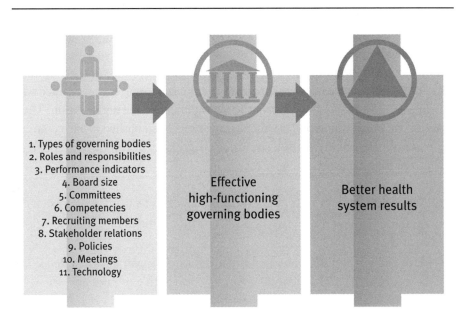

EXHIBIT 10.3
Infrastructure
of 11 Elements
for Good Board
Work

1. Types of governing bodies
2. Roles and responsibilities
3. Performance indicators
4. Board size
5. Committees
6. Competencies
7. Recruiting members
8. Stakeholder relations
9. Policies
10. Meetings
11. Technology

Effective
high-functioning
governing bodies

Better health
system results

Source: Adapted from Global Health Learning Center (2018).

3. The services provided are not of high enough quality or convenience to satisfy the beneficiaries.
4. The scarce resources of the organization are not as well used as possible.
5. The organization has difficulty attracting and retaining health workers needed to serve the population.

To govern in a manner that minimizes these risks, governing bodies must embrace and master a defined set of competencies, which will be discussed in the section on element 6.

Organizational Types

Health systems are composed of many organizations across a variety of venues:

- Hospitals
- Clinics
- Diagnostic centers
- Surgery centers
- Birthing centers
- Health insurance companies
- Health quality accreditation agencies
- HIV and AIDS programs
- Sexual and reproductive health programs

- Health and fitness companies
- Pharmacy shops
- Medical supply companies

All of these types of organizations are likely to have governing bodies charged with guiding, supporting, and overseeing the management of the organization. These roles can vary depending on how the organization is established in each country.

Governing bodies within countries' health sectors can be established by any of the following methods:

- Act of government (e.g., the governments of Kenya and Afghanistan)
- A country's laws for registration of for-profit entities or not-for-profit entities
- Actions by a nongovernmental organization (e.g., an informal decision by a group of rural residents to form a cooperative to raise and sell chickens to support a small village health post)
- Civil society organizations (e.g., in Uganda)
- Local CSOs (e.g., a group of South African health leaders linking their family planning organization to the International Planned Parenthood Association via its formal accreditation process)
- CSOs formed by advocacy groups that leverage the expertise and resources of global alliances (e.g., the Center for Victims of Torture, Alliance Myanmar)

Levels of Governance

Governing bodies can also be established to deal with health challenges at four basic levels, ranging from global to local. These levels are illustrated and described in exhibit 10.4.

Element 2: Roles and Responsibilities

Although legislation or regulations may guide the formation of a governing body, the terms of reference are often very general, with few concrete guidelines. Managers should expect to help draft these guidelines for the composition and work of their governing boards. The fundamental role of a governing board is to protect the mission of the organization by accomplishing certain essential oversight duties, as shown in exhibit 10.5.

Each board member's primary responsibility is to refine and serve the organization's mission by developing, monitoring, and enforcing specific guidelines in six key areas:

1. Quality performance
2. Financial performance

EXHIBIT 10.4
Levels of
Governance

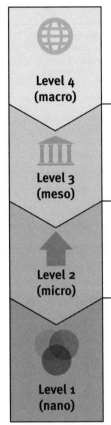

Governance across nation states, such as the World Health Organization (WHO), the World Trade Organization (WTO), and the Global Fund

Level 4 (macro)

Governance within the nation state—usually entrusted to a ministry of health, though some countries may have a mix of entities engaged in health matters (e.g., Ministry of Higher Education, Food and Drug Administration, Social Health Insurance Fund, Environmental Protection Agency)

Level 3 (meso)

Governance via oversight of institutions (public or private) within a country's health sector, such as governing bodies for hospitals, health centers, or provincial or district health councils; institutional or organizational bodies may be established by faith-based groups, local governments, or groups of interested citizens

Level 2 (micro)

Governance nested within different levels of an organization or institution (e.g., a hospital organization in South Africa might have governing bodies for each community hospital)

Level 1 (nano)

Source: Adapted from Global Health Learning Center (2018).

3. Planning performance
4. Management performance
5. Governance effectiveness
6. Community relations and advocacy

The governing body works with senior management to adopt specific outcome targets to measure the organization's vitality and overall performance. As members work to define and monitor progress toward these targets, they must be careful to remain in their governing role and not slide into trying to do management's job.

Element 3: Performance Indicators

The ultimate role of the governing body is to guide the organization to achieve key performance indicators related to health improvement. The organization's mission, goals, and strategic challenges should define this target list of performance indicators. Examples of organizational performance indicators for leadership and governance might include the following (WHO 2010)[13]:

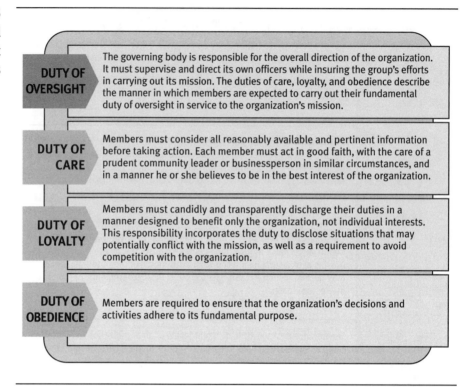

DUTY OF OVERSIGHT
The governing body is responsible for the overall direction of the organization. It must supervise and direct its own officers while insuring the group's efforts in carrying out its mission. The duties of care, loyalty, and obedience describe the manner in which members are expected to carry out their fundamental duty of oversight in service to the organization's mission.

DUTY OF CARE
Members must consider all reasonably available and pertinent information before taking action. Each member must act in good faith, with the care of a prudent community leader or businessperson in similar circumstances, and in a manner he or she believes to be in the best interest of the organization.

DUTY OF LOYALTY
Members must candidly and transparently discharge their duties in a manner designed to benefit only the organization, not individual interests. This responsibility incorporates the duty to disclose situations that may potentially conflict with the mission, as well as a requirement to avoid competition with the organization.

DUTY OF OBEDIENCE
Members are required to ensure that the organization's decisions and activities adhere to its fundamental purpose.

Source: Reprinted from Global Health Learning Center (2018).

- An up-to-date strategy linked to national needs and priorities
- Medicine policies specifying cost-effective options
- A national strategic plan for tuberculosis
- A comprehensive policy for maternal health
- A comprehensive plan for childhood immunization
- Mechanisms for obtaining patient input

Board members should discuss the importance of the various indicators, determine which ones are best for the organization, and consider the advantages and disadvantages of gathering data to track them. The indicators selected should influence the knowledge, skills, and attitudes needed within the governing body to successfully conduct its work.

Element 4: Board Size

Given the need for diverse competencies and the drive toward key performance indicators, how large does an organization's governing body need to be? No particular size will be ideal in every situation, but studies of group dynamics across various countries and cultures tend to suggest that 9 to 13 members is usually appropriate (see exhibit 10.6). If a group grows to more than 17

EXHIBIT 10.6
Ideal Size of a
Governing Body

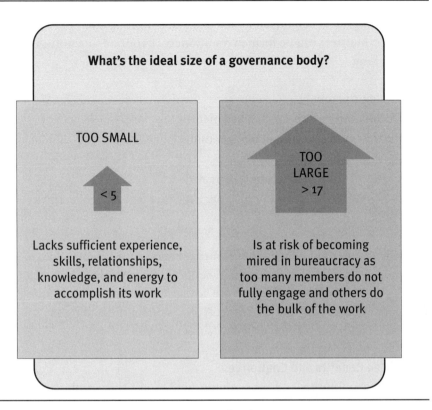

What's the ideal size of a governance body?

TOO SMALL

< 5

Lacks sufficient experience, skills, relationships, knowledge, and energy to accomplish its work

TOO LARGE
> 17

Is at risk of becoming mired in bureaucracy as too many members do not fully engage and others do the bulk of the work

Source: Reprinted from Global Health Learning Center (2018).

members, decision making can become cumbersome. If it has fewer than 7 members, it risks losing diversity of thought, political connections, and the wisdom needed to protect and pursue the organization's mission, plans, and goals.

In Zimbabwe, for example, the hospital management boards of the six central hospitals have an average of 8 or 9 members. The management board of Parirenyatwa Central Hospital, in Harare, has (1) a public health specialist; (2) an accountant, (3) an auditor, (4) a human resource management specialist, (5) a surgeon, (6) a representative of the medical school, (7) a lawyer, and (8) the hospital's CEO. Zimbabwe has eight provincial hospitals, which have hospital management boards similar to those of the central hospitals, and 60 district hospitals, governed by district health councils. Zimbabwe's 1,600 rural health centers have health center committees, each with about 12 members.

Element 5: Effective Committees

Many effective governing bodies rely on committees, councils, work groups, or task forces. These subgroups remain under the control of the governing body and are not independent, but they are often authorized to perform common duties to help cultivate underrepresented competencies and relationships, as well as to provide additional time and energy for the work of the board. Committee service can also be a good way for a member to prove her value to the group and to earn greater responsibility for expanded future roles.

Committees can be formed for a variety of routine functions, including the following:

- Strategic planning
- Community health needs assessment
- Finance, audit, and capital fundraising
- Quality assurance
- Continual governance improvement
- Designing new policies (e.g., policy for user fees and collections)
- Clinical audit

Committees are most effective when they function with a formal charge, follow an annual work plan, and receive staff support to accomplish their measurable objectives. Most of the subgroups are advisory to the overall governing body and work for a defined period of time. A provision for disbanding the subgroup after a certain point is often called a "sunset provision."

Committee Benefits and Challenges

Why form committees and other subgroups? Won't they create confusion or complexity for the board? Advantages of committees include the following:

- They enable a sharper focus on key areas of interest and importance to the organization.
- New experiences and insights improve decision making.
- Subgroup members may possibly serve as future governing body members.
- Political influence can be expanded through member reputations and relationships.

Committees, however, also have disadvantages:

- They lead to more meetings and more work for members.
- More staff work and time are needed to support the subgroups.
- Decision-making processes may be delayed.

Element 6: Competency-Based Governance

Competency-based governance—in which the people serving in the governing body bring a mix of competencies to decision-making processes—tends to yield higher performance. Attracting and retaining people with the appropriate competencies is more likely if they

- know their roles;
- are supported by staff;
- are encouraged to make transparent and ethical decisions;
- are proud to serve the organization; and
- work with leaders who respect and celebrate their efforts, time, and talents.

Good decision-making processes for a governing body demand solid structures and strategies that facilitate members' access to the right information and their ability to meaningfully engage in group decisions. This section of the chapter will discuss those structures and strategies related to competencies and recruitment.

Identifying Member Competencies

Good governance is both an art and a science. Studies of high-performing governing bodies suggest that they have a passion to identify a set of key competencies and then support those competencies' development. Such governing bodies consist of members who bring an optimal mix of the knowledge, skills, attitudes, experiences, and perspectives needed for successful work. No single member is likely to have all of the competencies needed to protect and pursue the organization's mission, but most of the desired attributes can be included in the collective balance of the group.

Examples of good competencies include the following:

- Is passionate and knowledgeable about the health and well-being of the people the organization serves
- Is respected by the communities served
- Has experience assessing the health needs of high-risk populations
- Is able to listen to others' ideas
- Is a logical thinker and problem solver
- Is knowledgeable of health risks and ways to address them
- Possesses community organization skills
- Has experience in medicine, nursing, or public health
- Is a champion for good teamwork
- Shows wisdom in mobilizing resources and relationships to support the mission and plans

Managers can use this sample list to take stock of the governance competencies in their own organization's governing bodies.

Building Diversity in the Governing Body

Governance for health is driven by the needs of the people the organization exists to serve. An effective governing body must make sound decisions about what people's health needs are, and then establish policies, plans, and programs to meet those needs. Therefore, good governance requires the engagement of diverse stakeholders who reflect the unique ages, genders, races, ethnicities, religions, and other characteristics of the beneficiaries. Members of the governing body should also reflect a diverse range of skills and experiences, possibly including such people as lawyers or businesspeople with no direct medical experience. Women, who are often major recipients as well as providers of health services, should be well represented in the governing process. Successful leaders work hard to invite, enable, and empower women to serve in governing bodies in the same capacities as men.

The following steps can help enhance the diversity of a governing body:

- Make a commitment to diversity in the governing body. Draft a simple diversity policy statement, and fulfill that commitment.
- Identify and remove barriers that might prevent members of certain groups—particularly those groups that are often marginalized, including youth, people with disabilities, ethnic minorities, and sexual minorities—from serving on the governing body. In selecting new members, consider representatives from the diverse communities being served. Ensure that the governing body membership reflects the diversity of the community.
- Maintain a governing body skills profile. Recruit new members based on the skills and characteristics that are currently lacking in the body as a whole—those skills and characteristics that are needed now or will be needed in the future.
- When recruiting for the governing body, consult with stakeholder constituencies about who might best represent their interests.

The next section offers practical approaches for recruiting and retaining diverse and effective board members.

Element 7: Recruiting Members with Governance Competencies

The recruitment of valuable members is essential for good governance. To support this goal, governing bodies are periodically encouraged and supported by chairpersons and their management to ask and answer the three questions shown in exhibit 10.7. The governing body should work with management and staff to blend the answers to these three questions into a single master list, which will clarify the set of desirable knowledge, skills, and attitudes that prospective members should have. The full governing body can then discuss the pros and cons of the various characteristics and prioritize them down to an essential 10 to 15. These competencies then become a guide for finding, recruiting, and appointing or electing members.

EXHIBIT 10.7
Key Questions
to Ask When
Recruiting
Governing Body
Members

Key questions to ask when recruiting governing body members

To accomplish our mission, what are the most important sets of knowledge, skills, and attitudes we need among our members?

What are the biggest challenges and obstacles we will likely face in the next two to three years? What experiences and competencies do we most need among our members?

To achieve our goals over the next three years, what actions, relationships, and investments will be most essential? What relationships and behaviors do we most need among our members to help lay these foundations?

Source: Adapted from Global Health Learning Center (2018).

Challenges to effective recruitment and retention can be overcome through three main strategies, as illustrated in exhibit 10.8 and described in the list that follows[14]:

Strategy 1: *Minimize obstacles to service.* The CEO and governing body leaders should develop an action plan to minimize common obstacles or challenges to recruiting competent board members. Common obstacles include the following:

- Discouragement resulting from the feeling that improvements in health will be impossible because of low resource availability

  Challenge: Many provincial and district health councils work in constrained resource settings, where provision of necessities is often difficult.

  Solution: Seek resources from diverse sources, including the local community and the people themselves. The search for funding must be driven by clear and well-developed strategic plans and budgets that explain how much funding is needed and how it will be wisely used. Be open to in-kind contributions of volunteer time and money for specific services or material needs. Requests for funding and in-kind

EXHIBIT 10.8
Strategies
to Overcome
Challenges with
Recruitment and
Retention

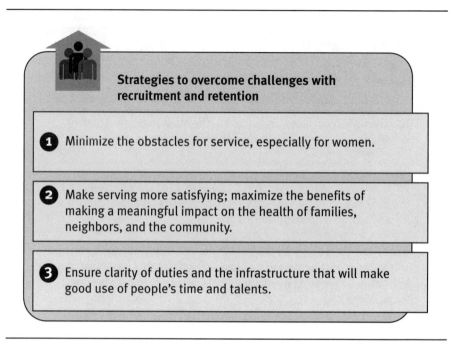

Strategies to overcome challenges with recruitment and retention

1 Minimize the obstacles for service, especially for women.

2 Make serving more satisfying; maximize the benefits of making a meaningful impact on the health of families, neighbors, and the community.

3 Ensure clarity of duties and the infrastructure that will make good use of people's time and talents.

Source: Adapted from Global Health Learning Center (2018).

contributions must be based on trust from citizens and beneficiaries; the organization and the governing body have to earn this trust through transparent decision making and results-oriented reporting of quality service delivery experiences.

- Concern that roles and responsibilities are not well defined or valued

    Challenge: People are more willing to work and volunteer their time and reputations if they understand what is expected of them and of others engaged in the same challenge.

    Solution: Develop, publish, and review job descriptions for membership in the governing body. Celebrate the good work of your organization so that people will be proud to be associated with the work it does in the community.

    Challenge: Many health sector governing body members are asked to give significant amounts of time and effort on a voluntary basis.

    Solution: Acknowledge the realities of service. Make it easier for people to be willing to provide this time by making sure that meetings are scheduled at convenient times, are well run, and are efficient. You may also advocate for some modest benefits, such as refreshments at meetings, easy-to-understand data for decision making, and a small stipend. Also, be up-front if time will not be compensated.

- Belief that meetings are confusing, ineffective, and not well managed

  Challenge: Good governing body members are often driven away by the feeling that their time and talents are wasted in boring or poorly run meetings, or by the belief that their reputation might become associated with members who are unethical or difficult to work with.

  Solution: Conduct periodic assessments of how your meetings are run, and identify ways to improve their functioning and results. Also, consider how attracting and retaining good governing body members helps to attract other talented people who are willing to serve, either on the board itself or on one of its committees.

Strategy 2: *Maximize the benefits of service.* Recruitment is easier when potential members can clearly see the benefits that will occur if they invest their time and talents. In addition to advocating for the role of the organization in promoting positive health outcomes, a good governing body can also yield the following key benefits:

- Decisions are more likely to reflect an understanding of key health risks and improvement needs in the community.
- Service improvement plans are more likely to be implemented, and significant and sustainable results and performance targets are more likely to be achieved.
- The resources needed to strengthen the organization are more likely to be mobilized and expanded.
- Communities are more likely to access and support the organization's health services if they see leaders serving as effective role models.
- The organization is more likely to reach target populations in a responsive and culturally appropriate manner.

High-performing governing bodies periodically show how their work maps back to these important benefits.

Strategy 3: *Reinforce clarity and support.* Among the most essential ways to support the recruitment and retention of talented members are the following:

- Regularly thank and publicly recognize members for their service, and remind them that their work yields meaningful results.

- Frequently remind members of their roles and responsibilities.
- Make it easier for members to participate by managing key factors that contribute to good decision making:
  - Provide accurate information to guide the organization's performance.
  - Provide practical staff support for member engagement.
  - Make sure meetings are reasonably scheduled, conveniently located, and efficiently run.
  - Establish processes that are transparent, open, and inclusive of service beneficiaries and vulnerable populations.
  - Rotate leadership to promote equity.

Element 8: Stakeholder Relations

Governing bodies contribute to the vitality of their organizations by leveraging members' relationships and contacts to support the organization's mission and work. As you take into account the key stakeholders with whom you would like to develop a better rapport, consider the following situation:

> You are the nurse executive director of a large maternal/child health program in Dhaka, Bangladesh. Your governing body chairperson has just informed you that her cousin, the deputy minister of health, is not happy with how politicians in your province receive progress reports about the reduction in maternal deaths. As a result, you must deliver a presentation next week to the Ministry of Health about how you and your board will commit to improving stakeholder relationships in the coming year.

Consider how the information in this section might help you prepare for such a challenge.

Wise governing bodies establish a culture that expects, encourages, and supports the development of positive working relationships among key stakeholder groups. These groups will vary from one organization to another, but they may include some or all of the following:

1. The ministry of health or other public institutions (e.g., Social Security, ministry of education)
2. Politicians and community leaders
3. Religious leaders
4. Major employers/businesspeople
5. Health workers
6. The media
7. Beneficiaries of the organization's services, who are also often financiers

8. Purchasers of health services, such as public or private insurance organizations

9. Financiers of the organization (e.g., investors, donors, public sector, public–private partnerships)

Most high-performing governing bodies see the following stakeholder activities as indicative of a good relationship:

- Knowing and supporting the organization's mission
- Identifying new ways to improve services
- Helping recruit and retain good health workers
- Helping secure political support
- Promoting increased use of services
- Fundraising to support the organization

To cultivate good stakeholder relationships, the board should seek to identify other groups in its district, county, region, province, or country with which it can build positive and sustainable outcomes.

Actions for Building Good Stakeholder Relations

A governing body is likely to achieve greater success if it employs the following five actions to develop positive relationships with stakeholders:

1. Clearly define why each group is important to the success of the mission.
2. Ask stakeholder groups for their ideas, and sincerely listen to their insights and comments; practice appreciative inquiry.[15]
3. Reach out to each group, and engage in collaborative governance planning meetings that are shaped by a clear recognition of the interdependencies among the social determinants of health.[16]
4. Earn trust by engaging in open, transparent, and honest two-way conversations about areas of mutual interest and need.
5. Develop transparent plans for collective action[17] to coproduce meaningful programs for health gains among target populations.

Avoid the following taboos:

- Acting and/or speaking inconsistently
- Seeking personal rather than shared gain
- Withholding information
- Lying or telling half-truths
- Being closed-minded

Building Trust

Trust is a major component of successful interpersonal relationships both inside and outside governing bodies. A commitment to building trust can help board members better connect with one another as well as with stakeholders and partners.

Consider the following five methods to build trust and cultivate positive relationships:

1. Be reliable.
    - Do what you say you will do.
    - Honor your promises.
    - Acknowledge the significance of a promise.
2. Be honest.
    - Tell the truth.
    - If you do lie, admit to it.
    - Speak from the heart.
3. Be open.
    - Volunteer information.
    - Do not omit important details.
    - Acknowledge secrets while protecting your privacy.
    - Do not mask truths.
    - Demonstrate that you expect reciprocal openness.
4. Keep confidences.
    - Avoid gossip—both telling and listening.
    - If you do break a confidence, apologize as soon as possible.
5. Be consistently competent.
    - Display loyalty.
    - Develop your skills.
    - Demonstrate a strong moral ethic.
    - Remain neutral in difficult situations.
    - Aim to be objective and fair.
    - Behave consistently.

Element 9: Governance Policies

Good governing bodies use written policies to guide the effectiveness and efficiency of their decision-making work. A set of written policies and procedures can be extremely useful in helping governing bodies carry out their responsibilities. Potential advantages include the following:

- The written set of policies and procedures quickly acclimates new board members to key responsibilities and processes.

EXHIBIT 10.9
Policies
for Good
Governance

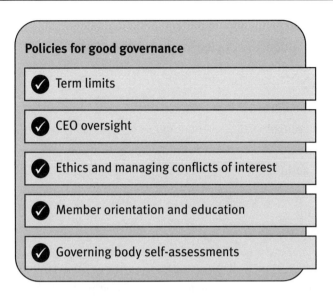

Policies for good governance

- ✓ Term limits
- ✓ CEO oversight
- ✓ Ethics and managing conflicts of interest
- ✓ Member orientation and education
- ✓ Governing body self-assessments

Source: Adapted from Global Health Learning Center (2018).

- It reminds seasoned board members of efficient practices.
- It enables transparent decision making.
- It helps build credibility with patients, clients, and beneficiaries.

In many organizations, the board has a manual of policies and procedures[18] that provides instructions for how the board should do its work, how it should receive compensation for expenses, and how it should make decisions in such areas as the following:

- Strategic visioning and planning, quality assurance, fiscal health, management, and relations with stakeholders and government agencies
- Descriptions, expectations, and performance reviews for the chairperson, members, committees, and senior managers
- Committee work plans
- Meeting calendars
- Meeting agendas
- Periodic governance assessments
- Plan for ongoing governance improvement

The manual may also contain policies on the following topics:

- Conflicts of interest
- Code of ethics and conduct

- Whistleblower protection
- Confidentiality
- Record retention and document destruction
- Member expenses
- Budgeting
- Capital expenditures
- Financial control
- Investments
- Financial audits
- Risk management
- Fundraising
- Sexual harassment

Five key areas of policy are highlighted in exhibit 10.9 and described in the sections that follow. These areas tend to be particularly important for health services organizations.

Term Limits

Term limits usually define the number of years a person is allowed to serve on a governing body. Not all boards use term limits, but, for public and nongovernmental organizations, common term lengths are one, three, and four years. Many organizations allow for consecutive terms. Term limit policies may apply to the governing body as a whole or just to the chairperson.

Term limits, whether for the chairperson or other members, can be beneficial for a number of reasons:

- *Graceful exit.* Term limits allow for people who are not performing effectively to retire gracefully. The downside is that an effective member or chair may have to be forced out early.
- *Recruitment.* Serving on a governing body can require an intensive commitment of time and energy. Prospective members are more likely to serve if they know their investment has an expiration date.
- *Leader development.* Boards that know they will need a new chair and members every few years will be more likely to recruit new people with an eye toward future leadership roles. Candidates who want to build their own leadership skills will be more likely to say yes if they know there are future opportunities.
- *Resource mobilization.* Board members are potentially the organization's most powerful connections with politicians, donors, health sciences schools, and government or private health purchasers. Leadership

transitions provide an opportunity to engage fresh avenues to resources that have relationships with the new leader.

- *Healthier governing bodies.* Term limits provide periodic injections of new energy and ideas, help prevent member and chair burnout, and reduce the likelihood that a few individuals will dominate discussions and decisions.

Chief Executive Oversight

One of the most important and delicate responsibilities of the governing body is to establish and nurture a positive relationship with the organization's managing director or CEO. The board is responsible for the oversight and review of performance across agreed-upon areas of authority, accomplished through routine CEO performance evaluations. The CEO performance review process is not an activity that many governing body members enjoy, but it is fundamental to good governance. It aligns the organizational mission, values, goals, and objectives with organizational and CEO performance.

Key actions for good CEO performance reviews include the following:

- Make performance evaluation an ongoing process, not just an annual occurrence.
- Focus on things that the CEO can actually control.
- Involve the CEO in the process, ensuring that he understands the evaluation objectives and elements.
- Make sure the performance criteria are agreed to by all parties.
- Pay attention to the CEO's personal leadership and management style, in addition to work activities.
- Focus on activities that fulfill the organization's mission and help accomplish its goals.

An effective evaluation should accomplish at least the following:

- It should clarify the board's expectations of the CEO.
- It should provide clear goals to help the CEO identify and prioritize tasks.
- It should educate the board about the nature of the CEO's roles and responsibilities.

An effective evaluation also benefits the CEO in a number of ways:

- It helps the CEO develop and upgrade her competencies and experiences.
- It gives the CEO an opportunity to engage in self-assessment.
- It provides the CEO with honest feedback, direction, and reaffirmation.

- It eliminates surprise—such as the evaluation pattern known as "Good job, good job, good job—gone!"

A good performance evaluation ultimately nurtures the growth and development of both the chief executive and the organization.[19]

Ethics and Conflicts of Interest

High-performing governing bodies establish policies concerning ethical behavior and conflicts of interest. Appropriate member behavior must be in accordance with the board's role and responsibilities. Members should know the difference between governance and management, consider service a responsibility of citizenship, and find enjoyment in such service.

Appropriate behavior should have several key characteristics:

- Respect for the organization, the management, the clinicians, the employees, and other members
- Openness in discussions and decision making
- Confidentiality—the more sensitive the issue under discussion, the more important the confidentiality

Conflicts of interest can arise in a variety of instances, including the following:

- When a board member's relative wants a job
- When a member has business dealings with the organization
- When a member has knowledge about the organization's planned new services, which could compete with a friend's business

The key challenge is not determining whether a conflict of interest exists but rather ensuring that it is managed carefully and in a disciplined manner. Some boards may decide that a potential conflict of interest precludes service; however, such a rule might not be necessary for effective governance. Policies addressing conflict of interest usually require members to disclose potential conflicts and, if necessary, to abstain from voting on matters related to the conflict.

Member Orientation and Education

High-performing governing bodies require members to receive a formal orientation to their roles and responsibilities, as well as ongoing education to help support their capacity development. The ability to bring new members up to speed quickly is a key determinant of board effectiveness.

All governing bodies need continuous education and development of competencies, and this process should begin when members are first approached to serve. At that point, members should be provided with a copy of their job description and a set of the board's values or code of conduct. Effective governing bodies conduct a structured orientation program within 30 days of a member's appointment. Large organizations may include a written orientation guide that covers such topics as the following:

- Mission and vision of the organization
- History of the organization
- Programs and services
- Staffing
- Strategies, plans, and planning processes
- Trends in service utilization and financial performance
- Funding (annual budget and funding sources)
- A candid SWOT assessment (i.e., an assessment of the organization's strengths, weaknesses, opportunities, and threats)
- Legal issues and risk management
- Terms of reference, expectations for participation, and code of conduct
- Board operations and policies
- Calendar of meetings
- Subcommittee work plans and opportunities for service

Wise, effective, and efficient governance does not just happen. Those who govern must invest individually and collectively to continuously improve their knowledge about how the organization functions and how its governance can be improved. Member education must be an ongoing process. The following strategies can help with the effective delivery of useful, current information in a relatively short amount of time:

- Develop and implement a new member orientation program.
- Begin each meeting with a brief (i.e., an education session that provides relevant background information about an issue on that meeting's agenda).
- Try to orient new members in time to attend the board's annual retreat.
- Establish a minimum number of continuing education hours for members.
- Conduct mini-retreats whenever all or most members attend the same education event.
- Create a leadership development/coaching framework within the existing board.
- Lay the groundwork for good quality of care and financial decisions by providing informal courses (possibly taught by an experienced member) for members who lack such expertise.

- Establish a "buddy system" in which experienced members are assigned to take new members under their wing.
- Have one operational area executive give an update at each meeting (rotating among all areas).
- Collaborate with other organizations to develop or present member education programs.
- Use self-assessments to measure progress and to help establish future education needs; ask members for their perceptions of the board's effectiveness and for suggestions on topics for future education or discussion.

Qualitative responses from governing body self-assessments have indicated that members benefit from professional development training in the following areas (University of Kansas Community Tool Box 2018):

- Resource mobilization and the role of members in raising funds
- Legislation applicable to for-profit of nonprofit organizations and their governing bodies, as appropriate
- Leadership succession and the role of the board
- Board member duties as individuals
- Funding sources, financial management, and the fiduciary role of the board
- Human resources (including staff compensation and benefits) and the role of the board in human resource management
- Strengthening accountability and transparency
- Measuring organizational impact
- Risk analysis and management
- The role of the governing body in supporting the chief executive

Governing Body Self-Assessments

A high-performing governing body continuously improves its own performance by periodically conducting self-assessments—organized quantitative evaluations of the board's satisfaction with all aspects of its performance. A self-assessment combines positive statements about the governance environment, processes, focus, and progress with member recommendations to improve performance. Done correctly and consistently, the process enables the board to accomplish several key goals:

- Setting measurable objectives for improving governance to boost the organization's performance

- Assessing the board's effectiveness in improving the organization's performance
- Developing and implementing governance improvement strategies
- Evaluating performance to support sustained improvement

In addition, an excellent governing body self-assessment process will achieve several major outcomes:

- It will define the most critical governance success factors.
- It will secure confidential, broad-based member input on the critical aspects of successful governing leadership.
- It will create an opportunity to address major issues and ideas in a nonthreatening, collaborative manner.
- It will clearly demonstrate where the governing body is either in or out of alignment with leadership fundamentals and issues.
- It will objectively assess the degree of common understanding, expectations, and direction for the governing body among its members.
- It will assess deficiencies that might affect the governing body's ability to fulfill its fiduciary responsibilities.
- It will identify opportunities for meaningful leadership improvement.
- It will help administration better understand and respond to the governing body's leadership education and development needs.

Self-assessment is an ideal way to engage members in an anonymous, confidential evaluation of the board's overall performance, while at the same time inviting them to consider their own personal contributions. However, conducting the self-assessment is only the first step toward improving governance performance. To be successful, the assessment must serve as a catalyst to engage board members in a discussion of findings that highlight performance gaps and areas where members lack consensus. Additionally, it must facilitate the development of an action plan for better decision making, with responsibilities, time frames, and projected outcomes.

Ideally, governing bodies should assess their performance annually. Many boards conduct their self-assessment as part of an annual educational and planning retreat, in which they set aside time to discuss the results and explore ways to improve board and leadership performance. Some boards are able to design and conduct their own self-assessments, compile and analyze the results, and facilitate the development of an action plan using internal resources. Other boards rely on outside consultants who offer tested and proven tools and techniques.

Consider following this ten-step plan for conducting your own governing body self-assessment:

1. Determine the unique objectives and projected outcomes of your assessment.
2. Design draft evaluation criteria and a measurement methodology (e.g., a scale from 5, for "very satisfied," to 1, for "very dissatisfied").
3. Print a draft questionnaire and test the criteria and methodology for relevance and completeness in meeting your assessment needs.
4. Distribute your self-assessment questionnaire to all trustees with a stamped, self-addressed envelope, ensuring both anonymity and confidentiality. Alternatively, you can develop a web-based self-assessment that can be administered online.
5. Compile the results and produce a report. The report should include graphs that depict areas in order of priority, from highest to lowest average score. Include verbatim comments and a brief analysis of key themes and findings.
6. Hold a special governing body meeting or retreat to review the assessment results and discuss their implications for all aspects of board activities and performance.
7. Appoint a committee or task force to develop specific recommendations for improvement. Then prioritize the most important areas of governance focus, and determine the resources required for success.
8. Implement the recommendations. Assign responsibilities, and determine outcomes.
9. Document and regularly report on the progress of the approved governance improvement initiatives.
10. Continually reassess governing body performance.

Element 10: Effective Meetings

Because much of the work of a governing body is conducted in meetings, those meetings need to be well planned and managed to ensure optimal results. As you explore this section, consider the challenges in the following situation:

> You and the governing body chairperson want to improve your work by improving the effectiveness and efficiency of your meetings. How can you achieve this goal? What are the characteristics of excellent meetings, and what infrastructure is needed to support them?

Excellent meetings require a combination of dedicated participants, useful agendas, relevant information, convenient venues, and a commitment to continual improvement.

Meeting Participants

Most governing body meetings include only members of the body and a few of the organization's senior leaders. If the group becomes too large, productive conversations can be difficult. However, occasional guest speakers can add valuable information and perspective to the decision-making process. The guests themselves also benefit because they can observe the work of the governing body and better support its plan and decisions.

The following are some examples of valuable meeting guests:

- Clients with positive or negative stories about their experiences
- Health workers focused on new trends or issues that the organization is likely to face
- Politicians or media representatives interested in supporting the organization's programs and services
- Governing body members from a similar organization
- Business leaders from other high-performing service providers (e.g., people from the hotel or airline industry)
- Visiting or diaspora health experts
- Donors, philanthropists, and funders

Meeting Agenda

The agenda provides an essential road map for a good meeting. The chairperson and the managing director or CEO should develop the agenda well in advance of the meeting. Every community and culture has different views and requirements for meetings and discussion. However, certain topics are common to most board meetings:

- Welcome and introduction of guests or new members
- Review of the last meeting's minutes
- Reports on subgroups
- Identification and discussion of current action items
- Other business
- Closing comments and agreement on the next meeting's priority topics
- Adjournment

The meeting agenda should include a clear-cut purpose and objectives, and it should be circulated to attendees in advance of the meeting. If the design of a meeting agenda remains unchanged for a long period, recipients may look at it less closely and have difficulty distinguishing between important and unimportant topics. Therefore, the design should be refreshed periodically.

During the meeting itself, the progress of agenda items should be tracked carefully. The chair of the governing body should limit extraneous input, comments, and personal agendas. A question-and-answer or "other business" section should be built into the agenda to encourage participants' involvement and to address outstanding issues that members might have.

Most high-performing governing bodies meet five to seven times a year, with each meeting lasting two to three hours. Longer meetings tend to burn out member enthusiasm and make discussion less productive. More frequent meetings may be necessary if the organization is addressing a health crisis or facing political or financial challenges. If a board is required by law or regulation to meet more frequently (e.g., monthly), consider hosting guest speakers, continuing education workshops, or strategic planning retreats.

Meetings should be structured so that about 80 percent of the time focuses on the future and strategies for dealing with expected problem areas and 20 percent of the time is devoted to a review of past history.

Meeting Information

Effective decision making requires good information that drives discussion and supports the consensus needed to take action. Unfortunately, too many governing bodies encounter five fatal information weaknesses, as shown in exhibit 10.10. In considering the information to be provided, remember that a governing body has limited time. If it spends hours sorting out unnecessarily complex information, it might not have time to address other significant and strategic matters.

As the meetings occur, someone needs to take minutes to ensure that key actions, information, and conclusions are captured and stored for the future. The following practical guidelines can help ensure that the minutes are taken in a form that is accessible and usable for future decision making:

- A staff person should be assigned the role and the resources to take notes on information flows and decisions made by the board.
- The minutes should capture key points, but they should not be so detailed that they inhibit open discussion or become too long to read.
- Where applicable, the minutes should include charts or graphs to help visualize activities.
- The minutes should be made available in digital formats.
- Members should be given the opportunity to challenge or edit any errors in the minutes.

Meeting Venues

Meetings can be more interesting and more productive if they occasionally occur in different settings. Almost any location can serve as a meeting venue as long as it meets the following basic criteria:

EXHIBIT 10.10
Five Fatal
Information
Weaknesses

Information is . . .	Practical ways to deal with each of these challenges
. . . nonexistent	Ask management for regular reports on client/patient care, service delivery trends, and current finances.
. . . not provided with enough time for members to digest it	Ask experts to provide clear and easy-to-understand information at least three to five days in advance of each meeting. Request a short interpretation of data messages and trend implications.
. . . not provided in a way that is easy to understand	Data should tell a clear story if shown in charts, pictures, or graphs. If accompanied by footnotes, trends and implications should be summarized.
. . . too verbose or complicated	Ask management for one-page summaries of all data reports. Trust leaders and subcommittees to do deeper analysis of complex data.
. . . inaccurate or even dishonest	Be very clear about expectations for timely and accurate data. Ask for second opinions. Praise reports that are transparent, honest, and clear. Replace staff who cannot provide information that meets these criteria.

Source: Adapted from Global Health Learning Center (2018).

- The location is comfortable and safe.
- It is easily accessible, even for vulnerable and marginalized participants.
- It is located close to where health services are provided.
- It provides audiovisual capabilities.
- It offers basic refreshments.

Meetings that occur once or twice a year can be scheduled in different venues to add interest and energy. Alternative locations to consider may include schools, hospitals, government buildings, health centers or screening clinics, and even buses or mobile settings that visit various organization sites (e.g., clinics, satellite offices) and carry out discussions on the road.

Continual Meeting Improvement

As with all practices and processes, good governance is enhanced when members remain ready to continually improve what they do and how they do it. Specific suggestions for meeting enhancement are provided in exhibit 10.11.[20]

EXHIBIT 10.11
Suggestions
for Enhancing
Meetings

Suggestions for enhancing meetings

Board publishes a clear agenda with expected time limits.

Chairperson encourages all members to participate in discussions and decisions.

Governing body culture encourages open and candid disagreements in pursuit of consensus.

Staff members support discussions but do not dominate.

Chairperson periodically solicits ideas about how meetings could be more valuable to members and stakeholders.

Source: Adapted from Global Health Learning Center (2018).

A governing body will often work for a consensus decision, but it may need to settle for a simple majority vote. In health services organizations, members do not "vote their shares," with one individual being able to outvote the rest. Instead, they reach a common understanding of the issues and hopefully achieve near-unanimous support of the final decision. At the same time, disagreement can have value, in that it can help the board to explore many facets of an issue before arriving at a wise choice. A governing body that is always in agreement may be suffering from **groupthink**—a condition in which the group weakens its decision making by inappropriately reaching consensus without considering alternative approaches or assumptions.[21] Groupthink can stifle member enthusiasm and result in missed opportunities for smarter problem solving and service innovations.

groupthink
A condition in which the group weakens its decision making by inappropriately reaching consensus without considering alternative approaches or assumptions.

Element 11: Board Work Technology

To make good decisions, boards must have easy access to essential information about the various topics under discussion. This information must be accurate, honest, easy to understand, and readily available. This section examines the role of technology in developing, managing, and using information in decision-making processes to support effective governance.

Benefits of Information Technologies

The governing body needs accurate, accessible, and appropriate information to support all five of its essential practices, and it needs to establish policies and make investments in information technology (IT) to ensure access to information for strategic planning, performance assessments, and improvement targets. Good information through effective IT helps board members and organizational leadership objectively understand

- the context in which their organization works,
- policy and strategy options that affect decision making, and
- advantages and disadvantages of alternate decisions and options.

Performance Dashboards

A variety of technologies are available to help governing bodies practice effective and efficient governance. **Performance dashboards** are an example of an intervention that can be used to support effective governance even in low-resource settings. A dashboard report (see exhibit 10.12) can be generated from a database to provide a display of key indicators across such areas as financial

performance dashboard
A display of key indicators across various areas to show progress toward goals and to support effective governance.

EXHIBIT 10.12
Example of a Performance Dashboard

QUALITY OF CARE

KEY: ■ Better than expected   ▦ Expected   ▨ Worse than expected   ▪ N/A

Q1	Q2	Q3	Q4	Year	SAMPLE PERFORMANCE METRICS
					Patient satisfaction
					Medication errors
					Patient felt fine
					Personal usage of pathways
					Total unadjusted mortality rate
					15-day readmission rate
					Primary cesarean birth rate
					Overall cesarean birth rate
					Vaginal birth after cesarean (VBAC) rate
					Cesarean birth surgical site infection rate
					Vaginal birth infection rate
					Newborn nosocomial infection rate—sepsis
					Nosocomial infection rate—surgical
					Critical care: central line bloodstream infections
					Critical care: ventilator-associated pneumonia
					Critical care: multi-drug resistant organism
					Peripherally inserted central catheter bloodstream infections
					Sentinel event
					Near-miss medical error
					Incident reports
					Total cases in litigation
					New lawsuits
					Total cases in litigation not previously identified

Source: Adapted from Global Health Learning Center (2018).

performance, operations, service to patients, human resources, quality of care, customer service, and patient safety. Dashboards are helpful for monitoring an organization's progress in fulfilling its mission and meeting its goals. The governing body typically receives an integrated quarterly report covering programs, operations, and financial issues, with a brief narrative summarizing the past quarter's performance and drawing attention to trends of note.

Web Portals

web portal
A basic website on which all the materials needed for a work function are stored.

As internet access has expanded in low-income countries, **web portals** have become more feasible as an option to support the work of governing bodies. A web portal is a basic website where the materials that members need for their work are stored. When used correctly by all parties, portals can improve the quality and efficiency of the information exchange between the board and management staff.

The benefits offered by web portals include the following:

- Time and cost savings (no need to print voluminous materials prior to meetings)
- Better-prepared members (round-the-clock access to relevant information)
- Better-educated members (access to helpful references and resources for capacity development)

In addition, portals can streamline the following tasks:

- Member and manager communication and document sharing
- Oversight procedures
- Staff updates to meeting information

Cell Phone Applications

The use of mobile phones and tablets is expanding worldwide, and these technologies are increasingly being used by boards to improve their work and make better decisions. A cellular phone or tablet can enable two-way communication among governing body members, managers, and health workers, which means that information can be pushed or pulled to enable more responsive and reliable decision making.

Information that can be pushed to members' devices includes the following:

- Meeting agenda reminders
- Progress reports tracking service utilization goals
- Community events to build stakeholder relations
- Monthly financial reports

- Stock-out reports
- Staffing vacancies

Information that can be pulled from members' devices includes the following:

- Responses to policy changes
- Board self-assessments
- Availability for special meetings
- Ideas to improve service utilization

As internet bandwidth and coverage continue to improve, new web-based applications are being adopted to move information for board decision making to and from members' phones. Management Sciences for Health has developed the Govern4Health software application to demystify health governance and provide practical tasks and activities for health leaders, managers, and people who govern. The app, which is free to download, offers evidence on why governance matters, a tool to assess gender responsiveness, and a variety of tips for continual governance enhancement.[22]

Summary

Good governance for health is a mission-driven and people-centered decision-making process carried out by a group of entrusted leaders who have the responsibility to protect, promote, and restore the health of the people being served. An organization's governing body—often known as a board of directors or a board of trustees—sets strategic direction and objectives; makes policies, laws, rules, regulations, and decisions; raises and deploys resources; and oversees the work of the organization. It seeks the best ways for the organization to achieve its strategic goals and objectives and enhance its long-term vitality.

This chapter has identified five essential practices of good governance: (1) creating a culture of responsibility, (2) engaging stakeholders, (3) setting a shared strategic direction, (4) stewarding resources responsibly, and (5) continuous improvement of the first four practices. The chapter has also explored 11 essential elements of a good infrastructure for effective board work: (1) types of governing bodies, (2) roles and responsibilities, (3) performance indicators, (4) board size, (5) effective committees, (6) competency-based governance, (7) recruitment of members, (8) stakeholder relations, (9) governance policies, (10) effective meetings, and (11) board work technology. Across these practices and elements, the chapter has presented a wide range of concepts, guidelines, and suggestions to support stronger health systems and better health outcomes.

Scenarios for Discussion

Rather than provide traditional discussion questions, we have provided a set of five scenarios that can be used for group discussion to support the application of SMART governance in realistic settings. Readers should work through the scenarios using the concepts presented in the chapter.

Scenario 1: Policy to Address a Global Health Problem

By 2025, sub-Saharan Africa will overtake the rest of the world in prevalence of and mortality from noncommunicable diseases (NCDs). The double burden of HIV/AIDS and NCDs will exert a major toll in the region in terms of lost economic opportunities and slowed poverty-reduction initiatives, particularly because it will largely affect the most productive age group (i.e., people between 20 and 45 years of age). HIV and NCDs share similar health system challenges and also disease screening and management algorithms. How can good governance prepare sub-Saharan African countries to address this expected double challenge?

Scenario 2: Role of Local Health Organization Boards

Imagine you are a senior staff member of the Strathmore University program in health services management in Nairobi, Kenya, and Kenya's Ministry of Health has contracted with your program to develop a training program for the decentralized county health boards. With a new constitution enacted in 2010, Kenya created a devolved system of government with 47 counties, each headed by an elected governor. Health services were devolved to the counties, with the national government, through the Ministry of Health, retaining the functions of policy formulation and the setting of quality standards. Transition to the devolved system of government posed some challenges for health service provision, particularly in terms of the following leadership, management, and governance issues:

- Problems with redeployment of health workers to the counties (e.g., lack of harmonization of terms of services, lack of training for health workers on new leadership and management responsibilities)
- Lack of training for the various boards of management on their key roles
- Lack of clarity regarding the roles of the national and county governments in purchasing and deploying vital diagnostic and treatment equipment

The Parliament has asked each county to form its own governing body from civic and business leaders. The terms of reference for these new bodies must be drafted within two months for consideration as a regulatory act in Parliament. What are the key considerations you would weave into this proposed new policy? What should be the essential roles and responsibilities of the county health boards?

Scenario 3: Conflicts of Interest

As a local restaurant owner, you have served on the Western Cape Provincial Health Council in South Africa for the past three years. You and the chairperson have become increasingly nervous that the behavior of a small number of your colleagues on the governing council might be unethical and that conflicts of interest might be affecting their decision making at meetings. One of the board members has a construction company and seems to be steering the procurement to build two new health centers to his friends. You have organized a meeting with the hospital's CEO and chairperson to discuss ways to update policies and procedures for the coming year. How should you best prepare for this meeting?

Scenario 4: Board Education

The Parliament of the Czech Republic wants to improve the quality of pharmaceuticals available for elderly patients with chronic disease. Low-quality generic drugs for diabetes have been coming into the country from India and need to be better regulated. You are serving on the new National Board for Quality of Essential Medicines, and you have been asked to prepare a comprehensive educational program for the board. The program needs to cover the board members' roles and the challenges they face in overseeing the manufacture and distribution of safe and effective pharmaceuticals for diabetes. You have 90 days to recommend your approach. How would you develop the work plan for this challenge, and what forms of educational materials and experiences would you consider?

Scenario 5: Board Meetings

Your private hospital has monthly board meetings that now last more than five hours. Discussions drift between considerations of quality of care, loss of money, changes in the supply of health workers, and bickering about the lack of diversity on the board. Board members also complain about the poor quality of information provided to the board by management just two days before the meetings. The morale among board members and managers is low, and frustrations are building to an unhealthy level. You have been asked to form a three-person committee to assess the situation and suggest ways to improve meeting quality. How would you evaluate the scope of the problems? What types of changes do you think the committee should consider to ensure that board members and managers feel their time and talents are being well used to serve the mission of the hospital?

Notes

1. Terms of reference (TOR) are documents used by multinational aid and finance organizations to define the scope of responsibilities for leaders, boards, and organizations that are expected to deliver value for money in defined contracts. For more information, see the World Bank's *Writing Terms of Reference for an Evaluation: A How-to Guide*, available at http://siteresources.worldbank.org/EXTEVACAPDEV/Resources/ ecd_writing_TORs.pdf.

2. Civil society organizations (CSOs) exist in all countries as a "third sector" between public-sector government and private-sector commercial companies. The terms *CSO* and *nongovernmental organization (NGO)* are often used interchangeably.

3. The organization Transparency International has called for good governance of healthcare organizations across the globe. For more information, see www.transparency.org.uk/wp-content/plugins/ download-attachments/includes/download.php?id=1407.

4. The authors recognize that nongovernmental and private-sector health systems in low- and middle-income countries today are playing a more significant role in health services delivery. For insights into the growing role of private health services organizations, see the World Health Organization (WHO) paper available at www.who.int/bulletin/ volumes/91/3/12-110791.pdf.

5. See www.usaid.gov/sites/default/files/documents/1864/HSS-Vision. pdf to review the health systems strengthening policy framework presented by the US Agency for International Development.

6. Per correspondence with Mahesh Shukla, Management Sciences for Health, and meetings with the African Union in Addis Ababa, Ethiopia, in summer of 2015.

7. *Managers Who Lead* can be accessed at www.msh.org/sites/msh.org/ files/mwl-2008-edition.pdf.

8. A discussion about Six Sigma in healthcare can be accessed at www. isixsigma.com/industries/healthcare/six-sigma-powerful-strategy-healthcare-providers/.

9. The Global Fund's governance policies can be found at www.theglobal fund.org/en/governance-policies/. Recommendations from the World Health Organization can be accessed at www.euro.who.int/__data/ assets/pdf_file/0019/171334/RC62BD01-Governance-for-Health-Web.pdf. Information from the World Bank is presented at www1. worldbank.org/publicsector/anticorrupt/Corruption%20WP_78.pdf, and information from the Organisation for Economic Co-operation

and Development is at www.oecd.org/els/health-systems/governance-health-systems.htm. The Center for Healthcare Governance of the American Hospital Association presents a governance tool kit at http://trustees.aha.org/boardeval/archive/tools/competency-based-governance-tool-kit.pdf.

10. For evidence that good governance matters, see the sources provided by the US Agency for International Development (USAID) at www.hfgproject.org/governance-workshop/.

11. On July 23, 2014, the USAID Health Finance and Governance (HFG) project hosted a one-day workshop at the National Press Club in Washington, DC, about generating evidence of governance contributions to health outcomes (see the website in the previous note). The event brought together health and governance professionals from USAID, prominent external organizations such as the WHO and the World Bank, and implementing partners to discuss key evidence gaps and to develop an action plan to address them. A list of participants is available at www.hfgproject.org/wp-content/uploads/2014/09/July-23-2014-USAID-HFG-Governance-Workshop-Participant-List.pdf.

12. The model guiding these practices was developed by colleagues in Management Sciences for Health in a USAID-funded Leadership, Management, and Governance Project, under cooperative agreement No. AID-OAA-11-00015; used by permission.

13. The WHO lists a variety of indicators in *Monitoring the Building Blocks of Health Systems: A Handbook of Indicators and Their Measurement Strategies*, which can be accessed at www.who.int/healthinfo/systems/WHO_MBHSS_2010_full_web.pdf. In addition, USAID's *Vision for Health Systems Strengthening* report, available at www.usaid.gov/sites/default/files/documents/1864/HSS-Vision.pdf, offers a number of illustrative indicators on page 21.

14. Concepts in this discussion have been adapted from a presentation by James Rice for the Management Sciences for Health (MSH) Leadership, Management, and Governance Project meeting accompanying the 13th World Congress of the World Federation of Public Health Associations in Addis Ababa, Ethiopia, in 2012.

15. For insights into the concept of appreciative inquiry (AI), see the materials provided by the AI Commons at https://appreciativeinquiry.case.edu/.

16. See www.who.int/social_determinants/en/ for resources provided by the WHO about the social determinants of health.

17. The Collaboration for Impact offers a variety of resources about collective impact at www.collaborationforimpact.com/collective-impact/.

18. A complete sample policy from the Global Fund can be accessed at www.theglobalfund.org/en/governance-policies/. A policy from the International Planned Parenthood Federation (IPPF) can be accessed at www.ippf.org/sites/default/files/ippf_code_of_good_governance.pdf.

19. Additional information about the CEO performance review process is available at www.integratedhealthcarestrategies.com/Library/KnowledgeCenter/articles/executive-consulting-strengthening-the-ceo-performance-review-process.

20. For another perspective on meeting enhancement, see the *Fresh Tracks* article at www.freshtracks.co.uk/ten-reasons-why-meetings-fail/, which identifies a set of ten meeting problems that should be avoided. Another set of suggestions, drawn from the work of school boards, is available from Charter Board Partners at www.publiccharters.org/wp-content/uploads/2014/09/Paper-Goverance-Best-Practices-for-Highly-Effective-Charter-School-Boards.pdf.

21. For more information about groupthink, see the *Psychology Today* resource at www.psychologytoday.com/basics/groupthink.

22. See www.lmgforhealth.org/Govern4HealthApp for more information and access to the Govern4Health app.

References

Ciccone, D. K., T. Vian, L. Maurer, and E. H. Bradley. 2014. "Linking Governance Mechanisms to Health Outcomes: A Review of the Literature in Low- and Middle-Income Countries." *Social Science and Medicine* 117: 86–95.

eManager. 2013. "How to Govern the Health Sector and Its Institutions Effectively." Published March. www.lmgforhealth.org/sites/default/files/files/eManager_How%20to%20Govern%20the%20Health%20Sector_4_11_13_FINAL.pdf.

Global Health Learning Center. 2018. "Governance and Health." Accessed June 29. www.globalhealthlearning.org/program/governance-and-health.

International Federation of Public Health Associations. 2012. "Insights from Those Who Govern: Factors That Facilitate and Frustrate Good Governance for Health." Roundtable discussion at the 13th World Congress of International Federation of Public Health Associations, Addis Ababa, Ethiopia, April 25.

International Planned Parenthood Federation. 2007. *Code of Good Governance.* Accessed June 28, 2018. www.ippf.org/sites/default/files/ippf_code_of_good_governance.pdf.

Kickbusch, I., and D. Gleicher. 2012. *Governance for Health in the 21st Century.* World Health Organization. Accessed June 29, 2018. www.euro.who.int/__data/assets/pdf_file/0019/171334/RC62BD01-Governance-for-Health-Web.pdf.

Management Sciences for Health. 2005. *Managers Who Lead: A Handbook for Improving Health Services.* Cambridge, MA: Management Sciences for Health.

National Leadership Council. 2012. *The Healthy NHS Board: Principles for Good Governance.* Accessed June 29, 2018. www.leadershipacademy.nhs.uk/wp-content/uploads/2012/11/NHSLeadership-TheHealthyNHSBoard.pdf.

Savedoff, W. D. 2011. "Governance in the Health Sector: A Strategy for Measuring Determinants and Performance." World Bank policy research working paper. Published May. http://documents.worldbank.org/curated/en/812751468158068363/pdf/WPS5655.pdf.

United Nations (UN). 2018. "Sustainable Development Goal 3: Ensure Healthy Lives and Promote Well-Being for All at All Ages." Accessed June 28. https://sustainabledevelopment.un.org/sdg3.

United Nations Economic and Social Commission for Asia and the Pacific. 2018. "What Is Good Governance?" Accessed June 28. www.unescap.org/sites/default/files/good-governance.pdf.

University of Kansas Community Tool Box. 2018. "About the Tool Box." Accessed July 2. http://ctb.ku.edu/en/about-the-tool-box.

US Agency for International Development (USAID). 2015. "USAID's Vision for Health Systems Strengthening." Accessed June 28, 2018. www.usaid.gov/sites/default/files/documents/1864/HSS-Vision.pdf.

———. 2014. "Accelerating Evidence Generation for Governance Contributions to Health Outcomes." Accessed June 29, 2018. www.hfgproject.org/governance-workshop/.

World Health Organization (WHO). 2010. "Leadership and Governance." In *Monitoring the Building Blocks of Health Systems: A Handbook of Indicators and Their Measurement Strategies.* Accessed June 29, 2018. www.who.int/healthinfo/systems/WHO_MBHSS_2010_section6_web.pdf.

———. 2000. *The World Health Report—Health Systems: Improving Performance.* Geneva, Switzerland: WHO.

MANAGING THE ORGANIZATION–ENVIRONMENT INTERFACE

HEALTH POLICY DESIGN

Suzanne Babich, DrPH, Irene Agyepong, DrPH, Egil Marstein, PhD, and Francisco Yepes, MD, DrPH

Chapter Focus

This chapter is designed to help health managers develop the knowledge and skills needed to understand, effectively influence, and adapt to global health policies. It focuses on key concepts in the design of health policies around the world that are of particular importance for health managers and organizational leaders.

Learning Objectives

Upon completion of this chapter, you should be able to

- discuss the relevance of global health policy design and analysis for health managers,
- describe key concepts in global health policy design and analysis,
- explore the implications of sociocultural factors on global health policy and management practice, and
- apply knowledge of these issues to managerial decision making and actions.

Competencies

- Advocate for and participate in healthcare policy initiatives.
- Interpret public policy, legislative, and advocacy processes within an organization.
- Describe the roles and relationships among the entities influencing global health.
- Analyze context-specific policymaking processes that influence health.

Key Terms

- Allocative or redistributive policies
- Global health policy
- Policy

- Policy analysis
- Policymaking
- Regulatory policies
- White paper

Key Concepts

- Global health policy
- Government policy
- Health policy analysis
- Health policy circuit

- Health policy design
- Sociocultural context
- Step method for policy analysis
- Transnational health policy

Introduction

global health policy
The complex web of rules, both formal and informal, that police vested interests in the attainment of the highest level of health possible for all people.

Global health policy can be described as a complex web of rules, both formal and informal, that police vested interests in the attainment of the highest level of health possible for all people (World Health Organization [WHO] Regional Office for South-East Asia 2016). This description acknowledges the role of various stakeholders as key players in these systems that determine who gets what health services and with what level quality, length of wait, and cost. The description also goes beyond personal health services to include policies that directly or indirectly affect health—whether those policies are rules that allocate or reallocate important resources (e.g., food, medicines) or regulations that control the behaviors of individuals and organizations (e.g., food companies, drug and device manufacturers, coal-burning power plants).

The health policy landscape includes macro-level, transnational policies; country-level government policies; and micro-level policies in smaller units of governance or in individual organizations. Examples of macro-level, transnational policies include the doctors' directive in the European Union (EU), which aims to promote the free movement of healthcare professionals, as well as EU laws targeting issues that directly or indirectly affect health or health services delivery (e.g., bovine spongiform encephalopathy, genetically modified foods). Often, different levels of health policy overlap. Some country- or local-level policies, for instance, have a global reach and should therefore be of vital interest to health managers globally. Examples might include policies to limit the spread of Zika virus, H1N1/avian influenza, chikungunya, or Ebola. Although national health policies often focus on domestic health services allocation, they may also call for specific actions in response to global health issues, including transnational initiatives on such topics as climate change or the treatment of refugees and migrants. Policies also exist at the organizational level, of course, with organizations located all over the world. An organization might prescribe health services for employee groups in conjunction with country-specific national health services.

The professional arena for many health managers today includes opportunities in global organizations, where significant cultural differences require new knowledge, skills, and abilities. Competent managers need to be knowledgeable and flexible enough to adapt to these organizational differences. Chapter 6 focused on the leadership principles necessary for managers undertaking that challenge; this chapter, meanwhile, focuses specifically on the health policies that are relevant in today's global context. This chapter focuses not on the policies that exist at the organization level but rather on the politically structured, institutionalized frameworks that govern the allocation of health resources for population groups. Such policy frameworks are largely shaped by national, regional, and transnational interest groups, and they come about through a process of stakeholder intervention, with each group representing a stake in the outcome, to determine health services procurement practices and distribution. Stakeholder interest groups include powerful corporations, nongovernmental organizations, charitable foundations, and competing political institutions seeking to safeguard their capacities to influence the impact and outcomes of health policies.

Making sense of any health policy issue requires an understanding of the social and political factors that dictate a policy's shape, pace, and direction. Many health managers possess extensive knowledge and experience in the country in which they work, and a high level of insight into many of the factors that influence health policies close to their locus of control and practice. They often have great familiarity with environmental conditions, including the social, political, economic, and organizational factors that provide the backdrop for the development and implementation of local policies. However, given the increasing interdependence of health systems and policies around the world, today's health managers—regardless of where they practice—must be proficient in analyzing and understanding health policies that span geographic boundaries and cultures.

Key Concepts in Health Policy Design and Analysis

Policies are rules that can be either formal or informal, written or unwritten. **Policymaking** is the process of creating those rules. **Policy analysis** involves examining those rules, the problems the rules are meant to address, the goals of the rules, and the criteria used to evaluate the efficacy of the rules. Typically, policy analysis also assesses alternatives to current policy and, based on results of the comparisons, makes recommendations from among the alternatives.

policy
A rule, whether formal or informal, written or unwritten.

policymaking
The process of creating the rules of policy.

policy analysis
The act of examining rules, the problems the rules are meant to address, the goals of the rules, and the criteria used to evaluate the efficacy of the rules.

Health policies have many sources, with governance structures that vary depending on where in the world the policies originate. Policies may be made at the federal, state, provincial, or local levels via legislative or elected bodies, administrative agencies, boards, commissions, courts, and so on. Health policymakers may include legislators, elected officials, agency members, board or commission officials, judges, and the like.

The forms that health policies take also vary. They may be set out in national, state, or provincial constitutions, or they may be put forth in doctrines, statutes, ordinances, rules and regulations, operational or judicial decisions, and other forms specific to the governance structure of the country in which they were created. As a general rule, federal or country-level policies tend to wield the most power, state or provincial policies have somewhat less power, and local-level policies have the least amount of strength or authority. As a result, top-level policies tend to be the slowest and most difficult to change, whereas local-level policies tend to be the easiest to influence.

Health policies can serve any number of purposes, but most fall into one of two broad categories:

allocative or redistributive policies
Policies that determine the way public goods or resources are shared.

regulatory policies
Policies that are designed to affect the behavior or actions of others through rules that dictate what can and cannot be done.

1. **Allocative or redistributive policies** are policies that determine the way public goods or resources are shared. Such policies typically give more resources to some groups and less to others. Examples include policies that provide free or reduced-cost services only to people who fall under a specified income level.
2. **Regulatory policies** are policies that are designed to affect the behavior or actions of others through rules that dictate what can and cannot be done.

The Global Health Policy Circuit

The model in exhibit 11.1 provides a visualization of the complexity of global health policy processes. The model highlights the following:

- The interconnectedness of public health policy, starting from the point of policy inception (political initiative)
- The shaping of rules and regulations (governance policies), perhaps establishing a new policy/reform paradigm
- The introduction of policy premises subsequent to implementation and sector administration
- Renewed stakeholder initiatives, perhaps engaging in strategic ploys, drawing attention to a preferred revision, potentially with the result of new political initiatives—completing the policy circuit

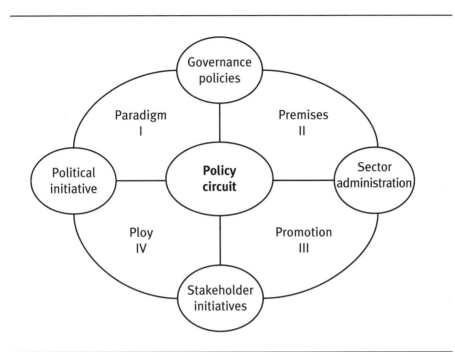

EXHIBIT 11.1
The Global
Health Policy
Circuit

Governing structures vary among countries. In a social democracy, like those common in Western nations, policy initiation and implementation emerge following some level of national debate. Emerging policies commonly reflect the paradigm that governs knowledge development at a given time. Policies that break with established epistemology or generally accepted philosophy about a given topic may be seen as radical proposals, setting the stage for intensified policy debates.

In a top-down approach to policymaking, policies are formalized at the more central health system levels and then passed down to peripheral governance structures responsible for implementation. The ultimate performance or output of any policy will be shaped by how these peripheral governance structures actually translate the policy into programs. Their actions and inactions—decisions and nondecisions—can effectively shape the public face of the policy. Whatever public service or good a policy is intended to govern, the relevant sector stewards promote that policy.

Ministries of health in many countries may have a hierarchical structure, with a central or national-level ministry responsible for agenda setting, policy formulation, and health sector coordination and more peripheral levels, especially district level and below, responsible for policy implementation. Plans, budgets, and programs for health services, education, and other areas may or may not completely reflect the established policy premises, depending on the extent to which centrally designed policies are modified peripherally in implementation.

Regardless of how complete and well-intended policies may be, they may, over time, be contested. A policy might not work as well as hoped, stakeholders might become unhappy, or public opinion might shift. Changing conditions in the policy environment might favor a new paradigm that prompts review of the policy. The discourse that subsequently takes place includes the ploy section of the exhibit—when actor agents might mask their actions for whatever gains may be sought. The potential for new political initiatives at this point illustrates the circular nature of the policy circuit.

In societies that lack well-functioning governance and legal structures, policy development and execution practices might be significantly different from what the model describes. In general, the practices of corrupt or incomplete policy development are beyond the scope of this chapter. However, in seeking to understand the policymaking contexts of those situations, the identification of key stakeholders and their policy goals and practices is critical.

Analyzing Health Policy

Health policy design and analysis are inherently social and political exercises. The environmental context in which policies play out may be shaped by a variety of changing conditions, including such factors as the economy, public opinion, election and budget cycles, and organizational interests. All of these factors can influence the shape, pace, or direction of a particular policy at a given time. Throughout the world, the conditions shaping policy environments, including governance structures and the power of stakeholder influences, vary widely.

At the top levels—the national, state, or transnational levels, such as within the EU—policy initiatives are approached systematically, often calling for complex structures and decision-making processes. At these levels, groups seeking to promote trade and regional development—such as the Association of Southeast Asian Nations (ASEAN), the European Free Trade Association (EFTA), the Latin American Free Trade Association (LAFTA), and the Southern African Development Community (SADC)—play an important role in determining how health policies are shaped and how they work once approved.

white paper
A comprehensive yet concise report that summarizes a position on a complex and often controversial or difficult issue; it aims to increase stakeholders' understanding of the issue to support the development of policy.

In Western countries, policy papers known as **"white papers"** are often drafted by governments as a first stage in a parliamentary process for establishing a future policy. White papers provide policy analysis as depicted in exhibit 11.2, with an emphasis on the following:

1. Formulating a problem statement and underscoring its relevance
2. Recognizing budgetary implications; identifying financial options
3. Identifying all resources considered necessary to determine a capacity to enact, following an assessment of critical prerequisites

EXHIBIT 11.2
Analysis of
Health Policies

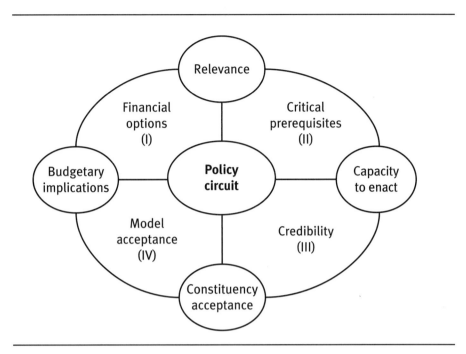

4. Reflecting on the policy's presumed credibility with regard to key stakeholders (constituency acceptance)
5. Concluding its analysis of the policy initiative as summarized in a model acceptance

Despite this complexity—or, indeed, in recognition of it—health managers should put forth the effort to understand the basic concepts and steps of policy analysis, because such knowledge can foster better organizational decision making and strategic planning. Performing a thorough analysis of a complex health policy can be extremely time consuming, however, and organizations will often be limited by time and other resources. Therefore, in organizational settings, analyses of health policies may be limited to relatively quick reviews or abbreviated studies, with certain steps in the process skipped or addressed in only a cursory way.

Given the time-consuming nature of policy analysis, it may be practical for analysis to be conducted by individuals who have prior knowledge of the policy in question. Even though such individuals might not be as objective as an analyst who has no prior knowledge of the case, the amount of time and energy needed for a newcomer to get familiarized with the necessary background may be too great (Patton, Sawicki, and Clark 2012).

No single, correct approach exists for conducting a policy analysis; in fact, the activity is as much an art as a science. Nevertheless, a number of approaches have been described in the literature, each attempting to apply a structure to a complex, multidimensional situation that typically evolves even as it is being studied. One of the most popular approaches—the step method—is widely taught in university courses, in part because it is easy to explain and intuitive to grasp.

The Step Method for Health Policy Analysis

The step method for the analysis of health policies follows a systematic sequence of logical activities that comprehensively examine a problem, the policy designed to address it, the intended consequences of the policy, the policy's outcomes, and the variants of the policy that could potentially improve the results. The analysis may include a recommendation for a "best choice" from among the suggested alternatives, plans for advocating for the preferred variant, and plans for evaluating the outcomes of the policy alternative.

The number of steps included in the model can vary depending on the source, but it typically includes five to eight steps. The core of the analysis—without including advocacy or evaluation plans—generally includes the following five activities:

1. *Defining the problem and its corresponding policy.* Think of the old adage, "There ought to be a law." This step consists of several linked components: A problem has to be identified; it has to be deemed sufficiently significant in magnitude, scope, cost, or some other criteria; and it has to draw the attention of policymakers. Once the problem has met these requirements, a policy may be created to address it.

2. *Collecting evidence.* In this step, a policy analyst becomes educated— often quickly—on as many facets of the problem as possible within time and other resource constraints. Evidence includes information from diverse sources, potentially including reports, news articles, governmental proceedings, published papers, financial records, scientific data, and input from stakeholders, including opinions and anecdotes. The evidence may be objective or subjective.

3. *Determining the policy goals and evaluation criteria.* The goals and evaluation criteria are often one and the same. In other words, once an analyst determines what the policy is meant to accomplish, assessment of how well the policy is working can be done by comparing the actual and intended outcomes.

4. *Laying out the alternatives.* The next step includes brainstorming several evidence-based variations of the current policy that might reasonably be expected to yield improved results. A "do nothing" option should be one of the alternatives, with the status quo serving as the standard

against which other alternatives are compared. The alternatives should be sufficiently diverse that meaningful differences can be discerned among them. Once several alternatives have been identified, the list should be culled to the three or four strongest options.

5. *Playing out the options and picking one.* For each potential policy alternative, the analyst extrapolates the likely results, assigning scores for each of the evaluation criteria. Matrixes, spreadsheets, grids, and charts can help illustrate the comparisons among the alternatives. This step should lead to the selection of the best option.

After the best option has been selected and the recommendation completed, the analysis may end, or it may continue with development of an advocacy plan or a plan for evaluating the new policy, should it be adopted.

Policy analyses are iterative. At any point in the analysis, if the results are unclear, the analyst can and should return to earlier steps and repeat the processes until the results enable a move to the next step.

Given the complex and time-consuming nature of policy analysis, most analyses, in reality, are incomplete or at some point deemed to be "good enough for now." Analysts may be forced to cut short or skip entire steps in the process if faced with time or resource constraints, meaning that a decision has to be made based on information that is less than ideal.

Exhibit 11.3, using an example from a major capital city in Western Europe, illustrates one way in which a policy analysis might be set up. In this example, the problem is that the city's hospitals are receiving large numbers of pregnant migrant women who present for delivery without having received adequate prenatal care, resulting in costly complications and adverse outcomes for infants and mothers. The policy alternatives represent ways in which the hospitals might provide prenatal care free of charge for pregnant migrant women who come to on-site outpatient clinics. Based on the comparison presented in the exhibit, the fourth policy alternative appears to be the best choice among those presented.

As noted in chapter 6, cultural competence is a crucial aspect of effective leadership, but the concept is equally important in the context of global health policy. Policies that do not take into consideration the community's unique social and cultural needs and characteristics risk underperforming or failing to meet their goals. Policies that are culturally incompetent might, for example, result in intended beneficiaries losing interest in a program or failing to use services intended to help them.

Background about the sociocultural factors pertinent to a particular policy context can be collected during the evidence-gathering phase of policy analysis. In many cases, it can be acquired through document reviews or discussions with stakeholders. Ideally, though, health policies should be conceived

EXHIBIT 11.3
Comparing
Projected
Effectiveness
of Policy
Alternatives
Based on
Evaluation
Criteria

	Criterion 1: Cost	Criterion 2: Time to Implement	Criterion 3: Effectiveness
Alternative 1: Maintain status quo	Poor	Good	Poor
Alternative 2: Increase the number of hospital-based outpatient prenatal clinics	Poor	Good	Fair
Alternative 3: Provide free transportation to hospital outpatient prenatal clinics	Fair	Good	Fair
Alternative 4: Move clinics to community-based sites in migrant neighborhoods	Good	Good	Good

and constructed with the active involvement and leadership of representatives of the community at which the policy is aimed. Participatory approaches to community engagement that are considered standard for health services research are equally relevant to the design and analysis of health policies. Policies are most valuable when they respect and respond to the health beliefs, practices, and cultural needs of the diverse populations being served.

Summary

Global health policy is a complex web of rules that police vested interests to promote the attainment of the highest level of health possible for all people. Health policies can be either formal or informal, and either written or unwritten. The health policy landscape includes macro-level, transnational policies; country-level government policies; and micro-level policies in smaller units of governance or in individual organizations. Health policies come from a variety of sources and take a variety of forms, but they typically can be divided into two broad categories: (1) allocative or redistributive policies, dealing with the way goods or resources are shared, and (2) regulatory policies that dictate what can and cannot be done. Health policy analysis involves examining the various rules, the problems the rules are meant to address, the goals of the rules, and the criteria used to evaluate the efficacy of the rules. One of the most popular approaches for health policy analysis is the step method, which follows a systematic sequence of activities to comprehensively examine a problem, the policy designed to address it, the policy's intended consequences, the policy's outcomes, and the variants of the policy that could potentially improve the results.

Discussion Questions

1. Define *global health policy*.
2. Identify the steps in the policymaking process. How does the process differ from one country to another? How is it similar?
3. Analyze the impact of sociocultural and political factors on the establishment and implementation of health policy. How does national health policy affect organizational management practice?
4. Describe the health policy process in your country. Analyze the impact that redistributive policy and regulatory policy have on your organization. How does this affect your approach to strategic planning?
5. As a healthcare leader or manager, what steps could you take to influence national health policy? How open is your ministry of health, or similar organization, to policy analysis emanating from the grassroots level? How can you work through the national political process to influence policy?

Case Study: The Global Policy to Immunize Against Human Papillomavirus

Human papillomavirus (HPV) is a necessary cause, though not the only cause, of several sex-related cancers, capable of leading to cancers of the uterine cervix, anus, penis, and pharynx. Of the more than 150 types of HPV, 15 are carcinogenic, and two are responsible for 70 percent of cases (Tomljenovic, Spinosa, and Shaw 2013).

After completing phase I, II, and III studies, three HPV vaccines have been approved by the US Food and Drug Administration (FDA), with the first—Gardasil—having been approved in 2006. The HPV vaccine has been endorsed by several major health authorities worldwide, including the World Health Organization (WHO), the European Medicines Agency (EMA), the US Centers for Disease Control and Prevention (CDC), and the ministries of health of more than 100 countries. However, despite its effectiveness and safety assurances, growing scientific controversy surrounds the use of the

(continued)

HPV vaccine, with a number of case reports suggesting serious adverse effects (Nicol et al. 2016; Brinth et al. 2015). The global health policy supporting HPV vaccination meets the generally accepted criterion of having a basis in a preponderance of scientific evidence. However, debate focuses on the potential for overestimation of vaccine effectiveness and the underestimation of vaccine safety risks. In addition, some have raised ethical concerns related to possible conflicts of interest on the part of scientists who have vested economic interest in the pharmaceutical industry (Cochrane Nordic 2016).

Health organization acceptance and advocacy of the HPV vaccine policy varies from country to country. Although the WHO, FDA, EMA, CDC, and most ministries of health continue to support widespread HPV vaccination for girls, some countries have changed course. Japan suspended public financing for the vaccine after adverse effects were reported (Wilson et al. 2015). The Danish Health and Medicines Authority (2015) submitted a report to EMA based on the Japanese findings and similar observations in Denmark. Similarly, the American College of Pediatricians (2016) sent a notice of alarm to its associates, and an important Canadian physician asked the government for a moratorium on the vaccination (Dyer 2015). Finally, Cochrane Nordic (2016), a center in Denmark, denounced EMA for ethical breaches.

Clearly, the HPV vaccine represents a complex and challenging area of global health policy. The vaccine policy is purportedly based on evidence, with application through ministries of health, health insurers, and health providers, with the intention of preventing cancers but with the possibility of causing adverse, unintended health consequences for the population it was meant to protect. Health administrators must be aware of the implications and ethical dilemmas associated with compliance or noncompliance with the global policy, and they must encourage serious and balanced discussions within their organizations.

Case Study Discussion Questions
1. What problem does the policy aim to address? State the problem in a sentence or two.
2. Describe the pros and cons of the current global policy.
3. Who has a stake in HPV vaccine policy? What are the interests of the primary stakeholders in the case, and how might these interests place practical limits on evidence-based standards for global health policy?
4. What are the ethical considerations associated with compliance or noncompliance with the policy?

5. What is the role of health managers in implementing HPV vaccination policy?
6. Should informed consent be required for application of the HPV vaccine?
7. Does the principle of *primum non nocere* (first do no harm) have any practical consequences in the application of this policy?

Case Study: The Ghana Arm of the 2015 Global Phase II Ebola Vaccine Clinical Trial

by Irene Akua Agyepong

Learning outcomes addressed by this case study include the following:

- Identification of contextual factors that affect policy implementation
- Analysis of how and why contextual factors affect given situations
- Analysis of the effect of health system complexity on intended and unintended policy outcomes
- Synthesis of the information to guide and justify possible response alternatives

Introduction

This case involves the contentious policymaking process used to address vaccine development in response to the Ebola virus disease (EVD) epidemic in West Africa in 2014 and 2015. Vaccines are effective public health tools that can bring about dramatic declines in the incidence and attributable mortality of various communicable diseases. Vaccines have been successful for such diseases as measles, whooping cough, diphtheria, and tetanus; in the case of smallpox, vaccines were key to the global eradication of the disease.

New vaccine development is a long and expensive process that involves science and epidemiological research in the form of clinical trials. Because clinical trials involve human subjects, strict national and international standards and best practices are in place to ensure that the trials are conducted in an ethical manner. Given the lengthy and expensive nature of the vaccine development process, priority in the use of public funding is given to diseases that affect large numbers of people. In instances where private organizations finance clinical trials, profitability of the new product is also an important concern.

(continued)

The Ebola Virus Disease Emergency

EVD became a global public health emergency in 2014 and 2015. Following a case that occurred in December 2013 in a remote rural area of the West African country of Guinea, the disease spread across borders into Sierra Leone and Liberia. The three countries soon faced an epidemic, affecting more than 22,000 people, with case fatality rates of at least 50 percent (Ohimain 2015). Panic spread globally with media reports and images of overflowing hospitals, dead bodies on the streets, health workers in protective suits, and the already-stressed health systems of Guinea, Liberia, and Sierra Leone seemingly caving in.

All the countries of the Economic Community of West African States (ECOWAS) recognized that they were at high risk. The disease was carried into Nigeria by an air traveler and into Mali and Senegal by people crossing the border by road. Imported cases were also found in Europe and the United States. The cases in Nigeria, Mali, Senegal, Europe, and the United States were quickly contained, and the disease did not spread in any of those areas. In Ghana, as in the rest of the West African subregion, the health institutions and the general public were on high alert. People were doubly concerned because of the country's relatively under-resourced health system.

The only tools available to fight Ebola were isolation, quarantine, and supportive treatment. No vaccine or medicines were available for use, although candidate vaccine products were at various stages of development. The epidemic and the declaration of a public health emergency of international concern led to a global acceleration of Ebola vaccine development and massive international funding to support the process. Phase I clinical trials were conducted, mainly in Europe and the United States, and some promising candidate vaccines were identified. Phase II clinical trials were planned, with coordination by the WHO, to be carried out in several countries in Europe, North America, and sub-Saharan Africa.

Clinical Trials in Ghana

Ghana has an extensive research infrastructure at the health and demographic sites of the Ghana Health Service, as well as at universities. The country has laboratories, clinical trials expertise, and well-established ethical review processes. Successful clinical trials in Ghana had informed the development of meningitis vaccines, and clinical trials for malaria vaccine development had been ongoing in the towns of Navrongo and Kintampo. Therefore, Ghana was one of the countries in sub-Saharan Africa that had been identified for the Ebola vaccine trials. Two Ebola candidate vaccines were to be tested in Ghana. The vaccines to be tested did not have Ebola virus (dead or alive) but rather had components of the identifying protein of Ebola attached to the common cold virus, to stimulate the body to produce antibodies against Ebola.

Part 8 of Act 851 of the Parliament of the Republic of Ghana, known as the Ghana Public Health Act, provides for clinical trials to be conducted in Ghana. The act also provides for the legal backing of the Clinical Trials Advisory Committee, which operates under the Ghana Food and Drugs Authority (FDA). Under section 151 of the law, the committee is tasked with providing the Ghana FDA with "ongoing and timely medical and scientific advice on current and emerging issues related to clinical trials" (FAOLEX Database 2012). The advisory committee is an independent, multidisciplinary panel of experts from various relevant specialties. The law specifies that it should include a clinical pharmacologist, a social scientist, an internal medicine practitioner, a clinical pharmacist, an epidemiologist, a pharmacologist, and a biostatistician, among other specialists. Before any clinical trial can be conducted in Ghana, it must undergo a review not only by the ethical review committee of the Ghana Health Service but also by the Clinical Trials Advisory Committee.

The Ghana Public Health Act, in section 156, maintains that "an applicant who is aggrieved by a decision of the Authority as regards the grant of an authorisation for the conduct of a clinical trial may make a representation to the Minister within sixty days" (FAOLEX Database 2012). Under Ghana's law, the FDA is the body with the authority to stop or suspend clinical trials. Section 160 (subsection 1) of the law states: "If at any stage during the authorised clinical trial of a medicine, herbal medicinal product, cosmetic or medical device the Authority is satisfied that considering the initial risks, discomforts or any other adverse event caused to a person or an animal taking part in the trials, it is in the public interest to stop or suspend the trial, the Authority shall order the person conducting the clinical trial to stop or suspend the trial immediately." Section 160 (subsections 2 and 3) adds: "Without limiting subsection (1), the Authority may for any other reasonable cause suspend, vary or stop a clinical trial . . . The Authority shall notify the person conducting the trial of its decision immediately and the reasons for the decision."

The principal investigators and collaborators on the Ghana clinical trials of the Ebola vaccine developed their protocol and subjected it to all the review mechanisms required by law. Given the global nature of the collaboration for Ebola vaccine development, the protocols were also subject to international review within the WHO. The investigators and collaborators,

(continued)

however, did not organize any national media education or discussions about the proposed clinical trials. In their experiences with previous clinical trials, they had found that following the law and educating the trial participants had always been enough. Ebola turned out to be a special case.

Controversy and Delay

Just as the clinical trials were set to begin, newspapers and radio stations broke the news that an Ebola vaccine trial was taking place in Ghana. The news reports suggested that participants were being bribed to take part in a dangerous undertaking that could potentially introduce the Ebola virus into the country. The stories prompted heated discussions on social media, in the press, and among the public and led to debates in Parliament and within the medical and academic communities. Clinical trials are a specialized area of research, and general understanding of what they entail is often low, even within parts of the medical community.

A section of the Ghana Academy of Arts and Sciences (GAAS) revealed that it had presented a position statement to the government advising caution in deciding to conduct Ebola vaccine trials in Ghana, and it made available a series of sophisticated questions to which it felt the government had not provided adequate answers. The group also stressed the need of the communities and individuals taking part in the trials to be adequately informed of the relevant benefits and risks. Ultimately, it advised that, "considering the gaps in our knowledge and state of preparedness, it would be unsafe to undertake the proposed EVD vaccine clinical trials in Ghana" (Osam 2015).

Whereas the researchers had focused on science and adherence to law, the GAAS proved adept at engaging national politics and the general public, making their concerns widely known through a press statement. The concerns voiced by the GAAS carried significant weight, because the GAAS is a prestigious body of eminent academics highly respected by the government and the public. The researchers involved in the clinical trials, on the other hand, did not engage the public or become involved in politics beyond the study sites because the rules for clinical trials did not allow them to "advertise" before receiving ethical approval. For the public, much of the medical community, and politicians, the perception that experts in the sciences were divided over the clinical trials further raised anxiety and doubt about the trials' wisdom and safety.

The Minister for Health and Parliament called a halt to the trials until the concerns about safety could be adequately addressed. If the concerns were not adequately answered, the trials were to be totally cancelled. The researchers put out rebuttals challenging the perception that the trials were dangerous, and they tried to address the key concerns through press conferences (*Graphic Online* 2015a; *Daily Guide* 2015). The Ghana Medical Association also organized a seminar on clinical trials and the Ebola vaccine trials, specifically.

Several months later, the concerns had been laid to rest, and Parliament gave permission for Ghana's Ebola vaccine trials to go ahead (*Graphic Online* 2015b). The horse, however, had already left the stable. Because the phase II trials were an international process involving several countries with agreed-upon time lines, the process had moved on without Ghana's participation. A phase II Ebola vaccine trial in Ghana was no longer relevant.

Case Study Discussion Questions

1. What is the global policy issue of concern in this case study?
2. What contextual issues affected the decision-making and implementation processes? Why do you think that previous clinical trials in Ghana, such as those for the meningitis and malaria vaccines, did not have such a stormy experience?
3. What do you think could have been done differently by the national investigators and by the global team of which they were a part?
4. What lessons or insights do you take away with regard to context-specific policymaking, the complexity of health systems, the intended and unintended effects on outcomes, and the roles and relationships of entities influencing global health?

Additional Resources

Hamowy, R. 2007. *Government and Public Health in America*. Northampton, MA: Edward Elgar Publishing.

Holland, W., E. Mossialos, P. Belcher, and B. Merkel (eds.). 1999. *Public Health Policies in the European Union*. Farmham, UK: Ashgate.

Kay, A., and O. D. Williams (eds.). 2009. *Global Health Governance: Crisis, Institutions and Political Economy*. London: Palgrave MacMillan.

Nichter, M. 2008. *Global Health: Why Cultural Perceptions, Social Representations, and Biopolitics Matter*. Tucson, AZ: University of Arizona Press.

People's Health Movement, Medact, Medico International, Third World Network, Health Action International, and Asociación Latinoamericana de Medicina Social. 2014. *Global Health Watch 4: An Alternative World Health Report*. London: Zed Books.

Rosanvallon, P. 2011. *The Society of Equals*. Cambridge, MA: Harvard University Press.

References

American College of Pediatricians. 2016. "New Concerns About the Human Papillomavirus Vaccine." Published January. www.acpeds.org/the-college-speaks/position-statements/health-issues/new-concerns-about-the-human-papillomavirus-vaccine.

Brinth, L., A. C. Theibel, K. Pors, and J. Mehlsen. 2015. "Suspected Side Effects to the Quadrivalent Human Papilloma Vaccine." *Danish Medical Journal* 62 (4): A5064.

Cochrane Nordic. 2016. "Complaint to the European Medicines Agency (EMA) over Maladministration at the EMA." Published May 26. http://nordic.cochrane.org/sites/nordic.cochrane.org/files/public/uploads/ResearchHighlights/Complaint-to-EMA-over-EMA.pdf.

Daily Guide. 2015. "Ebola Vaccine Trials Not Harmful—Experts." Published July 9. www.ghanaweb.com/GhanaHomePage/health/Ebola-vaccine-trials-not-harmful-Experts-367470.

Danish Health and Medicines Authority. 2015. "Report from the Danish Health and Medicines Authority for Consideration by EMA and Rapporteurs in Relation to the Assessment of the Safety Profile of HPV-Vaccines." Published September 4. http://sundhedsstyrelsen.dk/~/media/0A404AD71555435BB311CD59CB63071A.ashx.

Dyer, O. 2015. "Canadian Academic's Call for Moratorium on HPV Vaccine Sparks Controversy." *BMJ* 351: h5692.

FAOLEX Database. 2012. "Public Health Act, 2012." Food and Agriculture Organization of the United Nations. Accessed July 6, 2018. http://extwprlegs1.fao.org/docs/pdf/gha136559.pdf.

Graphic Online. 2015a. "Noguchi Boss Criticises Suspension of Ebola Vaccine Trials." Published June 14. www.graphic.com.gh/news/politics/noguchi-boss-criticises-suspension-of-ebola-vaccine-trials.html.

———. 2015b. "Parliament Approves Ebola Vaccine Trials in the Country." Published November 14. www.graphic.com.gh/news/general-news/parliament-approves-ebola-vaccine-trials-in-the-country.html.

Nicol, A. F., C. V. Andrade, F. B. Russomano, L. L. S. Rodrigues, N. S. Oliveira, and D. W. Provance Jr. 2016. "HPV Vaccines: A Controversial Issue?" *Brazilian Journal of Medical and Biological Research* 49 (5): e5060.

Ohimain, E. I. 2015. "How the Spread of Ebola Virus Was Curtailed in Nigeria." *International Journal of Medical and Pharmaceutical Case Reports* 4 (1): 11–20.

Osam, E. I. 2015. "Gov't Was Warned Against Ebola Vaccine Trial—Academy of Arts and Sciences." *CitiFMOnline.* Published June 12. http://citifmonline.com/2015/06/12/govt-was-warned-against-ebola-vaccine-trial-academy-of-arts-and-sciences/.

Patton, C. V., D. S. Sawicki, and J. J. Clark. 2012. *Basic Methods of Policy Analysis and Planning*, 3rd ed. New York: Routledge.

Tomljenovic, L., J. P. Spinosa, and C. A. Shaw. 2013. "Human Papillomavirus (HPV) Vaccines as an Option for Preventing Cervical Malignacies: (How) Effective and Safe?" *Current Pharmaceutical Design* 19 (8): 1466–87.

Wilson, R., P. Paterson, J. Chiu, W. Schulz, and H. Larson. 2015. *HPV Vaccination in Japan: The Continuing Debate and Global Impacts*. Center for Strategic and International Studies. Published April. https://csis-prod.s3.amazonaws.com/s3fs-public/legacy_files/files/publication/150422_Wilson_HPV Vaccination2_Web.pdf.

World Health Organization Regional Office for South-East Asia. 2016. "Our Mission, Our Work." Accessed November 16. www.searo.who.int/about/mission/en/.

GLOBAL DEMOGRAPHICS AND THE MANAGEMENT OF LONG-TERM SERVICES AND SUPPORTS

Mary Helen McSweeney-Feld, PhD, Carol Molinari, PhD, Min Cole, Serif Esendemir, PhD, and Xiaomei Pei, PhD

Chapter Focus

Global healthcare delivery systems in the twenty-first century face serious challenges related to the aging of the population, the prevalence of chronic and disabling conditions, and the growing demand for long-term services and supports across a variety of care settings. In this chapter, we will provide an overview of the demographic, historical, and cultural forces that affect the demand for long-term care, while also exploring key issues related to the supply of long-term care services. Sections of the chapter will focus specifically on staffing issues and the use of technology for effective long-term care management. Finally, the chapter will highlight five countries at varying stages of aging—Japan, Sweden, China, Turkey, and the United States—and examine their unique experiences, challenges, and solutions.

Learning Objectives

Upon completion of this chapter, you should be able to

- explain global trends in aging and disability in both developed and developing countries;
- identify the historical and cultural forces influencing the growing demand for long-term services and supports;
- describe the roles of formal and informal caregivers in providing long-term services and supports;
- discuss common management challenges related to long-term services in various developed and developing countries; and
- understand solutions for addressing gaps in the delivery of long-term services and supports.

Competencies

- Advocate for and participate in healthcare policy initiatives.
- Advocate for the rights and responsibilities of patients and their families.
- Demonstrate commitment to self-development, including continuing education, networking, reflection, and personal improvement.
- Contribute to the advancement of the profession of healthcare management by sharing knowledge and experience.
- Develop others by mentoring, advising, coaching, and serving as a role model.
- Demonstrate an understanding of the interdependency, integration, and competition that exist among healthcare sectors.

Key Terms

- Active life expectancy (ALE)
- Activities of daily living (ADLs)
- Aged society
- Aging in place
- Aging society
- Assisted living facility
- Chronic health condition
- Continuing care retirement community (CCRC)
- Direct care worker
- Disability
- Filial piety
- Health-adjusted life expectancy (HALE)
- Healthy life years (HLYs)
- Home and community-based services
- Hyper-aged society
- Instrumental activities of daily living (IADLs)
- Long-term services and supports
- Means-tested
- Medical home
- Memory care unit
- Population aging
- Skilled nursing facility

Key Concepts

- Coordination of care
- Dementia care
- Demographic shift
- Emerging technologies
- Epidemiological transition
- Formal and informal caregivers
- Integrated care
- Long-term care
- Mandatory insurance
- Public spending
- Universal coverage
- Workforce shortages
- Workforce turnover

Introduction

Healthcare systems throughout the world are facing mounting pressures from growing numbers of older adults, many of whom have complex care needs associated with chronic or disabling conditions. As people live longer, they are more likely to require **long-term services and supports**, whether at home or in various care settings, to help manage their regular life activities. In this chapter, we will examine many of the long-term care challenges that today's global healthcare managers face; the demographic and cultural forces that have contributed to those challenges; unique features of the long-term care workforce; and the technological advances that are likely to shape the delivery of long-term services and supports in the years ahead. The chapter concludes with a discussion of long-term care approaches employed in five specific countries—Japan, Sweden, China, Turkey, and the United States. Spending on long-term care, as a percentage of gross domestic product, is anticipated to increase in the years ahead, especially in countries with rapidly aging populations. Current levels of public spending on long-term care for various countries of the world are shown in exhibit 12.1.

long-term services and supports
Care, services, and assistance provided across various settings to help people address difficulties in performing their activities of daily living.

Demographic and Cultural Forces Affecting Demand for and Supply of Long-Term Services and Supports

The Aging of Populations

Population aging is a global demographic shift whereby older adults are making up an increasing proportion of the overall population (Takagi and Molinari 2017). This trend reflects both increased longevity and lower fertility across the various regions of the world. Between 2025 and 2050, the older adult population is expected to almost double to 1.6 billion globally, whereas the total global population will increase by just 34 percent (He, Goodkind, and Kowal 2016).

Population aging is a global trend, though the speed with which the process occurs is uneven from one region to another. Many developing countries, including China and Turkey, are considered **aging societies**, meaning that their older adult populations are growing rapidly, to the point that people aged 65 years or older make up between 7 and 14 percent of the population (Takagi and Molinari 2017). A number of more developed countries—including the United States and many European nations—are regarded as **aged societies**, meaning that the population of older adults has already reached 14 to 21 percent of society. Some countries, such as Japan, are categorized as **hyper-aged societies**, meaning that older adults make up more than 21 percent of the population (Coulmas 2007). Growth among older populations in developed countries is expected to continue in the coming years but at a slower rate than

population aging
A global demographic shift whereby older adults are making up an increasing proportion of the overall population.

aging society
A society in which people aged 65 years or older make up 7 to 14 percent of the total population.

aged society
A society in which people aged 65 years or older make up 14 to 21 percent of the population.

hyper-aged society
A society in which people aged 65 years or older make up more than 21 percent of the population.

EXHIBIT 12.1
Public Spending
on Long-Term
Care (health
and social
components)

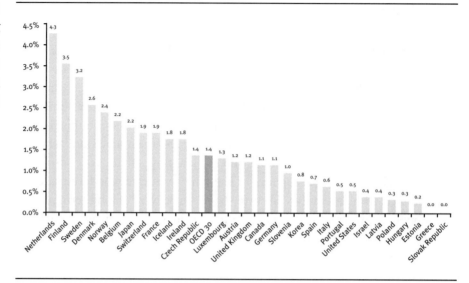

Notes: Figures are for 2014; OECD 30 = Average of 30 members of the Organisation for Economic Co-operation and Development.

Source: Reprinted with permission from Organisation for Economic Co-operation and Development (2018).

in developing or emerging nations, especially those in Asia and Latin America (He, Goodkind, and Kowal 2016).

The epidemiological transition toward older populations is largely the result of declining fertility rates, as well as lower mortality rates stemming from the medical advances of the twentieth century. In some countries, inflows of immigrants have affected population aging. In Italy and Spain—European countries with relatively old populations—immigration has slowed an overall decline in population numbers. Population aging may also be influenced by government policies, such as China's one-child policy, which will be discussed later in the chapter. In the coming decades, a number of countries, including China, South Korea, and Thailand, are expected to experience population aging coupled with overall decline in total population (He, Goodkind, and Kowal 2016).

Individuals with Chronic and Disabling Health Conditions

chronic health condition
A condition that lasts three months or longer and affects an individual's health or independence.

disability
A physical, sensory, cognitive, or intellectual impairment, or type of chronic disease, that limits a person's ability to function in a given social context.

Another factor driving the increased demand for long-term services and supports is the growing numbers of adults with chronic and disabling conditions. In considering this factor, we need to first establish the definitions of key terms. **Chronic health conditions** are those conditions that last three months or longer and affect an individual's health or independence. A **disability** can be a physical, sensory, cognitive, or intellectual impairment, or a type of chronic disease. A disability, as explained by Kunkel, Brown, and Whittington (2014, 111), reflects "a combination of an individual's health and social circumstances that determines one's ability to function within a given social context."

Levels of disability can be assessed based on a number of measures, including the individual's ability to function and carry out **activities of daily living (ADLs)** and **instrumental activities of daily living (IADLs)**. ADLs include routine and fundamental activities such as eating, bathing, and dressing, whereas IADLs include activities—such as cleaning, shopping, and managing finances—that enable people to live independently (McSweeney-Feld and Molinari 2017). Levels of disability may also be assessed using such measures as **active life expectancy (ALE)**, or disability-free life expectancy, and **healthy life years (HLY)**. **Health-adjusted life expectancy (HALE)** is a measure that adjusts for the severity of an individual's disability impairments (Kunkel, Brown, and Whittington 2014).

Measuring and estimating growth in the global population of adults with disabilities can be difficult, given that reliable data for many developing countries are unavailable. Furthermore, in some countries, functional measures such as ADL limitations may have different interpretations or not be culturally appropriate. Consequently, we need to look at developed and developing nations separately when considering this factor.

Among developed nations, people born in some Western European countries—notably, Denmark and Malta—can be expected to live nearly 70 HLYs, on average. People in the Baltic states of Estonia, Latvia, and Lithuania, however, have an average of only 48 to 50 HLYs (Kunkel, Brown, and Whittington 2014). Among developing nations, those with greater economic growth tend to have lower rates of disability, though some exceptions to this rule have been observed. The Philippines and Malaysia, for instance, are not as economically advantaged as Russia or Ukraine but have greater HALEs (Kunkel, Brown, and Whittington 2014).

The future of global disability rates is difficult to predict. Some types of disability may decline in response to improvements in medical services, though others may increase as a result of demographic trends or lack of sufficient services and supports, especially in developing economies. Global rates of Alzheimer's disease and other dementias are increasing, and sensory impairments, such as loss of hearing or vision, affect millions of people worldwide. According to the World Health Organization (WHO), more than 253 million people worldwide live with vision impairment, and 81 percent of that group is aged 50 years or older (WHO 2017). Disabling loss of hearing affects approximately one-third of adults aged 65 or older (WHO 2018). The percentages of people with sensory impairments are likely to grow as the population continues to age.

Supply Issues Affecting Long-Term Services and Supports

In the United States and the advanced global economies of Asia and the European Union, the importance of long-term services and supports for older adults and people with disabilities is well recognized. Many models of long-term care delivery in these nations have focused on the role of the acute care or curative

activities of daily living (ADLs)
Routine and fundamental life activities, such as eating, bathing, and dressing.

instrumental activities of daily living (IADLs)
Life activities—such as cleaning, shopping, and managing finances—that enable people to live independently.

active life expectancy (ALE)
The portion of total life expectancy during which an individual is not affected by disability; also called *disability-free life expectancy*.

healthy life years (HLYs)
The estimated number of years an individual will live without disability-related limitations on daily activities.

health-adjusted life expectancy (HALE)
A measure of life expectancy adjusted for the severity of an individual's disability.

sector, where individuals receive assistance from professionals in hospitals or other institutional settings. In other nations—particularly developing nations with fragile healthcare systems—long-term services and supports have remained the responsibility of family members and informal caregivers. Some countries have passed laws and regulations to formally establish the responsibilities of family caregivers.

In traditional societies, families have long provided care for their older members. Since the start of the twentieth century, however, declining fertility rates, the rise of industrialization, and changes in family structures have limited the ability of family members to provide the bulk of this support. As a result, a number of countries have established government-sponsored programs to provide services to complement the family's traditional role.

The United States and many other developed nations have experienced a trend toward independence in family relationships across the life cycle. As a result, many older adults in those countries live alone or just with a spouse so that their care needs are not a burden on family members who might be supporting younger dependent children. The number of "elder orphans"—individuals living alone without a family member available to provide care—in the United States is likely to increase as the baby boomer generation (those born between 1946 and 1964) ages. Ianzito (2017) reports that approximately 23 percent of US boomers will eventually be without family caretakers.

In developing nations, where the norms of family caregiving tend to remain strong, the co-residence of multiple generations continues to be a common living arrangement for older adults (Kunkel, Brown, and Whittington 2014). With further economic growth, however, alternative approaches to the delivery of long-term services and supports will be necessary to enable younger members of the population to pursue careers while still providing for older family members.

Vignette: Dementia Care

A major challenge in the provision of long-term services and supports worldwide involves the growing number of older adults with cognitive impairment due to Alzheimer's disease and related dementias. According to Alzheimer's Disease International (2015, 2016), approximately 47 million people worldwide were living with dementia in 2016, and experts have predicted that this number will roughly double every 20 years—up to 75 million in 2030 and to 131 million in 2050. Much of the increase will be in developing countries. In 2015, about 58 percent of people with dementia were living in low- and middle-income countries; this number is expected to increase to 68 percent by 2050 (Alzheimer's Disease International 2015). The growth in the proportion of older adults with Alzheimer's diagnoses is especially significant in China, India, and other countries of South Asia and the western Pacific (Alzheimer's Disease International 2015).

In many countries, the traditional model for caring for people with dementia has emphasized care provided in the home by unpaid, family caregivers. In countries with established residential long-term care communities, traditional models have involved **memory care units**, secure areas within nursing homes that focus specifically on dementia care. In recent years, however, newer models of care have emerged, particularly in European countries. In the Netherlands, Hogeweyk—a "dementia village"—allows individuals with dementia to live in a small town where conditions reflect their earlier lifestyles, while at the same time being observed by trained staff around the clock (Hogeweyk 2018). In the United Kingdom, the Butterfly model of care emphasizes emotional connection and emotional intelligence, as individuals live in small homes of six to seven beds and receive specialized care from dedicated, trained personnel (Sheard 2013). The Iris Murdoch Center of the University of Stirling, in Scotland, has a virtual care home, with the aim of demonstrating dementia-friendly design features and promoting the integration of new design ideas and concepts into existing long-term care communities (Dementia Services Development Centre 2012).

> **memory care unit**
> A unit in a nursing home that focuses specifically on dementia care.

Workforce Challenges in Long-Term Care

Long-term care is highly labor intensive, and the global delivery of long-term services and supports depends on both formal, trained professionals and informal, unpaid caregivers. **Direct care workers**, especially aides, represent the largest component of the long-term care workforce, and the development of this workforce segment has been identified as a key concern facing healthcare in the twenty-first century (Institute of Medicine 2008; Molinari and Zhang 2015). Many countries, including China, are facing a shortage of facilities and trained professionals ready to provide formal care (Kunkel, Brown, and Whittington 2014). Globally, the majority of long-term care is provided by family members, friends, and other informal caregivers.

Although demand for direct care workers is increasing, turnover is high and recruitment is difficult, in large part because of noncompetitive wages and benefits, negative industry image, and inadequate training (Stone and Harahan 2010). In the United States, turnover among home health aides ranges between 40 to 60 percent (National Direct Service Workforce Resource Center

> **direct care worker**
> An individual in the health workforce who provides care and personal assistance to individuals who are frail, sick, or injured or who have physical or mental disabilities.

2008), whereas turnover for nursing assistants in assisted living facilities was 29 percent (National Center for Assisted Living 2012).

Workforce studies have indicated that about 45 percent of direct care workers live below 200 percent of the federal poverty level and that, in 2009, 28 percent of direct care workers were uninsured (PHI 2011). The long-term care occupations often offer limited opportunities for career advancement, and many workers receive inadequate training and preparation for the evolving roles and responsibilities they must take on (Stone and Harahan 2010; Stone and Wiener 2001). Nursing, home health, and home care aides report that they do not feel their jobs are respected and valued (Bishop et al. 2009). Media reports that highlight stories of poor-quality care by providers can exacerbate the sense of low prestige felt by workers in the field. Furthermore, rules and regulatory policies in long-term care focus primarily on protecting consumers, not on addressing workers' concerns (Stone and Wiener 2001).

As individuals grow older and develop chronic conditions, many strongly prefer to **age in place** in their homes and communities rather than move into institutional settings. As a result, the **home and community-based services** provided by direct care workers have come to encompass an increasingly broad and complex array of physical and mental health needs, requiring skills in such areas as medication management, palliative care, and dementia care (Stone and Bryant 2012). Given the nature of these responsibilities, the relatively minimal training and preparation provided for people in direct care positions seem increasingly incongruent (Stone and Bryant 2012). In the United States, for instance, a person can become a Medicare- or Medicaid-certified home health aide with less than two weeks of training if they pass a competency test (Molinari and Zhang 2015).

The direct care workforce will be best positioned to meet today's challenges if it is given comprehensive training, effective supervision, and continued empowerment. Training and education are especially vital today, given the need for direct care workers to work with new, consumer-centered service delivery models and information technology systems that help better coordinate care. Furthermore, significant cost savings can be achieved when home care aides' scopes of practice are expanded and nurses have greater ability to delegate tasks to well-trained workers (Molinari and Zhang 2015). Effective training in many areas, however, is hampered by shortages of personnel able to educate and prepare people for careers in long-term care.

aging in place
The practice of remaining in one's own home and community during old age.

home and community-based services
Health-related services and assistance that are provided in the home and community in which an individual is already living.

The Evolving Role of Technology

Some of the challenges associated with shortages of trained providers can be addressed through the increased use of technology in the provision of services.

For instance, delivery of long-term care can be enhanced by telehealth capabilities and other health-enabling and ambient assistive technologies that collect data and provide communication in the home. Robotic devices may also provide some basic services at affordable prices.

According to McWilliams (2015), the global market for elder-care technology products was valued at $4.4 billion in 2015 and is expected to grow to $10.3 billion by 2020. Broadly speaking, such products include basic assistive items (e.g., eyeglasses, canes, walkers) as well as wearable technologies, safety monitoring systems, and applications for smartphones, tablets, social media, and other internet-based features.

In developed countries, technology has helped to extend life through a variety of devices and services, as well as through the use of high-technology medicine. In developing economies, too, portable technologies have enabled the inexpensive collection of healthcare information and improved communication between healthcare providers and people living in remote areas. Personal response systems can benefit individuals affected by serious health conditions, enabling faster emergency response and, therefore, reduced hospital utilization and mortality (De San Miguel and Lewin 2008).

Technological improvements can make a product or an environment more accessible to people with disabilities, while also benefiting others as well. For example, an automatic door opener benefits not only individuals using walkers and wheelchairs but also staff and family members carrying meal trays, supplies, or other items. The use of health information technology to make home environments "smart" and responsive, to automate buildings, and to maintain patient information in electronic health records can help providers improve care coordination as well as quality of care.

Emerging technologies have the potential to significantly improve care, as long as the costs are affordable and the human element of care is retained. Such technologies should be seen as a complement to, as opposed to a substitute for, personal long-term services and supports.

Models for Care Management and Care Transitions: International Frameworks and Perspectives

Throughout the world, long-term services and supports are provided in a wide variety of settings—from institutional and well-defined residential settings to people's own homes in the community—and across several types of delivery systems. Under universal coverage systems, national and local governments fund and administer long-term care coverage for all citizens. Under mandatory insurance programs, the government requires people of certain age groups or employment statuses to pay premiums toward insurance for long-term care.

means-tested
Having eligibility
criteria based on
income or financial
need.

Some countries have mixed systems, in which public **means-tested** elements
and private insurance both play important roles. In other countries, services
may be provided with few public funds or with no formal system (Niles-Yokum
and Wagner 2015). A summary of government policies and services in selected
countries is provided in exhibit 12.2, with further discussion in the sections
that follow.

Japan

History and Demographics

With high life expectancy, a low fertility rate, and a strikingly low number of
immigrants, Japan stands at the forefront of the population aging trend. In
2015, people aged 65 or older represented 26.6 percent of Japan's population, making it the oldest country in the world (He, Goodkind, and Kowal
2016). Experts believe that older adults may represent as much as one-third
of Japan's population by 2025.

filial piety
A cultural norm,
prevalent in
much of Asia,
emphasizing
that younger
family members
are expected to
take care of their
elders.

Traditionally, Japanese culture has emphasized **filial piety**, the idea that
younger family members have an obligation to take care of their elders. As a
result, families have taken on significant caregiving responsibilities, and care
through the hospital system has been used for more serious illnesses. In recent
years, however, changing family structures have caused a growing number of
older adults to live separately from their families, necessitating the restructuring of service networks.

In 2000, Japan introduced a national long-term care policy that redefined
the role of the government in providing care for older adults. The country
established a national long-term care insurance program, known as *Kaigo
Hoken*, that is administered separately from the national health insurance policies and is funded by general tax revenues as well as insurance premiums. The
policies are mandatory. All citizens older than age 40 must contribute (Yong
and Saito 2012), and the insurance covers long-term care services for people
aged 65 years or older with severe disabilities (Applebaum, Robbins, and Bardo
2014). Eligibility for services is determined through a standardized care needs
assessment questionnaire. Depending on level of eligibility, individuals may be
entitled to such benefits as home care services, house cleaning, meal delivery,
day care, and institutional care services (Takagi and Molinari 2017).

The Long-Term Care Delivery System
Residential Care
Residential care is covered under Japan's long-term care insurance plan, with
three types of nursing home settings available: (1) facilities, or residence homes,
that serve older or frail adults; (2) facilities that provide more institutional care

EXHIBIT 12.2
Long-Term Care Policies and Services in Japan, Sweden, China, Turkey, and the United States

	Japan	Sweden	China	Turkey	United States
Percentage of population 65+ (2014)	25.8%	19.8%	9.6%	8%	14.5%
National long-term care system	Universally available as a mandatory insurance program	Universally available as part of welfare system (but varies by municipality)	No formal long-term care system	Available to low-income and alone older adults through national security system	Available to low-income older adults through means testing
Home and community-based services	Widely available	Widely available	Available, but no specific programs exist and reimbursement is limited	Mostly available to urban aged; limited for countryside aged	Available through programs for low-income individuals
Support for informal caregivers	Local cities and nonprofit organizations offer support group, consulting, and respite care services	Each municipality offers its own financial payment program, respite care, consultation, and training programs	Rarely available	The Ministry of Family and Social Policies supports informal caregivers to help older adults to age in place	Financial payment is limitedly available in some states; local offices offer support group, consulting, training, and respite care services
Reforms and future direction	Emphasis on prevention to control cost of services; revision of eligibility criteria to improve finance and quality of services	Improvement of medical care and social service agencies; reduction of discrepancies in service quality and availability across municipalities	Expansion of service network to support community-based care; goal of adding more than 3 million institution-based beds	Movement toward services to encourage older adults with low income to age in their communities; gradual increase in private institutional care for older adults with high income	Emphasis on community-based services through innovative programs, such as the Program of All-Inclusive Care for the Elderly (PACE)

Sources: Adapted from Takagi and Molinari (2017). Data from Applebaum, Robbins, and Bardo (2014); KPMG International (2013); US Census Bureau (2015).

for people with significant medical needs; and (3) facilities that provide dementia care (Yong and Saito 2012). Studies of the plan have shown that utilization rates are high, especially for private institutional care, where move-in fees, or *nyuknokin*, are significant. Public nursing homes are also available, though potential residents face a long wait list. Japan's plan also provided funding for start-up nursing home construction, so a number of private, lower-cost homes have emerged to provide services in more remote areas, though quality levels tend to vary (Brasor and Tsubuku 2014).

Local governments also provide special facilities for individuals with limited financial means, including people with mental or physical disabilities. These "care houses" often attract low-income older adults who are given a room and sometimes meals in exchange for signing over their welfare payments. (Brasor and Tsubuku 2014).

Home and Community-Based Services

A community-based integrated care system was created under Japan's long-term care insurance plan, and it provides for the delivery of home and community-based services. Two key initiatives were introduced in 2012. The first initiative provided for regular and as-needed home visits, with close collaboration between long-term care and nursing staffs. The second initiative involved the creation of a composite service, adding healthcare to the "small-scale multifunctional in-home care" service that was established in 2006. Under both initiatives, local authorities hire service providers for a fixed monthly fee (Morikawa 2014).

Future Directions and Challenges

Filial piety remains part of Japanese culture, and family caregivers still play an important role in the lives of the country's older adults. However, the availability of younger family members to provide long-term services—as well as their desire to provide such care—has changed, shifting the balance between private and public caregiving entities (Takagi and Molinari 2017). At the same time, restrictive immigration policies have limited the number of workers available for caregiving services. The country has sought to develop leading-edge technology, including sophisticated robotics, to alleviate some of its workforce shortage issues.

Sweden

History and Demographics

Sweden has long been recognized as the first European country to have a long-term care plan and a publicly funded welfare state, and it ranks among the top European nations in investment in long-term services and supports as a percentage of GDP (Eurostat 2018). Life expectancy in Sweden ranks among the longest in the world—79.1 years for men and 83.2 years for women, as of 2010 (Swedish Institute 2013). People aged 65 or older represent 18 percent of the country's inhabitants, and this number is projected to rise to 23 percent by 2030, partly because of the large number of people born during the 1940s (Swedish Institute 2013). More than 5 percent of Sweden's population is aged 80 or older (Statista 2018).

The Long-Term Care Delivery System
Residential Long-Term Care Services

Swedish municipalities planning housing and residential areas are required to ensure that they meet the needs of all types of individuals with disabilities, regardless of age. These accessibility requirements have been given greater prominence in legislation over the years. A growing number of older adults want to live in "senior housing," ordinary homes for people aged 55 and over where accessibility is a priority. Some are newly built, while others are regular homes that have been made more accessible as part of conversion or renovation work. Long-term care services are organized at the local level, with municipalities purchasing care from both public and private providers, and many recipients have the possibility of choosing across competing providers. There has been limited measurement, however, of the effectiveness and safety of care, and few mechanisms for guaranteeing quality standards for services of the type found in healthcare.

Home and Community-Based Services

When a person with disabilities is no longer able to live independently, that person can apply for assistance from municipally funded home-help services (Swedish Institute 2013). The extent of care provided is determined by each municipality based on an assessment of need. In some cases, around-the-clock assistance enables older people with disabilities to keep living in their homes throughout their lives. Additional services include adult day services for individuals with dementia or other cognitive impairments, as well as transportation service in taxis and vehicles adapted for people with disabilities. In 2010, 11 million such journeys were completed, representing a national average of 34 per eligible person (Swedish Institute 2013). Sweden also pays for preventive care for its citizens and supports the use of health coaches. In addition, Swedish healthcare providers often provide prescriptions for healthy activities (sometimes in combination with medication) and monitor such activities on an ongoing basis (Swedish Institute 2013).

Caregivers and Care Coordination

Given that much of the care and treatment formerly provided in hospitals is now being provided in people's homes, the work of qualified, coordinated, multiprofessional teams is essential. To ensure high standards, the government, from 2011 to 2014, invested a total of 1 billion Swedish kronor (SEK) in additional training programs for staff working with older adults (Swedish Institute 2013). The Swedish government also invested SEK 4.3 billion in measures aiming to "improve coordination of home health care, elderly care, hospital care and health-center care provided to elderly people" (Swedish Institute 2013).

Future Directions and Challenges

Meagher and Szebehely (2012, 55) point out that the traditional Swedish system is undergoing significant change. They explain:

> There has been some retrenchment in eldercare evident in falling coverage and stronger targeting of people with higher levels of need. This development has led to the informalization of care for some groups of older people. In disability care, there has been a considerable expansion of services, perhaps most notably in the introduction of a personal assistance scheme for people with severe disabilities. These divergent trends in services for older people and people with disabilities have coincided with a convergent development across both care fields: the marketization of services and the emergence of large, corporate, for-profit providers.

Between 1995 and 2005, the number of private companies in Sweden's social services sector increased fivefold (Swedish Institute 2013). However, media investigations have unearthed alarming shortfalls at several such companies, and some critics have argued that organizations are allowing profit to have a negative impact on the standard of care (Paul, Schaeffer, and Coustasse 2017).

China

History and Demographics

China is an aging society with changing social structures, and it faces daunting challenges in meeting the demand for long-term services and supports. China's older adult population is growing rapidly, up to 136.9 million in 2015. Older adults represent 10.1 percent of China's total population, and this percentage is projected to increase to 17.2 percent by 2030 (He, Goodkind, and Kowal 2016). Additionally, the number of Chinese adults aged 85 or older is expected to grow at a rate of 1 million per year until 2025 (Wu and Dang 2013).

One reason for the rapid aging of China's population is the one-child policy that the country's Communist government introduced in 1979 in response to concerns over excessive population growth. The policy called for each family to have only one child, though some exceptions were allowed. The one-child policy was eventually phased out and replaced with a two-child policy in 2016, but by that time the number of children available to care for elderly parents had been significantly reduced. The number of available caregivers was further affected by the migration of young Chinese families to urban centers during the 1990s, which left many older adults in rural areas without family members to provide care and support.

Along with the dramatic growth in China's population of older adults will come commensurate growth in the number of older adults with physical and mental disabilities and chronic diseases such as cardiovascular disease, diabetes, hypertension, and stroke. These conditions—and their impact on the demand for long-term care—will require the attention of China's policymakers in the years ahead (Whitman and Burns 2017).

Of China's older adult population, 52 percent reside in urban areas, and 48 percent are in rural areas (National Bureau of Statistics of China 2017). Generally, rural nursing homes offer lower levels of care than urban ones. Many rural older adults remain in their villages taking care of their grandchildren while their adult children work in larger cities. Older adults in urban areas, meanwhile, often must contend with environmental concerns—such as a lack of elevators or ramps in older apartment buildings—that create barriers for people with mobility issues and increase isolation. Compounding these challenges is the fact that nearly a quarter of older adults in China have income levels below the poverty line (Keck 2013). Cases of suicide and abuse among older adults have been increasing (Wu and Dang 2013).

Many of the challenges faced by China's older adults run contrary to key aspects of China's cultural history, which is based on Confucianism, with a strong emphasis on the role of the family and filial piety. In an attempt to reinforce these principles, filial piety has been codified into Chinese law (Wong 2013). The Law on the Protection of the Rights and Interests of Elderly People, which came into effect in 2013, is part of an effort to bring aging-related issues into the national strategy; reinforce the family caregiving role; regulate long-term care; create a basic structure for aging services; emphasize the lifestyle, well-being, and spiritual needs of older adults; and support livable community development regulation (Wu and Dang 2013).

The Long-Term Care Delivery System

China has two broad systems that provide care to older adults: (1) a social welfare system of community-based elder services, residential facilities, and nursing homes and (2) a medical system consisting of physicians, hospitals, and primary care clinics (Whitman and Burns 2017). The services provided include long-term institutional care in nonacute settings, with significant levels of medical and support services, as well as noninstitutional "senior care services," encompassing a wide range of home and community-based services (Whitman and Burns 2017).

Home and Community-Based Services

With its tradition of filial piety, China has a strong commitment to family and community support. Younger relatives are required by law to visit older adults at least once a year. Most individuals with disabilities receive assistance in their homes either from family members or from live-in housemaid, or *bao mu*, services. More formal community-based services are also being developed, including large numbers of community service centers (Chu and Chi 2008).

In 2001, the Chinese government started the Starlight program to build new community service centers using national and local welfare lottery funds. By 2004, 32,490 Starlight homes for seniors were built, but the program became unsustainable because it lacked systematic policies for eligibility, regulation, and evaluation. Most of the Starlight centers remain open but are not used by people who need the services (Cao and Liu 2013).

Long-Term Care Services

As of the end of 2013, China had 42,475 senior facilities with 4.9 million beds, and about 72 percent of the total facilities were owned by the government (Whitman and Burns 2017). Long-term care communities are supported by government funding but may also receive money through medical insurance plans and private (out-of-pocket) expenditures. About 87 percent of China's facilities provide basic daily living supportive services, 10 percent provide nursing care at a high dependency level, and 3 percent provide hospice care (Wu and Dang 2014). The privately owned facilities are primarily in urban and metropolitan areas, whereas most of the government-owned facilities are in rural areas. Unequal competition for financial resources between privately owned facilities and government-owned facilities has led to low rates of profit for many private institutions (Wu and Dang 2014).

In 2008, China's senior housing industry sought to address the ongoing demographic challenges and the movement of younger family members to urban areas, and housing developers adopted the **continuing care retirement community (CCRC)** concept, which originated in the United States. Under the CCRC model, a comprehensive range of nursing and housing options are available within a single community, and services can be modified as individuals age and their needs change (McSweeney-Feld 2017). China's adoption of the model led to the development of large-scale senior housing complexes with varying levels of care across hospital, nursing, and rehabilitation components.

The move to adopt the CCRC model was influenced by reforms in the real estate market that started in 1998 (Yu 2016). Local governments became willing to provide land for senior housing development, and thus an incentive was created for private developers to develop senior housing and CCRCs. Chinese CCRCs primarily target high-income seniors such as scholars, professionals, people successful in business or entertainment, and individuals supported by their children in China or overseas. Key challenges faced by Chinese CCRCs have involved difficulties identifying the actual needs of older adults at each project location and measuring the financial aspects of providing care (Wu and Dang 2014).

continuing care retirement community (CCRC)
A model for long-term care in which a comprehensive range of nursing and housing options are available within a single community and services can be modified as individuals age and their needs change.

Post-Acute Services and Care Coordination

China continues to encourage the use of hospitals for any medical need. Often, older adults have long hospital stays, either because of a lack of available post-acute care facilities or because of the expectations of patients and providers (Whitman and Burns 2017). Most rehabilitation, medical, and nursing services facilities are located in the eastern part of China; often very few are available in the western areas (Wu and Dang 2014).

To better address the growing needs of older adults, China's central government, starting in 2013, launched a series of policy directives to support the delivery of "integrated care" (*yiyang jiehe*) in communities. Local governments have responded to the directives with plans and pilot projects, leading to the emergence of integrated service networks in large cities, where both older adults and the necessary resources are concentrated.

China's move to integrated care has involved the consolidation of social and health resources at the community level. For example, community health centers in the city of Shanghai have expanded their services to include nursing, rehabilitation, and palliative care. The centers have reached out to older residents in the community, and residents' access to the services is supported under existing medical insurance schemes.

Future Directions and Challenges

As part of its national strategic plan, the Chinese government has made strides to establish a long-term care system with comprehensive social care as the foundation, supported by institutional care. Its institutions have added millions of new beds to better meet the demands of the population (Feng et al. 2013). Nonetheless, the nation still lacks a comprehensive strategic and visionary plan, and the relationship between the government, the market, clients, families, and communities is not clearly defined. In addition, China's long-term care workforce has severe shortages in administrative, professional, and frontline caregiving roles across all levels and settings of care.

Turkey

Demographics and History

Like many other developing countries, Turkey faces a variety of concerns related to population aging and sociodemographic transition. According to the Turkish Statistical Institute (TÜİK), adults aged 65 years or older represented 8.2 percent of the Turkish population in 2015—doubling the percentage (4.1 percent) from 1975. The number is expected to reach 20 percent by 2050 (TÜİK 2013, 2016).

Historically, elder care services in Ottoman-Turkish society evolved, in parallel with the Western experience, over the course of four periods. The first was the traditional late Ottoman period (1832–1895). The earliest skilled nursing homes were built during this time, though they were similar to the rough almshouses of Western nations (Esendemir and Ingman 2011). The second period (1895–1957) was a period of stagnation for the opening of nursing homes, as keeping older adults with their families remained the norm. The collapse of the Ottoman Empire in 1923 may have contributed to the stagnation. After 1957, nursing homes became an alternative to home-based care, ushering in a transitional period (1957–1980). Finally, in the modern period (1980–present), institutional care became prevalent in large cities. Nonetheless, home-based care provided by families is still dominant.

The preference in Turkey for family- or home-based care can be tied to religious beliefs that emphasize traditional filial values, even though the family structure has weakened somewhat over time. Elder care is still considered to be primarily the responsibility of family members, particularly the elder's son's wife (Aytaç 2002). In addition, economic conditions may contribute to the predominance of family-based care, given that many families are unable to afford separate houses for parents. Finally, many people in Turkey are influenced by the negative perceptions of nursing homes seen in many countries around the world (Moody 1992). When family members institutionalize their parents, they often feel guilty or are labeled as such by society.

The Long-Term Care Delivery System
Long-Term Services and Supports

Turkey has no long-term care insurance system. Metropolitan cities such as Istanbul, Ankara, and İzmir have somewhat better services available than other parts of the country, but the country in general struggles to meet the needs of its growing population of older adults. In 2013, Turkey's General Directorate of Disabled and Elderly Services published a set of quality standards intended to guide institutional reform (Karadeniz 2014).

Turkey does have a program for compensating caregivers. If a person with a disability, regardless of age, receives care from a family member while living at home, the family member receives a means-tested monthly payment of the net minimum wage from Turkey's Ministry of Family and Social Policies (ASPB). If the person receives services in a care home, the ASPB payment is double the minimum wage (Karadeniz 2014).

Efforts to establish a long-term care insurance scheme have begun, including a draft report and projections prepared by ASPB. A reform introduced in 2014 enables ASPB to assist needy people aged 65 or older by purchasing care services under the Public Procurement Law. In addition, ASPB can finance care services provided by other public institutions and municipalities, which helps stimulate local governments and municipalities to offer care services (Karadeniz 2014).

Turkey has also taken steps toward integration of care, including elder care services. The Ministry of Health and the Ministry of Family and Social Policies, for instance, have begun working with city administrations on a common information network to support better coordination.

Caregivers

Because elder care in Turkey is still based primarily on informal care provided by family members, the professional system for long-term care is largely undeveloped. Typically, informal caregivers lack the education and expertise to effectively deal with problems related to such demanding conditions as Alzheimer's disease or Parkinson's disease. Educated nurses are generally only available for work in hospitals, and they generally lack the extra gerontological and geriatric education to meet the specific needs of the older population. To address this issue, a number of universities have opened aging care departments to prepare nursing students.

Future Directions and Challenges

Providing needed services for Turkey's rapidly aging population will be a challenge in the years ahead. Although the number of old-age institutions has increased in recent years, the institutionalization of older adults is unlikely to be the solution. More likely, the future direction—and future opportunities—will emphasize services and supports to help older adults more successfully age in place or age in their communities.

The United States

History and Demographics

The United States, like the other countries discussed in this chapter, is undergoing a significant demographic shift with major implications for the delivery of long-term services and supports. As Americans live longer and members of the baby boom generation grow older, the number of older adults in American society is increasing at a rapid pace. In 2013, the 65-or-older population in the United States was 44.7 million—representing 14.1 percent of the total population—and 6 million of those people were older than 85. By 2050, the number of older adults is projected to reach 89 million (CDC 2013).

From the early 1900s to the 1930s, almshouses—often regarded as "poor farms" for elderly "inmates"—provided some long-term care for people in need, though typically in harsh conditions. The Social Security Act of 1935 provided pensions for older people, and growing numbers of private boarding houses and nursing homes developed in the decades that followed. In 1965, the Medicare and Medicaid programs were established (McSweeney-Feld and Molinari 2017).

Long-Term Care Delivery System

Medicare provides nearly universal medical insurance for people aged 65 or older, but it does not cover nonmedical long-term services and supports. The only US public policy that offers coverage for nonmedical long-term care is Medicaid, which is limited to low-income individuals (Takagi and Molinari 2017). Eligibility for Medicaid's long-term care benefits—which generally cover services in nursing homes as well as at home on a limited basis—is determined via means testing, based on a set of guidelines concerning income level, household and family structure, and personal assets. Medicaid is funded jointly by tax revenues of the federal and state governments. People who are above the income eligibility level for Medicaid have to pay for their long-term care expenses either out of pocket or through private long-term care insurance.

Residential Services

Common residential arrangements available in the United States include **assisted living facilities**, where staff help residents with activities of daily living, and **skilled nursing facilities**, which also provide some medical, nursing, and rehabilitation services (McSweeney-Feld 2017). Various models and variations have emerged over time, including CCRCs (discussed earlier in the chapter), where independent living, assisted living, and skilled nursing services are combined on a single campus. Many of these residential options, however, are either primarily private pay (e.g., assisted living) or require a high entry fee (e.g., many CCRCs). The Affordable Care Act (ACA) of 2010 introduced incentives for individuals to receive care in their homes and communities, rather than in institutional settings. The ACA has thus contributed to an expansion of home care services and the development of other models for the provision of care at home, such as patient-centered **medical homes**.

Home and Community-Based Services

A growing number of initiatives in the United States seek to fund Medicaid home and community-based service waivers for low-income older adults who need nursing home–level care. The Money Follows the Person (MFP) program and the Program of All-Inclusive Care for the Elderly (PACE) are both aimed at enabling frail, low-income older adults to receive care in their own homes and communities. Newer technologies such as telehealth and remote patient monitoring systems are also being adopted for home and community-based care, and they have demonstrated the potential to prevent hospital readmissions, keep individuals out of institutional settings, lower the cost of services, and increase the quality of care.

assisted living facility
A facility in which staff help residents with activities of daily living and work to ensure residents' health and well-being.

skilled nursing facility
A facility that provides medical, nursing, or rehabilitation services on a residential basis.

medical home
A care approach in which a primary care physician works with other specialists and providers to enable coordinated access to services when and where they are needed.

Across every state, a not-for-profit network called the Aging Network provides care management and coordination of services for older adults with long-term care needs. The network includes Area Agencies on Aging (AAAs) and Aging and Disability Resource Centers (ADRCs). The network can provide information and referrals, as well as such services as nutrition assistance and transportation for lower-income individuals.

Caregivers

The Family Medical Leave Act of 1993 requires US employers with 50 or more employees to allow up to 12 weeks of unpaid family leave for employees who need to serve as caregivers (US Department of Labor 2016). Under this rule, caregivers still face the loss of wages, but they are at least able to keep their employment while attending to their family members' needs. Federal funding through the Older Americans Act of 1965 also supports the National Family Caregiver Support Program, which helps eligible informal caregivers access programs and services such as support groups, training, and respite care (Administration for Community Living 2017). Consumer-directed home care programs, another type of support for family caregivers, allow older adults in some states to employ their family members as paid caregivers (Ruggiano 2012).

Future Directions and Challenges

As the US population ages and the number of people with chronic conditions increases, the depth and scope of long-term services and supports will need to expand. Since the passage of the ACA, the US healthcare system has implemented a variety of new approaches to promote the health and safety of people who need long-term services and supports. Special attention has been placed on opportunities for better integration and coordination of services, as well as on potential innovations in service delivery and reimbursement (McSweeney-Feld and Molinari 2017). Additional trends include a heightened emphasis on preventive care and primary care services, attention to social and environmental determinants of health, and new uses for emerging technologies.

Summary

As populations of older adults and people with disabilities increase throughout the world, mounting pressures will be placed on healthcare delivery systems, and new approaches for addressing people's care needs will have to be developed and implemented. In this chapter, we have discussed the various historical and demographic forces that have brought us to the current situation, and we have examined the steps that health systems in several countries have taken to adapt to current and future challenges.

In developed nations, government pension systems and medical care systems are likely to benefit from solutions that encourage consumer self-help and education, as well as strategies that use emerging technologies to support individuals, families, and communities in new and innovative ways. In developing nations, changing demographics, family structures, and economic conditions may necessitate the creation of new long-term care delivery systems with residential care options to complement existing home and community-based service models. In both developed and developing nations, strategies and solutions need to reflect the appropriate cultural values and preferences of the individuals who need care.

As long-term care systems evolve, key service delivery issues will emerge. Workforce shortages remain a global concern. Integration efforts to facilitate seamless transitions of care—between acute care settings, rehabilitative services, people's homes and communities, and other care settings—will be essential. Promising new directions can be seen in applications of robotics, telehealth, and ambient assistive technology, as well as in the development of new dementia care models that are both safe and empowering. However, these and other solutions will require significant investments of money and labor and may be subject to economic and political uncertainties in the years ahead.

Discussion Questions

1. What are the key demographic forces affecting the provision and management of global long-term services and supports?
2. What are the key demand and supply issues affecting global long-term care?
3. Describe five models of long-term care service delivery.
4. Compare and contrast home and community-based long-term care with residential long-term care.
5. Define *disability*, and describe the various ways it can be measured.
6. What tends to be the predominant form of caregiving in developing nations?
7. What is the largest component of the long-term care workforce, and what are some of the challenges in developing and retaining these workers?
8. What is filial piety, and in what parts of the world is it an important concept for long-term service provision?
9. What are continuing care retirement communities? Where do they exist, and how have they evolved over time?
10. How does technology influence the delivery of global long-term care services, and what will be its role in the future?

References

Administration for Community Living (ACL). 2017. "National Family Caregiver Support Program." Updated December 13. www.acl.gov/programs/support-caregivers/national-family-caregiver-support-program.

Alzheimer's Disease International. 2016. *World Alzheimer Report 2016: Improving Healthcare for People Living with Dementia*. Published September. www.alz.co.uk/research/WorldAlzheimerReport2016.pdf.

———. 2015. *World Alzheimer Report 2015: The Global Impact of Dementia*. Published August. www.alz.co.uk/research/WorldAlzheimerReport2015.pdf.

Applebaum, R., E. Robbins, and A. Bardo. 2014. "Long-Term Services and Supports." In *Global Aging: Comparative Perspectives on Aging and the Life Course*, edited by S. R. Kunkel, J. S. Brown, and F. J. Whittington, 163–86. New York: Springer.

Aytaç, I. A. 2002. "Tradition or Need? Reasons for Coresiding with Elderly in Urban Areas." *Nüfusbilim Dergisi* 24: 23–36.

Bishop, C. E., M. R. Squillace, J. Meagher, W. L. Anderson, and J. M. Wiener. 2009. "Nursing Home Work Practices and Nursing Assistants' Job Satisfaction." *Gerontologist* 49 (5): 611–22.

Brasor, P., and M. Tsubuku. 2014. "Generation Gaps Filled by Brick and Mortar." *Japan Times*. Published June 2. www.japantimes.co.jp/community/2014/06/02/how-tos/generation-gaps-filled-brick-mortar/#.W2h9cdVKhhE.

Cao, J., and Q. R. Liu. 2013. *China Aging Development Overview*. Beijing, China: Hualing Press.

Centers for Disease Control and Prevention (CDC). 2013. *The State of Aging and Health in America 2013*. Atlanta, GA: Centers for Disease Control and Prevention, US Department of Health and Human Services.

Chu, L. W., and I. Chi. 2008. "Nursing Homes in China." *Journal of the American Medical Directors Association* 9 (4): 237–43.

Coulmas, F. 2007. *Population Decline and Ageing in Japan: The Social Consequences*. New York: Routledge.

Dementia Services Development Centre. 2012. "Iris Murdoch Building." Accessed August 7, 2018. http://dementia.stir.ac.uk/about-dsdc/iris-murdoch-building.

De San Miguel, K., and G. Lewin. 2008. "Personal Emergency Alarms: What Impact Do They Have on Older People's Lives?" *Australasian Journal on Ageing* 27 (2): 103–5.

Esendemir, S., and S. R. Ingman. 2011. "The Birth of the Nursing Home Phenomenon in Ottoman-Turkish Society: The Case of Darulaceze (Almshouse) in Istanbul." *Journal of Aging in Emerging Economies* 3 (1): 17–23.

Eurostat. 2018. "Healthcare Expenditure Statistics." Accessed August 6. http://ec.europa.eu/eurostat/statistics-explained/index.php/Healthcare_expenditure_statistics.

Feng, Z., C. Liu, X. Guan, and V. Mor. 2013. "China's Rapidly Aging Population Creates Policy Changes in Shaping a Viable Long-Term Care System." *Health Affairs* 31 (12): 2764–73.

He, W., D. Goodkind, and P. Kowal. 2016. *An Aging World: 2015.* Washington, DC: US Census Bureau.

Hogeweyk. 2018. "Hogeweyk, Living in Lifestyles: A Mirror Image of Recognizable Lifestyles in Our Society." Accessed August 6. https://hogeweyk.dementiavillage.com/en/.

Ianzito, C. 2017. "Elder Orphans: How to Plan for Aging Without a Family Caregiver." AARP Public Policy Institute. Accessed August 8, 2018. www.aarp.org/caregiving/basics/info-2017/tips-aging-alone.html.

Institute of Medicine (IOM). 2008. *Retooling for an Aging America: Building the Health Care Workforce.* Washington, DC: National Academies Press.

Karadeniz, O. 2014. "Country Document Update 2014: Pensions, Health and Long-Term Care: Turkey." European Commission. Published March. http://ec.europa.eu/social/BlobServlet?docId=12985&langId=en.

Keck, Z. 2013. "Poverty and Old Age in China." *Diplomat.* Published June 3. https://thediplomat.com/2013/06/poverty-and-old-age-in-china/.

KPMG International. 2013. *Uncertain Age: Reimagining Long Term Care in the 21st Century.* Published April. www.kpmg-institutes.com/content/dam/kpmg/governmentinstitute/pdf/2013/an-uncertain-age.pdf.

Kunkel, S. R., J. S. Brown, and F. J. Whittington (eds.). 2014. *Global Aging: Comparative Perspectives on Aging and the Life Course.* New York: Springer.

McSweeney-Feld, M. H. 2017. "Residential Settings for Long-Term Care Services." In *Dimensions of Long-Term Care Management: An Introduction,* 2nd ed., edited by M. H. McSweeney-Feld, C. Molinari, and R. Oetjen, 73–94. Chicago: Health Administration Press.

McSweeney-Feld, M. H., and C. Molinari. 2017. "Introduction to the Dimensions of Long-Term Care." In *Dimensions of Long-Term Care Management: An Introduction,* 2nd ed., edited by M. H. McSweeney-Feld, C. Molinari, and R. Oetjen, 3–20. Chicago: Health Administration Press.

McWilliams, A. 2015. "Technologies for Long-Term Care and Home Healthcare: Global Markets." BCC Research. Published September. www.bccresearch.com/market-research/healthcare/elder-home-healthcare-market-hlc079c.html.

Meagher, G., and M. Szebehely. 2012. "Long-Term Care in Sweden: Trends, Actors, and Consequences." In *Reforms in Long-Term Care Policies in Europe,* edited by R. Costanzo and E. Pavolini, 55–78. New York: Springer.

Molinari, C., and T. Zhang. 2015. "Long Term Care." In *Handbook of Healthcare Management,* edited by M. D. Fottler, D. Malvey, and D. J. Slovensky, 429–59. Northampton, MA: Edgar Elgar Publishing.

Moody, H. R. 1992. *Ethics in an Aging Society.* Baltimore, MD: Johns Hopkins University Press.

Morikawa, M. 2014. "Towards Community-Based Integrated Care: Trends and Issues in Japan's Long-Term Care Policy." *International Journal of Integrated Care*. Published February 26. www.ijic.org/articles/10.5334/ijic.1066/.

National Bureau of Statistics of China. 2017. *China Statistical Yearbook 2016*. Beijing, China: China Statistics Press.

National Center for Assisted Living (NCAL). 2012. *Findings from the NCAL 2011 Assisted Living Staff Vacancy, Retention, and Turnover Survey*. Published October. http://media.mcknights.com/documents/40/ncal_worker_survey_9854.pdf.

National Direct Service Workforce Resource Center. 2008. *A Synthesis of Direct Service Workforce Demographics and Challenges Across Intellectual/Developmental Disabilities, Aging, Physical Disabilities, and Behavioral Health*. Washington, DC: National Direct Service Workforce Resource Center.

Niles-Yokum, K., and D. L. Wagner. 2015. *The Aging Networks: A Guide to Programs and Services*, 8th ed. New York: Springer.

Organisation for Economic Co-operation and Development (OECD). 2018. "Long-Term Care." Accessed August 7. www.oecd.org/els/health-systems/long-term-care.htm.

Paul, D. P. III, K. C. Schaeffer, and A. Coustasse. 2017. "Long-Term Care Policy: What the United States Can Learn from Denmark, Sweden, and the Netherlands." Paper presented at the Business and Health Administration Association Annual Conference, Chicago, IL, March 22–24.

PHI. 2011. "Who Are Direct-Care Workers?" Published February. https://phinational.org/wp-content/uploads/legacy/clearinghouse/PHI%20Facts%203.pdf.

Ruggiano, N. 2012. "Consumer Direction in Long-Term Care Policy: Overcoming Barriers to Promoting Older Adults' Opportunity for Self-Direction." *Journal of Gerontological Social Work* 55 (2): 146–59.

Sheard, D. 2013. "Mattering in a Dementia Care Home: The Butterfly Approach." Dementia Care Matters. Accessed August 6, 2018. www.dementiacarematters.com/pdf/modern.pdf.

Statista. 2018. "Share of the Elderly Population in Sweden in Selected Years from 2000 to 2016, by Age Group." Accessed August 6. www.statista.com/statistics/525637/sweden-elderly-share-of-the-total-population-by-age-group/.

Stone, R. I., and N. Bryant. 2012. "The Impact of Health Care Reform on the Workforce Caring for Older Adults." *Journal of Aging & Social Policy* 24 (2): 188–205.

Stone, R. I., and M. F. Harahan. 2010. "Improving the Long-Term Care Workforce Serving Older Adults." *Health Affairs* 29 (1): 109–15.

Stone, R. I., and J. M. Wiener. 2001. *Who Will Care for Us? Addressing the Long-Term Care Workforce Crisis*. Urban Institute and American Association of Homes and Services for the Aging. Published October. https://aspe.hhs.gov/system/files/pdf/73111/ltcwf.pdf.

Swedish Institute. 2013. *Facts About Sweden: Elderly Care*. Published October. https://sweden.se/wp-content/uploads/2013/11/Elderly-care-high-resolution.pdf.

Takagi, E., and C. Molinari. 2017. "Global Trends in Long-Term Care Policies and Services." In *Dimensions of Long-Term Care Management: An Introduction,* 2nd ed., edited by M. H. McSweeney-Feld, C. Molinari, and R. Oetjen, 199–220. Chicago: Health Administration Press.

Turkish Statistical Institute (TÜİK). 2016. "Elderly Statistics, 2015." Published March 17. www.turkstat.gov.tr/PreHaberBultenleri.do?id=21520.

———. 2013. "Elderly Statistics, 2012." Published March 20. www.turkstat.gov.tr/PreHaberBultenleri.do?id=13466.

US Census Bureau. 2015. "International Data Base." Updated July. www.census.gov/population/international/data/idb/informationGateway.php.

US Department of Labor. 2016. "Employee Rights Under the Family and Medical Leave Act." Revised April. ww.dol.gov/whd/regs/compliance/posters/fmlaen.pdf.

Whitman, J., and L. R. Burns. 2017. "Providing and Financing Elder Care in China." In *China's Healthcare System and Reform,* edited by L. R. Burns and G. G. Liu, 269–88. Cambridge, UK: Cambridge University Press.

Wong, E. 2013. "A Chinese Virtue Is Now the Law." *New York Times.* Published July 2. www.nytimes.com/2013/07/03/world/asia/filial-piety-once-a-virtue-in-china-is-now-the-law.html.

World Health Organization (WHO). 2018. "Deafness and Hearing Loss." Published March 15. www.who.int/news-room/fact-sheets/detail/deafness-and-hearing-loss.

———. 2017. "Blindness and Visual Impairment." Published October 11. www.who.int/news-room/fact-sheets/detail/blindness-and-visual-impairment.

Wu, Y. S., and J. W. Dang. 2014. *Report on the Development of China's Elderly Care Industry.* Beijing, China: Social Sciences Academic Press.

———. 2013. *China Report of the Development on Aging Cause.* Beijing, China: Social Sciences Academic Press.

Yong, V., and Y. Saito. 2012. "National Long-Term Care Insurance Policy in Japan a Decade After Implementation: Some Lessons for Aging Countries." *Ageing International* 37 (3): 271–84.

Yu, H. 2016. "This Is Why China's Housing Market Is Such a Mess." *Fortune.* Published February 11. http://fortune.com/2016/02/10/china-housing-market-mortgage-down-payment/.

MANAGING THE HEALTH OF POPULATIONS

William Aaronson, PhD, Ellen Averett, PhD, MHSA, Thomas T. H. Wan, PhD, Bo Jordin, MD, Ana Maria Malik, MD, PhD, and Anatoliy Pilyavskyy, PhD

Chapter Focus

This chapter is designed to guide health managers as they develop the knowledge and skills necessary to understand, effectively plan for, and manage the health of a constituent population. It focuses on key concepts in the assessment of population health, the design of population health management strategies, and trends in population health management. The chapter's concepts are supported with examples from throughout the world with particular relevance for health managers. Population health management involves a reconceptualization of the role of health services. To effect the necessary strategic changes, managers must possess both innovative thinking and outstanding leadership.

Learning Objectives

Upon completion of this chapter, you should be able to

- understand the forces that are motivating health services organizations to shift their focus toward population health;
- explain the significance of managing population health as an aspect of the "triple aim";
- describe the methods and materials needed to assess and manage the health of populations;
- analyze the use of community health assessments and national health registries to estimate and respond to the health challenges facing constituent communities;
- evaluate the importance of social determinants of health in understanding the health needs of communities; and
- plan for expanding organizational support for improvements in community health status.

Competencies

- Promote ongoing learning and improvement in the organization.
- Respond to the need for change, and lead the change process.
- Encourage diversity of thought to support innovation, creativity, and improvement.
- Present results of data analysis in a way that is factual, credible, and understandable to decision makers.
- Demonstrate an understanding of system structure, funding mechanisms, and the ways healthcare services are organized.
- Promote the establishment of alliances and consolidation of networks to expand social and community participation in health systems, both nationally and globally.
- Establish goals and objectives for improving health outcomes, based on an understanding of the social determinants of health and the socioeconomic environment in which the organization functions.

Key Terms

- Community health needs assessment (CHNA)
- Determinant
- Epidemiology
- Health demography
- Health economics
- Health psychology
- Health registry
- Human ecology
- Medical sociology
- Population health management (PHM)
- Population health science
- Preventive medicine
- Social and managerial epidemiology
- Social determinants of health (SDOH)

Key Concepts

- Care management
- Chronic disease management
- Data analytics
- Health information technology
- Health research
- Morbidity and mortality
- Patient-centered care
- Population health
- Predictive analytics
- Triple aim

Introduction: What Is Population Health Management and Why Is It Important?

Healthcare managers around the world are under increasing pressure to demonstrate value in healthcare delivery. A report by the Economist Intelligence Unit describes a global shift toward value-based healthcare, noting that "European governments, like those in other parts of the world, are feeling the strain on their health budgets caused by an ageing population, a rise in the prevalence of chronic conditions and the acceleration of medical innovations that have increased demand for state-of-the-art treatment. As a result governments are looking to make their money stretch further" (Koehring 2015). The delivery of value is best achieved when healthcare organizations and national health systems meet the "triple aim" of "improving the experience of care, improving the health of populations, and reducing per capita costs" (Berwick, Nolan, and Whittington 2008, 759). Therefore, the management of population health is a prime objective for national health systems and health services organizations.

Population health management (PHM) is a crucial concept for the delivery of value-based healthcare, but consensus on the term's exact meaning has been elusive. Steenkamer and colleagues (2017) conducted a thorough review of the literature on the topic and concluded that the overall aims of PHM are to

- improve health and psychosocial well-being of a defined population or subpopulation;
- improve quality and health service delivery, including aspects of patient and provider satisfaction;
- reduce cost per capita (or reduce growth in cost per capita); and
- improve workforce productivity.

population health management (PHM)
The use of management strategies to improve the health and well-being of a defined population, to improve quality, to reduce costs, and to improve workforce productivity.

To understand population health, you must understand the nature of health and the factors that contribute to the health and well-being of the population. A key global trend affecting PHM in recent years involves the growing impact of chronic disease, which has supplanted infectious disease as a leading cause of morbidity and mortality. This trend presents both a challenge and an opportunity for healthcare managers. Whereas infectious disease prevalence tends to ebb and flow over time and within populations, chronic disease prevalence tends to be relatively steady and predictable. Therefore, with regard to chronic disease, healthcare managers are better able to measure, plan for, and manage the health needs of the population being served. At the same time, however, the multifaceted nature of chronic disease and the intersection of environmental, economic, and sociocultural influences create a host of challenges and complications. Effective PHM requires health managers to work

determinant
A factor that determines or contributes to an outcome.

epidemiology
The scientific discipline dealing with the distribution and determinants of disease and other health-related events in a population.

human ecology
The study of human adaptation and lifestyles in varying geospatial settings.

health demography
The statistical study of vital events such as fertility, morbidity, mortality, and disability.

medical sociology
A field of study dealing with social and environmental factors that influence the health of a population.

social and managerial epidemiology
A field of study that examines the patterns and trends of morbidity and mortality associated with social factors and health services.

collaboratively across educational institutions, nongovernmental organizations (NGOs), businesses, local governments, houses of worship, and other community organizations.

Infectious disease, of course, remains a concern. Although many of the most devastating infectious diseases have been controlled or eradicated, many countries—particularly low-resource countries—face local and regional epidemics. The 2014–2015 Ebola outbreak in West Africa provides one such example. The methods and techniques of PHM provide substantially stronger responses to infectious disease outbreaks than traditional medical approaches that are unsupported by systematic views of the population experience.

The hallmark of PHM is a shift in emphasis away from specialty-driven medical care and toward a holistic, interdisciplinary approach that takes into account the measurement of population health and the numerous **determinants** that can influence health. A population health approach emphasizes community-based primary care, with a focus on understanding and managing the health needs of the population. Effective PHM strategies extend beyond traditional medical care to encompass a wide variety of behavioral, sociocultural, and environmental elements.

Trends and Issues in Population Health Management

Health services and economics researchers have played a pivotal role in identifying and understanding the distributions, correlations, and consequences of health disorders or illnesses at the population level. The current emphasis on PHM strategies might be a relatively recent development, but the study of population health has roots as far back as ancient Greece. The discipline of **epidemiology**—which studies the distribution and determinants of disease and other health-related events in a population—can be traced back to Hippocrates in the fifth century BCE.

Historically speaking, a variety of disciplines have established research paradigms that bring a multidisciplinary perspective to health and healthcare. Population health concepts can therefore be linked to the fields of (1) **human ecology**, the study of human adaptation and lifestyles in varying geospatial settings; (2) **health demography**, the statistical study of vital events such as fertility, morbidity, mortality, and disability; (3) **medical sociology**, which deals with social and environmental factors that influence the health of a population; (4) **social and managerial epidemiology**, which examines the patterns and trends of morbidity and mortality associated with social factors and health services; (5) **health economics**, which addresses health services consumption and efficiency, as well as the financial arrangements that influence the delivery of healthcare services; (6) **health psychology**, which examines behavioral factors, such as attitude, perception, motivation, and preference, as they relate to health; and (7)

preventive medicine, which focuses on preventive strategies and interventions for the promotion of community and population health. Over time, collaborative health research has gradually evolved from *multidisciplinary* investigations to more integrative *transdisciplinary* investigations. This shift is evident in the systematic review of the scientific literature on diabetes care and management published in the *World Journal of Diabetes* (Wan, Terry, McKee, et al. 2017).

Furthermore, the new specialty area of **population health science** has emerged through the integration of human genetics, epidemiology, biostatistics, behavioral science, public health, policy science, medical geography, and health informatics. A notable example in this area is the Population Health Science division that operates under the National Health Research Institutes (2018) in Taiwan. There, scientists collaborate on inquiries into the causes, instances, and consequences of morbidity and mortality, with the aim of supporting the design, implementation, and evaluation of innovative population health policies and management programs.

Among countries that belong to the Organisation for Economic Co-operation and Development (OECD), four main factors are triggering the need for a population health focus: (1) the aging population; (2) the increased prevalence of chronic conditions; (3) the need to contain costs of care, improve efficiency, and strengthen organizational performance; and (4) the desire for patient-centered care. Numerous policy interventions to improve quality and efficiency have been developed and implemented throughout the world, particularly in the OECD countries. However, a one-size-fits-all strategy is neither desirable nor feasible for addressing health burdens associated with the provision of acute care, subacute care, and long-term care at the population level.

Disease management and use of care management technology tend to be central components of PHM programs (Wan, Terry, McKee, et al. 2017). Data science, particularly the exploration of "big data," can also help with the detection of patterns of morbidity and mortality for at-risk populations. However, a lack of specificities and conceptually grounded models can prevent the formulation of effective predictive analytics to guide policy interventions and changes. For instance, the adoption and diffusion of the medical home modality in primary care represents an alternative, patient-centered solution to population health problems, and some evidence suggests the modality's effectiveness (Rosenthal 2008; Nielsen et al. 2016); however, such structures are often inadequately conceptualized in their formation and implementation. The following fundamental questions should be raised when considering the underlying rationale for a patient-centered care initiative:

1. What are the mechanisms that lead to better patient outcomes and lower costs when patient-centered care is in place?
2. What are the causal paths for optimizing population health using a patient-centered care modality?

health economics
A field of economics that addresses health services consumption and efficiency, as well as the financial arrangements that influence the delivery of healthcare services.

health psychology
A field of psychology that examines behavioral factors, such as attitude, perception, motivation, and preference, as they relate to health.

preventive medicine
The area of medicine dealing with preventive strategies and interventions for the promotion of community and population health.

population health science
An interdisciplinary specialty area that integrates elements of human genetics, epidemiology, biostatistics, behavioral science, public health, policy science, medical geography, and health informatics.

3. To whom should the innovative care modality be targeted?

4. What is an optimal amount of clinical and self-reported data to be collected longitudinally and consistently for patients, providers, insurers, and other stakeholders for program evaluation?

5. How do we empower patients and the general population in the journey for optimal health?

Disease management programs represent the mainstream of the population health movement. Such programs take a proactive approach to the management of chronic conditions—such as heart failure, hypertension, coronary heart disease, diabetes, chronic obstructive pulmonary disease, asthma, and chronic kidney disorder—through the provision of coordinated and integrated care, with the aim of containing costs and improving patient care outcomes (Fiedler and Wan 2010; Kroneman et al. 2016). Disease management efforts should be integrated with health wellness management at both the individual and population levels. Such efforts can take a variety of forms. For instance, one hospital system, having been influenced by evidence from a systematic review about incentivizing wellness activities, launched an employee wellness incentive plan, in which all employees were encouraged to join in wellness center activities, with membership fees covered by the hospital (Wan 2016).

The use of innovative care management technology is a relatively new trend in population health. In the United States, the Centers for Medicare & Medicaid Services (CMS) plays an important role in shaping health reform and improving quality of care through the implementation of various initiatives and financial demonstration projects. The US government's meaningful use standards (discussed in chapter 5) support the expanded use of electronic health records (EHRs) and provide an impetus for new research infrastructures for data scientists and new avenues for improving the efficiency of health services.

Health information technology (HIT), coupled with medical care technology, can have a powerful impact on a variety of outcome measures, including patient satisfaction (a proximal outcome via improved patient–provider interactions and communications), adherence to medical regimens (an intermediate outcome via use of home monitoring devices), and the betterment of health status or health-related quality of life (a distal outcome via the HIT application). Advances in HIT also offer opportunities for transforming health and healthcare at the population level, as demonstrated by the innovative data-mining operations of Optum (2018).

The development of functional predictive analytics and decision support systems requires the integration of health and healthcare information from both the individual level and the population level. The use of integrated decision support software with the administrative, executive, clinical, and financial components combined in HIT—so-called "informatics integration"—is imperative, because integrated multifunctional systems have greater potential to enhance the efficiency and effectiveness of data use by scientists and healthcare managers (Wan 2002, 2006).

Factors Influencing Variability in Population Health Management

Careful inspection of healthcare trends and issues reveals ten important factors that influence variability in the design, structure, operation, and performance of PHM activities.

The first factor is the demographic shift that has occurred in recent decades across the globe, attributable to the transition from high to low fertility and mortality rates. With birth rates slowing and life expectancies extending, the shift has the effect of raising the average age of populations. This "fast-track aging" is particularly apparent in Asian countries such as China, India, Japan, Singapore, and Taiwan.

The second factor is that this aging population manifests diverse and demanding health needs for which many countries are unprepared or underprepared. Many older adults have multiple chronic conditions and complex health needs that require specific initiatives and facilities. Examples of programs that have emerged to meet these needs include memory care centers in the Netherlands for people with Alzheimer's and dementia-related diseases (Ramakers and Verhey 2011); the Effective Practice and Organization of Care (EPOC) Project in Europe (Grol et al. 2013; Wensing et al. 2011); the integrated care model for chronic kidney disease in Thailand (Jiamjariyapon et al. 2014); and the diabetes care nonprofit program in Bulgaria (Struckmann et al. 2017).

The third factor is that the methodologies for assessing population risks for various chronic diseases have evolved significantly. Such methodologies have ranged from the use of a simple screening index for multidisciplinary team referral (Hegarty et al. 2016) to a complex classification system for heart failure diagnosis and risk assessment (American College of Cardiology Foundation / American Heart Association 2013). Because of the heterogeneity of population health needs, multiple strategies for risk assessment, prevention, and reduction need to be designed and implemented.

Fourth, disparities in care management effectiveness contribute to variability in both objectively assessed and self-reported patient care outcomes. For example, inadequate use of digital technologies, such as EHRs, can lead to disparities in health status and healthcare. Better-integrated informatics can facilitate coordinated care and improved outcomes, regardless of disease.

The fifth factor is the critical cultural lag that can limit the promotion of comprehensive and preventive programs for specific population groups. Often, health promotion and disease prevention programs lack coherent behavioral change strategies, possibly because little information is available on the proper dose–response relationship to guide the execution of health education interventions. In addition, clinical science needs to develop a better understanding of the natural history of multiple chronic conditions, with better information on disease presence and progression. The data science field therefore should aim to assemble massive amounts of personal and ecological (contextual) data to help answer such questions as the following:

1. What are the transitional probabilities of one chronic disease leading to another chronic disease?
2. What are the mechanisms to bring about the compression of the disease?
3. How can preventive-oriented scientists or scholars use the information about transitional probabilities or change trajectories of chronic conditions to influence patients to modify the risk or public health professionals to formulate preventive programs for varying stages of the disease?

Future preventive efforts addressing multiple chronic conditions must strengthen the data collection system to gather pertinent information about the timing and number of interventions to compress impending morbidity and mortality risks.

Sixth, the adoption of medical technologies and devices that can monitor and evaluate health is on the rise. Wearable devices and sensors have the potential to collect relevant and timely data to pinpoint specific directions for health improvement, particularly as it relates to chronic care in the home or in community-based settings. Remote devices can enhance the delivery of telehealth across multiple settings, enabling physicians and other providers to offer value-added communications and services more efficiently.

The seventh factor involves health workforce issues related to teamwork, staff cross-training, and coordination of skills. Patients with chronic illnesses are often referred to multiple specialists for care, so teamwork is essential. Often, PHM efforts are hampered by a shortage of well-trained medical professionals capable of working together for chronic care; the field, therefore, needs to prioritize finding better ways to recruit and train the necessary medical and support staff. Furthermore, PHM has to effectively implement care management activities, starting from the systematic care assessment, to care plan development, to care monitoring, to care evaluation. The adequacy of PHM operations must be assessed not only in terms of cost savings but also in terms of actual performance, quality improvement, and patient care outcomes.

The eighth factor is social media, which has emerged as a popular mechanism for sharing new developments and interventions. The use of social media and other online tools to improve health education and to facilitate lifestyle change can have a substantial benefit for PHM efforts geared toward people with multiple chronic conditions. For instance, a collaboration of organizations—namely, the National Center for Creative Aging, the Pabst Foundation, and the University of Central Florida—has developed and supported a web-enhanced artistic tool kit to help relieve the stress and reduce the burden of caregivers for patients with dementia (Golden et al. 2017; Wan, Sun, and Golden 2016). Such efforts have great potential for global application.

Ninth, data scientists are interested in developing predictive analytics and decision support software based on logically constructed statistical algorithms. Such algorithms can transform data into useful information and evidence-based knowledge to guide practice changes or performance improvement at both the patient and organizational levels. The development of universally applicable predictive analytics for a specific chronic disease will require the collaborative efforts of a wide variety of health professionals across domestic and international partners.

The tenth factor involves the global genome collaborative project that has gathered massive health and genetic data from a large number of populations across multiple countries (Kosseim et al. 2014). Genome-wide analysis has been employed for the Chinese Longitudinal Health Longevity Study, an effort to identify biological/social/environmental signals that might influence the life span and health conditions of the "oldest-old" age group in China (Zeng et al. 2017). Systematic and causal analyses of genomes may have applications for improving therapeutic outcomes for diseases such as Alzheimer's disease, Parkinson's disease, and dementia with Lewy bodies that share common genes (Guerreiro et al. 2016). Thus, future population-based studies may provide more conclusive evidence to differentiate specific pathogeneses of multiple related diseases.

Mechanisms for Integrating Multiple Domains of Population Health Determinants

White, Williams, and Greenberg (1961), in their seminal work titled "The Ecology of Medical Care," discuss the key components of the healthcare delivery system and advocate for the expansion of health services beyond acute care to encompass preventive care. To optimize the effectiveness of curative-oriented services, we must develop a broader perspective in the promotion of population health. Wan (2010) argues that the integration of personalized care and population-focused care can be accomplished through translational, transformational, and transdisciplinary research. Furthermore, population health should be viewed as a joint function of contextual/ecological and individual factors that influence variability in health and healthcare.

Global health research investigates the determinants and consequences of population health problems. Epidemiological techniques have advanced this research, with applications for investigating factors that influence morbidity, disability, and mortality (Antecol and Bedard 2006; Jacobsen 2008; Wan 1995). Comprehensive prospective studies have gathered extensive data on the internal and external exposure factors that may influence healthcare outcomes and human development, either directly or indirectly. However, although strategies for promoting population health have been well documented in World Health Organization (WHO) publications (Lopez et al. 2006; Lu et al. 2007; Murray, Lopez, and Wibulpolprasert 2004; van Doorslaer, Masseria, and Koolman 2006), only a limited number of theoretical and substantively meaningful frameworks have been developed to illuminate how ecological correlates and their dynamics influence the health of different ethnic populations around the globe (Wan 2010).

An integrated perspective of contextual and personal determinants is useful for conducting systematic studies of population health, particularly as related to global health. The contextual domains represent four components, which can be remembered by the letters *POET*:

1. Risk identification of population health needs (P)
2. Innovative health organizational structure (O)
3. Design of healing environments (E)
4. Adoption and diffusion of technology (T)

These four components represent the ecological complex of macro-level determinants that may influence personal and population health. Micro-level determinants of health, meanwhile, include individual or personal attributes, such as predisposing factors (e.g., demographic characteristics, attitude, perception, behavior propensity, cultural preference), enabling factors (e.g., family income, health insurance coverage, access to primary care, health system–related factors), and need-for-care factors (e.g., health status, diagnostic conditions, severity of illness, perceived health).

The integrative approach to health determinants includes both micro- and macro-level factors that affect health services use and healthcare outcomes. Furthermore, the investigation of global health must consider the interaction effects of individual, ecological, and contextual factors. Analytically speaking, global health research should perform multilevel analysis of the determinants of health or illness from a transdisciplinary research approach.

Successful PHM requires a solid basis in evidence, incorporating experiential and scientific knowledge developed through experimentation. Such evidence is based on research that sheds light on what does and does not work. By conducting systematic reviews and meta-analyses about factors that influence patient care outcomes, researchers are able to gain valuable insight about how PHM should target the patient population and implement efficacious interventions (Wan, Terry, Cobb, et al. 2017). Ideally, PHM experiments should be conducted to yield replicable evidence to guide clinical care management and improvement. One promising approach is to couple expanded data-mining efforts, guided by a substantively meaningful framework (such as a transdisciplinary research perspective), with the design of graphic-user interface (GUI) decision-support systems. This approach enables researchers to validate and confirm predictive analytics with large databases for multiple population groups.

Social Determinants of Health

A major goal of PHM is to improve the health and psychosocial well-being of a defined population or subpopulation. As noted earlier in the chapter, health and well-being are influenced by a variety of factors, or determinants. Many people assume that the quality of healthcare services or access to healthcare services is the greatest influence on a population's health. In actuality, healthcare services have a relatively small impact on population health. The **social determinants of health (SDOH)**, on the other hand, play a much larger role. One estimate puts the impact of the social determinants of health on a population's health at 55 percent, with medical care at only 20 percent (Tarlov 1999).

> **social determinants of health (SDOH)**
> Factors found in living and working conditions that influence the health of a population; such factors are distinct from individual characteristics and behaviors.

What are these factors that represent more than half of the influence over a population's health? According to the US Centers for Disease Control and Prevention (CDC), SDOH are the "conditions in the places where people live, learn, work, and play [that] affect a wide range of health risks and outcomes" (CDC 2018). The WHO (2018) defines them similarly as "the conditions in which people are born, grow, live, work and age." The WHO extends the definition further to include factors that influence those conditions—specifically, "the distribution of money, power and resources at global, national and local levels."

Essentially, the SDOH are factors found in people's living and working conditions that affect health and are distinct from individual factors such as genetic propensities or vulnerabilities or sequelae of behaviors or choices. SDOH include such elements as adequate housing, safe neighborhoods, a clean environment, access to nutritious food, and access to education, in addition to access to good healthcare services. Although no universally agreed-upon list of SDOH is available, certain general categories can be identified. The Kaiser Family Foundation lists the following six (Artiga and Hinton 2018):

1. Economic stability (employment, expenses, debt, support)
2. Neighborhood and physical environment (housing, transportation, safety, recreation)

3. Education (literacy, language, vocational training, higher education)
4. Food (hunger, access to healthy options)
5. Community and social context (social integration and support, community engagement)
6. Healthcare system (health coverage, provider availability, cultural competency, quality)

Health inequities between and within populations are most often the result of SDOH. Typically, large numbers of SDOH exist together and interact with one another to produce an impact on mortality, morbidity, life expectancy, health status, quality of life, and other outcomes within a population. At a given time, an individual is likely to experience either multiple social determinants of poor health outcomes or multiple social determinants of better health outcomes. For instance, if a neighborhood is generally considered to be unsafe, it is less likely to be an area where people will want to exercise, travel, or play outdoors. Such an area is also less likely to have good schools and options for nutritious food. By contrast, if a neighborhood is generally considered to be safe, people are more likely to exercise, travel, and play in the community. Such an area is also more likely to have good schools and grocery stores stocked with nutritious foods. Thus, an individual rarely experiences just one poor or inadequate social determinant; SDOH tend to cluster together.

In using the word *determinant* to describe these factors, a distinction should be noted between the individual and the population. A specific factor might be a determinant of worse health for a population in general, but that factor might not be a determinant for a specific individual. For example, in a neighborhood where exercising or playing outdoors is regarded as unsafe, the population, on average, is likely to be heavier than the population of a safer area that is otherwise similar; however, not every individual in the less-safe neighborhood will be heavy, and not every individual in the safer area will be thin. The SDOH apply to the population as a whole, not necessarily to individuals. In fact, given that SDOH may influence but do not necessarily determine the health of individuals, some people have argued that *social influencers of health* would be a more appropriate term (Simon 2017).

Positive and negative SDOH among a population are often the result of public policies, or the lack of public policies. For example, in developed countries, government regulations aim to ensure not just access to water but also the cleanliness of the water being accessed. In the United States, the population's access to clean water is achieved through a combination of regulations and enforcement efforts at the national, state, and local levels (Environmental Protection Agency 2018). These policies aim to prevent pollution at water sources (e.g., rivers, wells) and to ensure potability at the point of consumption (e.g., water faucets in homes and offices).

In 2008, the WHO established a Commission on Social Determinants of Health, which produced a report with three overarching recommendations for addressing inequities caused by SDOH (WHO Commission on Social Determinants of Health 2008):

1. Improve daily living conditions.
2. Tackle the inequitable distribution of power, money, and resources.
3. Measure and understand the problem, and assess the impact of action.

These issues are of concern to all countries and to every entity trying to manage and improve population health.

In 2011, the WHO convened a World Conference on Social Determinants of Health in Rio de Janeiro, Brazil, which led to the adoption of the Rio Political Declaration on Social Determinants of Health. The declaration outlined five priority areas to be addressed (WHO 2011):

1. Adopt better governance for health and development
2. Promote participation in policymaking and implementation
3. Reorient the health sector toward reducing inequities
4. Strengthen global governance and collaboration
5. Monitor progress and increase accountability.

The declaration emphasized that health equity can only be achieved when the various SDOH are addressed in addition to equitable access to healthcare.

Health Informatics and Data Analytics to Optimize Population Health

Successful PHM depends on the conversion of data into information or knowledge. Health informatics research—an interdisciplinary investigation of how information can be integrated and used to guide clinical, administrative, and managerial decision making in healthcare—is a relatively new enterprise (Wan 2006). It helps transform massive amounts of data into usable information and valid knowledge to enhance clinical and managerial practices. The availability of digitized clinical and personal data enables the development of collaborative efforts from multiple disciplines—such as epigenetics, health services research, health demography, biostatistics, social and behavioral sciences, and clinical sciences—to detect causal paths relevant to the design of population-based intervention strategies. Ultimately, more efficient and effective care modalities, incorporating evidence-based practice, can be developed through the application of health informatics research (Wan 2002).

Critical to the application of health informatics and data analytics is the availability of large data sets constructed from the building blocks of individual health records, health registries, and demographics and population health data. Ministries of health in most countries collect such data for purposes of health improvement. Managers should be familiar with the health profiles of the countries where they work, and they should have a firm understanding of the important health challenges.

The advent of the electronic health record has opened new possibilities for population health research and management. Whereas previous data analyses might have been limited to a sample of medical records extracted by hand, today's researchers are able to extract data and build databases that allow for much more efficient and exhaustive study. The data can be aggregated to any level desired, subject only to limitations in the ability of the various systems to communicate. In countries with single-system interoperability, such communication is not an issue. In countries, including the United States, where data are collected by local health systems, interoperability challenges may arise, though they are generally becoming less of an obstacle. Patient-level data, when aggregated to the community level, provide a critical input into the evaluation of population health.

The WHO provides access to country-specific data through its annual *World Health Statistics* publication. The 2017 edition presents health statistics for 194 member states, highlighting countries that have had success in meeting major health challenges (WHO 2017). This type of macro-level health data provides a good starting point for determining the health needs of the population being served.

health registry
A collection of disease-, condition-, or procedure-specific information about individuals.

Health registries are another important source of information for healthcare managers. Registries are collections of disease-, condition-, or procedure-specific information about individuals, and they can be established by national governments, nongovernmental organizations, healthcare facilities, or private companies. The chief purpose of a health registry is to catalog treatments and outcomes for disease conditions to help identify best practices and to assess cost-effectiveness of procedures and early identification of adverse events. Nordic countries have been at the forefront of the effort to use national health registries to improve quality (Thygesen and Ersbøll 2011).

The Swedish registry of total hip arthroplasty, for instance, enabled a research team to extract and review data for one of the most common surgical procedures among OECD countries (Malviya, Abdul, and Khanduja 2017). Total hip replacement—which involves implanting an artificial ball-and-socket to replace the natural head of the femur—has been called "the operation of the century" because of the great impact it has had on improving the quality of life for countless men and women of all ages (Learmonth, Young, and Rorabeck 2007). The researchers in Sweden used the registry to conduct a data analysis across a full sample of Swedish implant procedures, ultimately reaching conclusions, with some degree of certainty, about the most effective prostheses and adhesive methods. The availability of real-time data through the registry facilitated the early identification of faulty prosthetics, preventing them from being used elsewhere.

Community health needs assessment (CHNA) is increasingly becoming recognized as a way to more effectively analyze and manage the health of a population. According to Wright, Williams, and Wilkinson (1998, 1310), CHNA "involves epidemiological, qualitative, and comparative methods to describe health problems of a population; identify inequalities in health and access to services; and determine priorities for the most effective use of resources." The CHNA process refocuses efforts from the level of individual patients to the level of the population (Rowe, McClelland, and Billingham 2001), and it requires the collection of large amounts of data and the assembly of data in large data sets. It also takes into account SDOH indicators, thereby providing a comprehensive approach to identifying the health needs of a defined population. Once a CHNA is complete, the next step is to engage in program planning to address the identified health needs. For health services managers, this step generally requires collaboration with NGOs and other community groups to address SDOH and the management of chronic disease.

CHNA takes a relatively long-term approach and facilitates planning for population-based health services and programs. The assessments can be used in combination with organization-level performance improvement to produce better and more cost-effective services.

community health needs assessment (CHNA)
A comprehensive process for examining the health problems of a population, identifying inequalities, and determining priorities to guide the use of resources.

Summary

Health managers and clinicians are increasingly being held accountable for the health of the communities and populations they serve. Previously, the accountability of managers and clinicians was largely confined to individual patient encounters and service delivery within organizational boundaries. Today, however, partly as a result of the rapid growth in chronic disease prevalence and obesity across the age spectrum, health services organizations need to approach care in the context of population health.

Population health management is an essential tool for meeting the "triple aim" of improving the experience of care, improving the health of populations, and reducing per capita costs. Improvements in technology and methodologies have given us enhanced data analytic capacity to meet these goals. The health manager plays a key role in refocusing efforts to meet the needs of communities being served—not just the needs of patients who come through the doors. This chapter has provided an overview of many of the PHM tools that are available to identify and address the critical health needs of the populations being served.

Discussion Questions

1. Define *population health management*. Analyze the importance of PHM in meeting national health goals to provide high-value, low-cost care to meet pressing health needs.

2. Briefly describe the key trends and issues in population health research. What evidence does the research provide regarding the value and effectiveness of PHM?

3. Propose a strategy by which your health services organization (or a health services organization with which you are familiar) can identify and better respond to the health needs of the community or population being served.

4. A variety of tools are available to help health managers address important community and population needs. Describe national health registries, disease management programs, and community health needs assessments. Analyze the relationship among them, and evaluate the usefulness of each in managing the health of the community.

Case Study: Community Health Management at a University Hospital in Brazil

A major public university hospital in Brazil, along with several other specialty institutes, has become concerned about long-stay patients. The patients are mostly located in cardiology, neurology, and orthopedics units, and several of them have remained in the hospital after they were considered able to be discharged. (Brazilian legislation does not allow institutions to forcibly remove discharged patients who do not leave on their own will.) In 2015, the hospital, seeking a better understanding of the situation, conducted a study of patients who did not leave after discharge.

The study revealed that children generally were not problematic; most left on discharge. Older age groups, however, remained after discharge at a higher rate. For patients who did not leave promptly after discharge, the most common causes were that (1) the family lacked means of transportation, (2) the hospital did not have available ambulances, (3) the health network in the patients' neighborhood lacked proper facilities, (4) the patients and/or family did not want the discharge, and (5) the patient's house lacked appropriate infrastructure. These findings differed from those in the international literature, which did not identify transportation issues and unsupportive health networks as the most common causes of overstays; this difference highlights the need to understand the unique features of national cultures.

Case Study Discussion Questions

1. How might a population health management approach assist the hospital in resolving the problem of hospital overstays?
2. What steps can the hospital take to reduce the likelihood of patients staying after discharge?
3. How might collaboration with social service organizations, as well as churches and other community-based groups, help to resolve this problem?

Case Study: Community-Based Primary Care in Ukraine

In the 1990s, as managed care took hold, many healthcare leaders in the United States expected that healthcare systems would become integrated around patient need. This expectation stemmed in large part from the pivotal and growing role of primary care services in care management. The US Agency for International Development (USAID) entered into a cooperative agreement with the American International Health Alliance to solicit proposals for developing community-based primary care.

Temple University, in Philadelphia, entered a partnership with Kyiv City Health Administration in Ukraine to pilot a demonstration. The project led to the establishment of a Family Medicine Center to provide family medicine and integrated behavioral health services in Darnitskiy Rayon, Ukraine. A key aspect of the project involved identifying the health needs of the rayon (district), in part through the use of a geographic information system (GIS) component that assessed health at a neighborhood level. The project required a considerable amount of effort, close collaboration between the center and neighborhood health centers and the rayon polyclinic (multispecialty clinic), and the retention of staff capable of data analysis and interpretation for program planning purposes.

During the period of the USAID-funded project, the Family Medicine Center's physicians, nurses, social workers, psychologist, and information systems staff received extensive training to support development of their roles within an innovative community-based primary clinic. Behavioral health integration and the collection and analysis of data were successfully implemented. The project demonstrated that primary care initiatives offer feasible and effective ways to improve the health of a constituent population. However, after completion of the project and the ensuing staff turnover, the clinic reverted to more traditional medical roles, though still based on delivery of high-quality primary care.

(continued)

Case Study Discussion Questions

1. Is a population health management approach to primary care sustainable? What kind of efforts are required to continually monitor the health of the population served? What resources are needed?
2. How should the Family Medicine Center use data collected from multiple sources to better serve the population in its geographic area?
3. Imagine you are the director of the Family Medicine Center. What steps would you take to sustain a community-based approach to managing the health of the population after the completion of the demonstration project?

Case Study: Identifying Problems with an Artificial Hip

In August 2010, the US Food and Drug Administration (FDA) recalled the DePuy Articular Surface Replacement (ASR) artificial hip because it had been associated with a high failure rate, resulting in significant pain and medical problems for patients. In many instances, a patient needed a second surgery to fix the problems resulting from the initial implant. The exact number of ASR devices implanted in the United States prior to recall is hard to come by, but by August 2011 more than 7,500 ASR complaints had been filed with the FDA (Meier and Roberts 2011). By contrast, Sweden had stopped using this type of artificial hip after implanting only 394 devices (Gray 2013).

Case Study Discussion Questions

1. How were authorities in Sweden able to discover the problems associated with the ASR artificial hip so much earlier than authorities in the United States?
2. As a health services manager, how would you prevent situations in which an innovative approach to surgery or treatment proves to be unsafe after it is put into use?

Case Study: Registries for Chronic Disease Management

More than 30 million people in the United States suffer from diabetes, a chronic disease that is usually managed in primary care (CDC 2017). The mortality and morbidity burden from diabetes is huge. Registries can help track how diabetes management compares to established standards of care, ultimately leading to improvements in the health of the diabetic population and possibly reducing costs (careful monitoring can be significantly less expensive than amputation). Sweden uses data from its diabetes registry to inform the development and improvement of its national guidelines for diabetes management.

Case Study Discussion Questions

1. Many countries use registries to track the prevalence of health conditions or medical incidents. How can registries help with population health management?
2. What is the value of implementing a disease management program? Conduct a search for information about disease management programs for diabetes. How might you deploy such a program at your organization?
3. In what ways can healthcare managers use registries to assess and promote health in the communities they serve?

References

American College of Cardiology Foundation (ACCF) / American Heart Association (AHA). 2013. "The 2013 ACCF/AHA Guideline for the Management of Heart Failure." *Journal of the American College of Cardiology.* Published October. http://content.onlinejacc.org/article.aspx?doi=10.1016/j.jacc.2013.05.019.

Antecol, H., and K. Bedard. 2006. "Unhealthy Assimilation: Why Do Immigrants Converge to American Health Status Levels?" *Demography* 43 (2): 337–60.

Artiga, S., and E. Hinton. 2018. "Beyond Health Care: The Role of Social Determinants in Promoting Health and Health Equity." Kaiser Family Foundation. Published May 10. www.kff.org/disparities-policy/issue-brief/beyond-health-care-the-role-of-social-determinants-in-promoting-health-and-health-equity/.

Berwick, D. M., T. W. Nolan, and J. Whittington. 2008. "The Triple Aim: Care, Health, and Cost." *Health Affairs* 27 (3): 759 69.

Centers for Disease Control and Prevention (CDC). 2018. "CDC Research on SDOH." Updated January 29. www.cdc.gov/socialdeterminants/.

———. 2017. "New CDC Report: More Than 100 Million Americans Have Diabetes or Prediabetes." Published July 18. www.cdc.gov/media/releases/2017/p0718-diabetes-report.html.

Environmental Protection Agency. 2018. "Water Topics." Updated March 5. www.epa.gov/environmental-topics/water-topics.

Fiedler, B. A., and T. T. H. Wan. 2010. "Disease Management Organization Approach to Chronic Illness." *International Journal of Public Policy* 6 (3/4): 260–77.

Golden, A., D. Gammonley, G. Hanna Powell, and T. T. Wan. 2017. "The Challenges of Developing a Participatory Arts Intervention for Caregivers of Persons with Dementia." *Cureus* 9 (4): e1154.

Gray, B. H. 2013. "Registries as a Knowledge-Development Tool: The Experience of Sweden and England." Urban Institute. Published July. www.urban.org/sites/default/files/publication/23791/412860-registries-as-a-knowledge-development-tool.pdf.

Grol, R., M. Wensing, M. Eccles, and D. Davis. 2013. *Improving Patient Care: The Implementation of Change in Health Care*, 2nd ed. New York: Wiley-Blackwell.

Guerreiro, R., V. Escott-Price, L. Darwent, L. Parkkinen, O. Ansorge, D. G. Hernandez, M. A. Nalls, L. Clark, L. Honig, K. Marder, W. van der Flier, H. Holstege, E. Louwersheimer, A. Lemstra, P. Scheltens, E. Rogaeva, P. St. George-Hyslop, E. Londos, H. Zetterberg, S. Ortega-Cubero, P. Pastor, T. J. Ferman, N. R. Graff-Radford, O. A. Ross, I. Barber, A. Braae, K. Brown, K. Morgan, W. Maetzler, D. Berg, C. Troakes, S. Al-Sarraj, T. Lashley, Y. Compta, T. Revesz, A. Lees, N. J. Cairns, G. M. Halliday, D. Mann, S. Pickering-Brown, J. Powell, K. Lunnon, M. K. Lupton, International Parkinson's Disease Genomics Consortium, D. Dickson, J. Hardy, A. Singleton, and J. Bras. 2016. "Genome-Wide Analysis of Genetic Correlation in Dementia with Lewy Bodies, Parkinson's and Alzheimer's Diseases." *Neurobiology of Aging* 38: 214.e7 214.e10.

Hegarty, C., C. Buckley, R. Forrest, and B. Marshall. 2016. "Discharge Planning: Screening Older Patients for Multidisciplinary Team Referral." *International Journal of Integrated Care* 16 (4): 1.

Jacobsen, K. H. 2008. *Introduction to Global Health*. Sudbury, MA: Jones & Bartlett.

Jiamjariyapon, T., A. Ingsathit, K. Tungsanga, C. Banchuin, K. Vipattawat, S. Kanchanakorn, V. Leesmidt, W. Watcharasaksilp, A. Saetie, C. Pachotikarn, S. Taechangam, T. Teerapornlertratt, T. Chanarojsiri, and V. Sitprija. 2014. "Effectiveness of Integrated Care on Delaying Chronic Kidney Disease Progression in Rural Communities of Thailand (ESCORT Study): Rationale and Design of the Study." *BMC Nephrology* 15: 99.

Koehring, M. 2015. "An Introduction to Value-Based Healthcare." Economist Intelligence Unit. Published April 22. http://perspectives.eiu.com/healthcare/introduction-value-based-healthcare-europe.

Kosseim, P., E. S. Dove, C. Baggaley, E. M. Meslin, F. H. Cate, J. Kaye, J. R. Harris, and B. M. Knoppers. 2014. "Building a Data Sharing Model for Global Genome Research." *Genome Biology* 15: 430.

Kroneman, M., W. Boerma, M. van den Berg, P. Groenewegen, J. de Jong, and E. van Ginneken. 2016. "Netherlands Health System Review." *Health Systems in Transition* 18 (2): 1–239.

Learmonth, I. D., C. Young, and C. Rorabeck. 2007. "The Operation of the Century: Total Hip Replacement." *Lancet* 370 (9597): 1508–19.

Lopez, A. D., C. D. Mathers, M. Ezzati, D. T. Jamison, and C. J. Murray. 2006. "Measuring the Global Burden of Disease and Risk Factors, 1990–2001." In *Global Burden of Disease and Risk Factors*, edited by A. D. Lopez, C. D. Mathers, M.

Ezzati, D. T. Jamison, and C. J. Murray, 1–14. New York: Oxford University Press and the World Bank.

Lu, J. F., G. M. Leung, S. Kwon, K. Y. Tin, E. van Doorslaer, and O. O'Donnell. 2007. "Horizontal Equity in Healthcare Utilization: Evidence from Three High-Income Asian Economies." *Social Science and Medicine* 64 (1): 199–212.

Malviya, A., N. Abdul, and V. Khanduja. 2017. "Outcomes Following Total Hip Arthroplasty: A Review of the Registry Data." *Indian Journal of Orthopaedics* 51 (4): 405–13.

Meier, B., and J. Roberts. 2011. "Hip Implants Surge, Even as the Dangers Are Studied." *New York Times.* Published August 22. www.nytimes.com/2011/08/23/business/complaints-soar-on-hip-implants-as-dangers-are-studied.html.

Murray, C. J., A. D. Lopez, and S. Wibulpolprasert. 2004. "Monitoring Global Health: Time for New Solutions." *BMJ* 329: 1096–100.

National Health Research Institutes. 2018. "Overview." Accessed July 9. http://english.nhri.org.tw/NHRI_WEB/nhriw001Action.do.

Nielsen, M., L. Buelt, K. Patel, and L. M. Nichols. 2016. *The Patient-Centered Medical Home's Impact on Cost and Quality: Annual Review of Evidence, 2014–2015.* Patient-Centered Primary Care Collaborative. www.pcpcc.org/resource/patient-centered-medical-homes-impact-cost-and-quality-2014-2015.

Optum. 2018. "Data and Analytics." Accessed July 10. www.optum.com/solutions/data-analytics.html.

Ramakers, I. H., and F. R. Verhey. 2011. "Development of Memory Clinics in the Netherlands: 1998 to 2009." *Aging and Mental Health* 15 (1): 34–39.

Rosenthal, T. C. 2008. "The Medical Home: Growing Evidence to Support a New Approach to Primary Care." *Journal of American Board of Family Medicine* 21 (5): 427–40.

Rowe, A., A. McClelland, and K. Billingham. 2001. "Community Health Needs Assessment: An Introductory Guide for the Family Health Nurse in Europe." World Health Organization European Region. Accessed July 9, 2018. www.euro.who.int/__data/assets/pdf_file/0018/102249/E73494.pdf.

Simon, G. 2017. "What's Wrong with the Term 'Social Determinants of Health'?" *Medium.* Published July 27. https://medium.com/@KPWaResearch/whats-wrong-with-the-term-social-determinants-of-health-8e69684ec442.

Steenkamer, B. M., H. W. Drewes, R. Heijink, C. A. Baan, and J. N. Strujis. 2017. "Defining Population Health Management: A Scoping Review of the Literature." *Population Health Management* 20 (1): 74–85.

Struckmann, V., F. Barbabella, A. Dimova, and E. van Ginneken. 2017. "Integrated Diabetes Care Delivered by Patients—A Case Study for Bulgaria." *International Journal of Integrated Care* 17 (1): 6.

Tarlov, A. R. 1999. "Public Policy Frameworks for Improving Population Health." *Annals of the New York Academy of Sciences* 896 (1): 281–93.

Thygesen, L. C., and A. K. Ersbøll. 2011. "Danish Population-Based Registers for Public Health and Health-Related Welfare Research: Introduction to the Supplement." *Scandinavian Journal of Public Health* 39 (Suppl. 7): 8–10.

van Doorslaer, E., C. Masseria, and X. Koolman. 2006. "Inequalities in Access to Medical Care by Income in Developed Countries." *Canadian Medical Association Journal* 174 (2): 177–83.

Wan, T. T. H. 2016. "Financial Incentives for Health Promotion and Behavioral Changes for Hospital Employees." *Review of Public Administration and Management* 4 (3): 1–3.

———. 2010. "Global Health Research Strategies." *International Journal of Public Policy* 5 (2/3): 104–20.

———. 2006. "Healthcare Informatics Research: From Data to Evidence-Based Practice." *Journal of Medical Systems* 30 (1): 3–7.

———. 2002. *Evidence-Based Health Care Management: Multivariate Modeling Approaches.* Boston: Kluwer Academic Publishers.

———. 1995. *Analysis and Evaluation of Health Care Systems: An Integrated Approach to Managerial Decision Making.* Baltimore, MD: Health Professions Press.

Wan, T. T. H., A. Sun, and A. Golden. 2016. "A Pilot Study on Health-Related Quality of Life and Caregiving Burden of Caregivers for Dementia: A Cross-Sectional Report on the Pre-test Assessment Results." *Jacobs Journal of Gerontology* 2 (1): 16–23.

Wan, T. T. H., A. Terry, E. Cobb, B. McKee, R. Tregerman, and S. D. S. Barbaro. 2017. "Strategies to Modify the Risk of Heart Failure Readmission: A Systematic Review and Meta-analysis." *Health Services Research and Managerial Epidemiology* 4: 1–16.

Wan, T. T. H., A. Terry, B. McKee, and W. Kattan. 2017. "A KMAP-O Framework for Care Management Research of Patients with Type 2 Diabetes." *World Journal of Diabetes* 8 (4): 165–71.

Wensing, M., A. Oxman, R. Baker, M. Godycki-Cwirko, S. Flottorp, J. Szecsenyi, J. Grimshaw, and M. Eccles. 2011. "Tailored Implementation for Chronic Diseases (TICD): A Project Protocol." *Implementation Science* 6: 103.

White, K., T. F. Williams, and B. G. Greenberg. 1961. "The Ecology of Medical Care." *New England Journal of Medicine* 265 (18): 885–92.

World Health Organization (WHO). 2018. "About Social Determinants of Health." Accessed July 11. www.who.int/social_determinants/sdh_definition/en/.

———. 2017. *World Health Statistics 2017: Monitoring Health for the SDGs.* Accessed July 11. www.who.int/gho/publications/world_health_statistics/2017/en/.

———. 2011. "Rio Political Declaration on Social Determinants of Health." Published October 21. www.who.int/sdhconference/declaration/Rio_political_declaration.pdf?ua=1.

World Health Organization (WHO) Commission on Social Determinants of Health. 2008. *Closing the Gap in a Generation: Health Equity Through Action on the Social Determinants of Health.* Accessed July 9, 2018. www.who.int/social_determinants/thecommission/finalreport/en/.

Wright, J., R. Williams, and J. R. Wilkinson. 1998. "Development and Importance of Health Needs Assessment." *BMJ* 316 (7140): 1310–13.

Zeng, Y., Q. Feng, D. Gu, and J. W. Vaupel. 2017. "Demographics, Phenotypic Health Characteristics and Genetic Analysis of Centenarians in China." *Mechanisms of Ageing and Development* 165 (Pt. B): 86–97.

LOOKING AHEAD IN GLOBAL HEALTH MANAGEMENT

FUTURE TRENDS IN GLOBAL HEALTH

14

Steven J. Szydlowski, DHA, Robert Babela, Benjamin K. Poku, DrPH, Terra Anderson, Vladimir Krcmery, MD, PhD, ScD, FRCP, Bruce J. Fried, PhD, Fevzi Akinci, PhD, Blair Gifford, PhD, Steven G. Ullmann, PhD, Afsan Bhadelia, PhD, and Felicia Knaul, PhD

Chapter Focus

This chapter identifies and describes key global health trends affecting healthcare managers and health system design. It addresses issues of health policy, technology, public health, human rights, workforce planning, health sector changes, catastrophic events, and consumer behavior, with a forward-thinking approach to critical issues affecting global health status.

Learning Objectives

Upon completion of this chapter, you should be able to

- apply concepts of health, disease, illness, and epidemiology as they relate to global population health status;
- demonstrate the skills, competencies, values, and points of view needed by global health leaders;
- project the impact of global trends on health service design;
- synthesize knowledge and concepts in an integrated view of global health management; and
- forecast the competencies that will be required for future healthcare managers in global settings.

Competencies

- Analyze problems, promote solutions, and encourage decision making.
- Encourage diversity of thought to support innovation, creativity, and improvement.

- Commit to competence, integrity, altruism, and the promotion of the public good.
- Demonstrate commitment to self-development, including continuing education, networking, reflection, and personal improvement.
- Be aware of one's own assumptions, values, strengths, and limitations.
- Use the established ethical structures to resolve ethical issues.
- Promote the establishment of alliances and consolidation of networks to expand social and community participation in health networks, both nationally and globally.
- Optimize the healthcare workforce around critical local issues, such as shortages, scope of practice, skill mix, licensing, and fluctuations in service.
- Promote the effective management, analysis, and communication of health information.
- Recognize the local implications of global health events and the interconnectivity of health systems.
- Demonstrate an understanding of the interdependency, integration, and competition that exist among healthcare sectors.

Key Terms

- Aggravated assault
- Bioterrorism
- Closed colony
- Community health worker (CHW)
- Connected health (cHealth)
- Continuous manufacturing
- Digital fabrication
- Disruptive innovation
- Herd immunity
- Human trafficking
- Just culture

- Mobile health (mHealth)
- Neoliberal economic policies
- Plasticity
- Point-of-care (POC) healthcare technology
- Poverty line
- Precision medicine
- Simple assault
- Social gradient in health
- Stalking
- Structural adjustment policy
- Telehealth

Key Concepts

- Communicable disease
- Consumer-directed care
- Data and analytics
- Electronic health records (EHRs)
- Globalization of health services
- Global partnerships and collaboration
- Health information technology
- Health workforce management
- Low-resource care settings
- Management competencies
- Medical tourism
- Nongovernmental organizations (NGOs)
- Personalized care and precision medicine
- Poverty
- Women's health
- Workplace violence

Introduction

Today's healthcare managers must continually monitor the impact of health policy on system design and assess the potential impact of infectious diseases, immigration patterns, and other critical global issues on population health and health status. Historically, government leaders and key influencers have focused on country-specific priorities that support the cornerstones of any healthcare system: cost, quality, and access. The intention—rightly so—has been to lower cost, improve quality, and increase access to care, thereby improving the health status of citizens within a given country. Today, however, leaders can no longer ignore the need to engage in global collaborations and partnerships. To achieve optimal health for citizens, health policy needs to consider both internal and external influences.

Senior healthcare executives have made the shift from managing organizations from an internal operations perspective to predicting and anticipating how the external environment will affect the institution. For the most part, however, these executives have not made the critical shift in thinking about how global factors influence the delivery system. Healthcare leaders within any given country need to be concerned about global health concerns that might influence the types of acute and chronic cases being presented in their organizations. This need is particularly vital as the potential for communicable and infectious diseases to spread internationally continues to grow.

Whereas public health entities previously could focus on preventing and managing local and regional epidemics, they now must also address the impact of global infectious and communicable diseases. Public health entities in recent years have clearly shifted closer to the forefront of forced engagement in global matters, as evident in the cases of Ebola, Zika, and bird flu, to name just a few.

Such events highlight long-standing concerns about the engagement between public health and medical delivery systems. How can the integration of these systems support population health and position the global community to better prevent illness and disease, ultimately improving the health status of the world?

Looking to the future, corporate social responsibility should be a guiding principle to ensure long-term environmental and financial sustainability, and ethical and moral decision making should remain a prominent competency for healthcare leaders. From a global health perspective, what is the role of the corporation in creating healthy populations? How do we instill and sustain universal best practices to protect the environment and prevent pollution? How can we increase the number of successful public–private partnerships that benefit local and regional economies while still maintaining reasonable profit margins? Organizations can contribute to global health through their efforts to support the health and well-being of citizens, to improve the environment, and to advance other social justice interests. Corporations can also support local economies through employment, the purchase of raw goods, and engagement in international trade, all of which contribute to healthier, more productive societies.

From a consumer perspective, we need to look beyond the perception that healthcare is a service available to treat an acute episode of illness, to address a surgical need, or to manage a chronic condition. This perception must be expanded to include such aspects as wellness and exercise, diet and nutrition, psychosocial well-being, genetics, individual lifestyles, holistic (i.e., emotional, physical, spiritual) health, and personal responsibility and accountability.

Health literacy efforts and consumer awareness appear to have initiated some shift in thinking. However, are we to the point where consumers of healthcare consider how epidemics and communicable diseases that have originated in other countries can affect their health? Are consumers considering how bioterrorism and the changing climate can affect their health? Should such considerations influence the selection of a health insurance carrier or healthcare provider? We argue that awareness and understanding of such topics as global health epidemics, natural disasters, bioterrorism, global warming, growing diversity in communities, and medical tourism, among other things, should be considered part of health literacy.

In light of all these issues—and all the topics discussed in this book's first 13 chapters—how do we prepare the global health workforce to work within complex health systems to address local needs that are unique to communities? Should management and clinical education involve both population health and global health as areas of curriculum and training beyond the discipline-specific content and competencies?

Some of our biggest challenges and opportunities involve health information technology. Rapid advances in technology have helped improve access to care through telemedicine and enabled the digital reading of lab work and X-rays from professionals across the globe. How can technology help serve people who are impoverished, at risk, and underserved? How can people in poverty gain access to the necessary technology? We have a global duty, rooted in principles of social justice, to ensure that basic health needs, including vaccinations and immunizations, sanitation, and clean water, are available to all.

Clearly, global partnerships will be needed to address the voluminous public health, population health, and medical needs identified by the United Nations (UN) in its Millennium Development Goals (UN Development Programme 2018). As governments, nongovernmental organizations, foundations, and public–private partnerships face increasing pressure to generate value, reduce costs, and improve access, synergy in partnership-based models is essential. How can we build a global framework for more effective collaborative models? How can we use existing, successful partnership models as a template for increased collaboration to address global health needs?

Meeting people's health needs and designing effective systems for care are complex tasks with rapidly changing targets and a broad mix of stakeholders—including consumers, providers, insurers, vendors, politicians, pharmaceuticals, and even nonhealthcare businesses that affect the environment. In this chapter, we will address some of the major trends and developments that will continue to influence health and healthcare in this century. Specific emphasis is placed on global problems, challenges, and opportunities.

The Future of the Pharmaceutical Industry

From a global perspective, healthcare is in a state of flux, and healthcare spending has been soaring. Several countries have introduced initiatives aiming to bring costs under control. Around the world, reforms have unleashed numerous disruptive innovations. The United States is still learning how to deal with the changes brought about by the Affordable Care Act of 2010. At the same time, growth in emerging markets is creating a large pool of prospective consumers.

Pharmaceutical companies are also dealing with challenges specific to their field. Ehrhardt (2015) explains:

> Patents for many drugs—some of them blockbusters, which have created billions of dollars in revenue—have expired, and more will do so in the coming years. Health systems are no longer willing (or able) to pay what they used to for pharmaceuticals. Regulators and the public are asking pharma companies to produce and deliver more complex product portfolios at a lower cost, in more and more markets—while continuing to meet stringent quality requirements.

We can expect major changes. Production innovations such as **continuous manufacturing** and **digital fabrication** are already having a major impact. Ehrhardt (2015) writes:

continuous manufacturing
A manufacturing process by which pharmaceuticals can be produced in a continuous, efficient process in a single facility, minimizing delays associated with previous methods.

digital fabrication
A technology for making small batches of medicines that previously had been considered too costly and impractical to produce.

> A new approach called continuous manufacturing is on the verge of transforming the pharmaceutical value chain. It will affect every company in this industry, from giant multinationals to the third-party manufacturers that small startups hire to make their products. This shift in production capability will rapidly become "table stakes" for leading pharmaceutical firms. It has the potential to make drug manufacturing more efficient, less expensive, and more environmentally friendly. It is not the only transformative innovation in this space. Digital fabrication—the so-called 3D printing of drugs—is also gaining traction as a viable technology for making small batches of medicines that have been too costly and impractical to produce.

The pharmaceutical industry will need to embrace these and other innovations if it hopes to adapt to the challenges it faces today (Ehrhardt 2015).

We can also expect that big data will play a more important role in therapeutic decision making with regard to pharmaceuticals, as well as in research and development; that personalized medicine will more strongly influence clinical decisions; that biosimilars (i.e., products that are nearly identical to products offered by other companies) will play a more important role within the pharmaceutical landscape; and that greater emphasis will be placed on cost-effectiveness. In a Brookings Institution paper, Rauch (2015) writes that a "cost-no-object, value-no-concern approach" has made the pharmaceutical industry "seemingly impervious to disruptive innovations" but that "a growing culture of disruptive entrepreneurship is gaining a foothold."

Ongoing Global Health Threats

Healthcare managers today must confront myriad medical, social, and public health issues at all times. Some of the most prominent health issues in the news today involve communicable disease, bioterrorism, violent crime, and human trafficking.

Communicable Disease Outbreaks

Vaccines have the ability to limit disease transmission and greatly improve population health. The World Health Organization (WHO 2018c) writes: "Immunization is a proven tool for controlling and eliminating life-threatening disease and is estimated to avert between 2 and 3 million deaths each year. It is one of the most cost-effective health investments, with proven strategies that make it accessible to even the most hard-to-reach and vulnerable populations."

Nonetheless, vaccine-preventable diseases remain a concern. Describing the situation in the United States, Buchbinder and Shanks (2017, 460) write: "Due to lack of immunization in other countries, porous borders, global travel, and parental refusals to vaccinate their children in this country, diseases we once thought we vanquished with vaccines are making a comeback, often in tragic ways." Parental refusals often stem from fears that injecting a child with a vaccine might cause the child to become sick, and such fears have been fueled by discredited reports linking the mumps, measles, and rubella vaccines to childhood autism.

Failure to vaccinate raises the global health risks associated with such diseases as measles, polio, pertussis, and influenza. Measles is highly contagious, and the virus can be transmitted via the air for up to two hours after an infected individual has coughed or sneezed. Pertussis, caused by the bacterium *Bordetella pertussis*, is another highly contagious disease that can be transmitted through the air. Polio virus can be spread through contact with the stool of an infected person and through droplets from a person's sneeze or a cough. It may also spread through objects, such as toys (Buchbinder and Shanks 2017).

The 2014–2015 Ebola outbreak in West Africa provides an example of the risks taken by healthcare workers who treat people with communicable diseases. The Ebola virus is transmitted through direct contact with bodily fluids, and health workers who interacted with sick, dying, or dead Ebola victims during the outbreak faced a much greater risk of infection. Appropriate personal protective equipment was not available in all facilities, and two nurses contracted the virus from a patient in 2014 because of the lack of protection (Buchbinder and Shanks 2017).

Exhibit 14.1 presents information about the various diseases discussed in this section. Measles, polio, pertussis, and influenza, put together, kill more

Disease	US Cases and Deaths	Global Cases and Deaths
Measles	173 cases in 21 states and the District of Columbia; 5 outbreaks in 2015	145,700 deaths in 2013; about 400 deaths daily, or 16 deaths every hour
Pertussis	10,000–40,000 cases each year; 10–20 children's deaths	16 million cases in 2008; 195,000 children's deaths
Polio virus	None; free of disease for 30+ years due to vaccine	416 reported cases in 2013; 1 out of 200 infections leads to irreversible paralysis, and 5 to 10 percent of such cases lead to death when the patient's breathing muscles become immobilized
Influenza	98,680 cases in 2014–2015; 125 pediatric deaths, 90 percent unvaccinated	250,000–500,000 deaths (all ages)
Ebola virus	4 cases, 1 death	20,272 cases and 7,953 deaths across 10 countries

EXHIBIT 14.1
Disease Cases and Deaths in the United States and Other Countries

Source: Adapted from Buchbinder and Shanks (2017).

herd immunity
A state in which most of a community is vaccinated against a disease, making the disease unlikely to spread throughout the group.

closed colony
A state in which everyone in a community is vaccinated, and no new people come in or out.

just culture
An organization approach that emphasizes truth, integrity, and responsibility rather than blame.

bioterrorism
The deliberate release of viruses, bacteria, or other germs to cause illness or death in people, animals, or plants.

people annually than Ebola did at the height of the 2014–2015 outbreak (Buchbinder and Shanks 2017).

Healthcare managers should be knowledgeable about various communicable diseases, and they must be prepared for potential outbreaks. Furthermore, they should promote immunization programs to minimize the health risks associated with vaccine-preventable diseases. When most of a community is vaccinated, **herd immunity** (sometimes called *community immunity* or *indirect immunity*) exists, meaning that a disease is unlikely to spread throughout the group even if certain individuals are unvaccinated. A **closed colony** exists when everyone is vaccinated, and no new people come in or out.

Healthcare managers should emphasize teamwork and a **just culture** when dealing with issues related to communicable disease (Buchbinder and Shanks 2017). A just culture approach emphasizes truth, integrity, accountability, and responsibility. In the words of Barnsteiner (2011), it puts the focus on "what went wrong, not who caused the problem." A just culture distinguishes between human errors (e.g., a slip, lapse, or inadvertent action); at-risk behavior (e.g., a behavioral choice that increases risk, where risk is either not recognized or mistakenly thought to be justified); and reckless behavior (e.g., consciously choosing to disregard a substantial risk) (Buchbinder and Shanks 2017).

Bioterrorism

A **bioterrorism** attack involves the "deliberate release of viruses, bacteria, or other germs . . . to cause illness or death in people, animals, or plants" (Centers for Disease Control and Prevention 2006). Biological agents can be spread through the air, through water, or in food. The agents used in bioterrorism are typically substances found in nature, but they may be altered to increase their ability to cause disease, to make them resistant to current medicines, or to increase their ability to spread in the targeted environment. Bioterrorism can happen at any moment, and health managers should have emergency response plans in place for a wide variety of scenarios.

Violence and Other Crimes in Healthcare Settings

The National Institute for Occupational Safety and Health (NIOSH 2014) defines *workplace violence* as "violent acts (including physical assaults and threats of assaults) directed toward persons at work or duty." It can range from threatening language to robberies to physical attacks or even homicide. An act of violence can happen to anyone—whether a doctor, a nurse, or even a patient—at any type of healthcare facility. Violence in healthcare settings is not always reported, in part because many workers feel that such risks come with the territory of the job. Of all healthcare workers, those in mental health settings face the highest rates of violent incidents. Many people assume that emergency room personnel would be at similar risk, though such expectations have not yet been fully supported by data (Buchbinder 2014a).

A Bureau of Justice Statistics report found that **simple assault** (which does not involve weapons or serious injury) and **aggravated assault** (which does involve weapons or serious injury) accounted for about 94 percent of violent incidents in the workplace (Duhart 2001). Simple assault was much more common than aggravated assault. Sexual assault and sexual harassment are serious concerns in healthcare, as they are in other fields. Some incidents in healthcare settings involve **stalking**, which the US Department of Justice (2018) defines as "a course of conduct directed at a specific person that would cause a reasonable person to fear for his or her safety or the safety of others or suffer substantial emotional distress." Forms of stalking may include targeting a victim with unwanted phone calls, text messages, letters, and emails; making posts and interactions on social media; giving unwanted items or gifts; following or spying on a victim; or appearing or waiting, without legitimate reason, at places where the victim will appear. Stalking is reported often by mental health professionals. One study found that 5 percent of counseling center staff members had been stalked by a current or former client and that 65 percent had experienced harassment (Buchbinder and Shanks 2017).

Workplace violence and abuse can cause physical injury and disability, as well as long-lasting psychological trauma. It can also lead to negative organizational outcomes, such as lost productivity, low morale, increased stress, and distrust of managers and coworkers (NIOSH 2014). Victims of violence may have to miss work because they are not physically or mentally able to perform their job, and organizations may face lawsuits stemming from violent incidents.

Healthcare managers must be prepared to guard against and respond to any instances of workplace violence. They must be able to identify hazards and risk factors, implement prevention strategies, ensure workplace security, and develop appropriate response plans. Managers have an obligation to protect their employees, and they must maintain a safe environment in which workers feel comfortable talking to the manager about personal and professional concerns.

A number of resources are available to help health leaders build an appropriate prevention plan. Examples include the Emergency Nurses Association's (2010) *Workplace Violence Toolkit*, which includes a step-by-step plan for addressing violence in an emergency department; the Occupational Safety and Health Administration's (2016) *Guidelines for Preventing Workplace Violence for Healthcare and Social Service Workers*; and the New York Department of Labor's (2009) *Workplace Violence Prevention Program Guidelines* (Buchbinder and Shanks 2017).

Human Trafficking

Another issue with significant implications for global health is **human trafficking**, or the trade of human beings for such purposes as forced labor or sexual exploitation. Human trafficking covers a wide assortment of crimes, especially against women and children. In 2000, the UN General Assembly

simple assault
Assault that does not involve weapons or serious injury.

aggravated assault
Assault involving weapons or serious injury.

stalking
Following, spying, or making unwanted contact with a specific person in a manner that is likely to cause fear or emotional distress.

human trafficking
The trade of human beings for such purposes as forced labor or sexual exploitation.

adopted a Protocol to Prevent, Suppress and Punish Trafficking in Persons, Especially Women and Children (also called, more simply, the Trafficking in Persons Protocol), which defines *human trafficking* as follows (UN Office on Drugs and Crime 2004, 42):

> "Trafficking in persons" shall mean the recruitment, transportation, transfer, harbouring or receipt of persons, by means of the threat or use of force or other forms of coercion, of abduction, of fraud, of deception, of the abuse of power or of a position of vulnerability or of the giving or receiving of payments or benefits to achieve the consent of a person having control over another person, for the purpose of exploitation. Exploitation shall include, at a minimum, the exploitation of the prostitution of others or other forms of sexual exploitation, forced labour or services, slavery or practices similar to slavery, servitude or the removal of organs.

Shelley (2010, 4) points out that reliable data about the scale of human trafficking are scarce, given "the covert nature of the problem" and the fact that "trafficking is often perpetrated by distinct ethnic groups that are hard for outsiders to penetrate." Nonetheless, nearly every expert on human trafficking and smuggling acknowledges that the problem is significant and growing, as both demand for people and supply of people rise.

Europe in recent years has struggled with the illegal migration of large numbers of people from Africa, the Middle East, and Asia, and the movement of illegal immigrants from Mexico has long been a concern in the United States. Many of the migrants in these instances pay human smugglers to move them and therefore cannot be considered victims of human trafficking (Shelley 2010). Often, however, the individuals who pay smugglers become victims of trafficking during the course of their journey, or upon arrival. Antitrafficking campaigns have had some success in countering certain forms of trafficking, but data collection and management—essential for monitoring country and regional trends, investigation information, and prosecution rates—continue to be a challenge.

Since 2000, the UN's Trafficking in Persons Protocol has sought to bring nations together in antitrafficking efforts aiming to protect human rights, with special attention to women and children. However, enforcement of the protocol has been lacking, and human trafficking is often overlooked by police. Some countries have signed the protocol in general but left certain spaces unsigned (Buchbinder 2014b).

The victims of human trafficking face serious health concerns. They typically are treated poorly, with little regard to their health and well-being. They generally receive no education or medical care during the trafficking experience and are simply tossed aside if they become sick. The harsh conditions can lead to a variety of physical and psychological problems, and the average life expectancy for a woman or child who survives the trafficking ordeal may be as low as seven years (Hauser and Castillo 2013). Global healthcare managers are in a position to help the survivors. Victims of trafficking should be treated with respect, provided with care, and pointed toward approriate education.

Consumer-Directed Healthcare and Disruptive Innovation

Healthcare, traditionally, has not been something that people shop for like they would for groceries. People have difficulty knowing what options represent the best value for their money, because the necessary information often is not available. For example, if your doctor recommends that you visit a particular specialist, are you confident that the specialist is the best expert available for your money? Or perhaps the doctor is simply looking out for the specialist, who is a personal friend. Consumers generally lack a clear idea of what options are best or how much they are paying for care. Callahan (2012, 134) points out that the traditional fee-for-service model "encourages patients to be ignorant of and indifferent to costs." Cowles (2011) argues that "the health care community, insurance industry and, of course, the government have worked together, perhaps unwittingly, toward a common goal: the disempowerment of the American consumer." These conditions are changing, however, with the shift toward consumer-directed healthcare and the more active engagement of individuals in their own care.

The new healthcare consumers emerging in recent years are internet-savvy individuals who will go online to look up symptoms and diagnose what they think the doctor will say. Many of these individuals have purchased their insurance through online shopping, and many use their phones and other mobile devices to monitor their health. Such technologies have given these consumers greater command over their healthcare journey. The new consumers might see nurse practitioners instead of primary care physicians, and they might select particular doctors they wish to see, often going to places where they have not been treated before. It is not just young consumers who are changing the way they approach their health; baby boomers are doing it as well.

Change is happening quickly and continuously in healthcare, and healthcare managers need to make sure that they and their organizations are strategically ready. **Disruptive innovation**, in the words of the Christensen Institute (2018), is "the phenomenon by which an innovation transforms an existing market or sector by introducing simplicity, convenience, accessibility, and affordability where complication and high cost are the status quo." In other words, it involves the introduction of a new, inexpensive, and straightforward way of doing things. In the United States, the Affordable Care Act provides an example of a disruptor of health insurance, offering cheaper insurance packages and helping consumers shop from among the various packages available in the

disruptive innovation
A new development that transforms an existing market or field by introducing new, inexpensive, and straightforward ways of doing things.

exchanges. Another example of a disruptor is CVS, which was formerly just a retail pharmacy but has now morphed into one of the largest players in the healthcare field. Through numerous acquisitions, CVS now operates more than 9,600 retail pharmacies and 1,100 walk-in clinics (*Seattle Times* staff 2016). Disruptive innovation is likely to continue in global healthcare, and managers must be prepared to capitalize on potential improvements.

Challenges in Health Workforce Management

Every country struggles with producing and maintaining a health workforce—and most fall short. According to estimates, anywhere from one billion to three billion people globally lack access to health services as a result of workforce shortages. In countries with aging populations, the health workforce often is poorly prepared for the multiple responsibilities associated with disease chronicity and the various long-term care arrangements. Some parts of the world fail to attain even minimum ratios of health workers relative to population. For example, the WHO reported that Africa has only 2.3 health workers per 1,000 people, whereas the Americas have 24.8 (WHO 2006b). Even among countries that do have a sufficient number of health workers, many face distributional challenges at the subnational level, with workers avoiding or abandoning less desirable locations, leaving the areas with chronic shortages. Many countries lack training capacity and qualified educators, and virtually all health systems—even those in high-income countries—suffer from inadequate training for managers and supervisors. An understaffed and stressful work environment, coupled with poor compensation, will often result in a demotivated and unstable staff. Furthermore, in many locations, including the United States, health workers are frequently subject to abuse and violence (Phillips 2016). Finally, in some countries, personnel systems are deficient or nonexistent, preventing the accurate counting and monitoring of workers.

The workforce is an essential building block of any healthcare system, and the challenges facing workforce management are daunting. These challenges expand in magnitude when we consider the broad range of professionals necessary for an effective health system. Every professional group—including nurses and midwives, physicians, dentistry workers, pharmacy workers, laboratory workers, environmental and public health workers, community and traditional health workers, and health management and support workers—presents its own unique challenges in such areas as training, deployment, compensation, continuing education, and supervision. The salient issues facing these professions vary across countries and within countries across regions.

Looking ahead, a key focus of global healthcare will be to disentangle these complex and interrelated challenges and develop uniformly applicable strategies for achieving a competent and stable health workforce. We recommend approaching human resources trends and challenges from four perspectives, which are not mutually exclusive: (1) issues related to a country as a whole; (2) subnational challenges affecting particular regions; (3) healthcare organization and management problems; and (4) cross-sectoral challenges facing the workforce in the country as a whole. As we examine present and future issues salient to each of these perspectives and potential avenues of amelioration, we need to recognize that profound differences exist between countries. For example, in Hungary, physicians are vastly underpaid relative to other professions, resulting in large-scale physician emigration. In contrast, Egypt faces a surplus of physicians and a critical shortage of qualified nurses. Further, in many countries, doctors and nurses report that they feel overskilled for their work, suggesting a waste of human capital. Determining how and why these trends emerge in various countries requires consideration of numerous economic, demographic, and social factors.

Countrywide Issues

Education and training will continue to be of paramount importance to all health systems. This need applies not only to health professionals engaged in "Western" medicine but also to **community health workers (CHWs)**. Despite their importance, community health workers remain a largely untapped resource. Further, as the nature of healthcare continues to evolve, we need to ensure that new healthcare workers are attuned to new technologies and provided with continuing education throughout their careers, ensuring that they remain capable of working effectively in ever-changing multidisciplinary team-based settings. Increasingly, health workers need to be flexible in their work and able to assume expanded responsibilities, particularly in low-resource settings.

community health worker (CHW) A worker who provides education and preventive care at homes and in villages away from the hospital.

Workforce shortages and maldistribution of professionals are chronic problems, and they may be related to training issues, migration, salary differentials, personal lifestyle preferences, and a host of other causes. Countries throughout the world are facing a scarcity of nurses prepared at advanced levels to serve as faculty in educational programs. Given that nurses and the workers they supervise provide about 85 percent of healthcare globally, the lack of educators severely restricts countries' ability to meet demands for care. One way to increase the supply of workers is to increase training capacity, although this approach typically requires years of development, often with the building and staffing of new training facilities. In addition, a number of countries face severe health worker emigration issues, meaning that investments in the training of health professionals may be lost when workers move away.

Workers emigrate for a number of reasons, which can generally be categorized as "push" or "pull" factors. Push factors are aspects of the current work environment that motivate people to leave—for instance, low compensation, poor working conditions, or little opportunity for advancement. Pull factors are aspects of work environments elsewhere that draw people away. Addressing these push and pull factors is a long-term proposition. In the short term, countries can consider instituting mandatory service requirements for new health professionals, such that certification or licensure is dependent on professionals having served in an under-resourced area for a specified amount of time.

In some countries, the health workforce might shift from a situation of shortage to one of surplus over a relatively short period. Health workforce planners have struggled for years to deal with this problem and to predict the timing and nature of the next workforce shortage or surplus. Workforce planning methods are useful but imperfect in predicting future workforce needs and supply (Fraher and Morrison 2015).

Cost and value are continuing concerns in all health systems. Demand for mid-level providers, as well as nonprofessional community and lay health workers, exists and will continue globally. In some instances, value has been demonstrated in bringing traditional healers into the formal healthcare system. The use of such individuals can help control costs and also create opportunities by freeing up highly trained professionals to take on the most complex cases. However, the use of nonprofessional healthcare workers requires investments in training and supervision, to ensure that they are effectively integrated into the health system.

A related workforce strategy is task shifting (discussed in chapter 4), which involves redistributing tasks among members of health workforce teams, typically from highly trained health workers to less highly trained health workers (WHO 2006a). Task shifting most commonly occurs between physicians, nurses, mid-level health professionals (e.g., nurse practitioners), and community health workers. The practice can be useful in expanding access to healthcare services, but it requires attention to a number of factors, including competencies, the scope of practice regulations, and professional autonomy.

Subnational Challenges

Specific, critical workforce challenges often confront particular regions within a country. Most commonly, these subnational challenges surface in rural locations where health professionals are less likely to settle. Many countries have sought to address these challenges by creating incentives for health professionals to practice in rural locations, and such strategies have found varying levels of success. Methods for attracting workers to rural settings may include educational initiatives, regulatory interventions, financial incentives, and personal and professional support (WHO 2010). Efforts within the educational domain may involve targeting certain students for admission to training programs, locating health professional training schools in rural locations, and working to expose medical students to rural practice.

In the area of regulation, governments may consider enlarging health professionals' scope of practice, based on the well-accepted premise that expanding one's tasks and responsibilities can increase job satisfaction and, ultimately, retention. Governments may also establish compulsory service requirements to work in rural or other remote locations. A relatively new approach for addressing workforce shortages involves the concept of **plasticity**. Similar to task shifting, this approach releases workforce planners from the traditional confines of professional disciplines and enables communities to use existing healthcare workers more efficiently. Because different health professionals often have overlapping scopes of practice, various configurations of professionals are possible to help meet a community's specific healthcare needs (Holmes et al. 2013).

plasticity
A workforce planning approach that loosens the traditional confines of professional disciplines and enables communities to use existing healthcare workers more efficiently.

Cross-Sectoral Challenges

A number of challenges that cross sectors have a profound impact on the health workforce. Perhaps of greatest importance is the state of the economy, which generally dictates the level of investment possible in any sector. Some locations also face increasing competition for talent. Healthcare organizations may compete among themselves for talent, but they may also find themselves competing with organizations in other sectors.

Technology presents both opportunities and challenges. On the positive side are advances in diagnosis and treatment and the growth of telemedicine, mobile health, and other communication modalities that allow for the efficient flow of information between patients and providers and among providers. Technology can also support teams of workers communicating in a virtual environment. Advances in information technology (IT) provide unique opportunities for the management of human resources. For example, well-managed data sets, whether at a country or organizational level, can provide useful metrics on the return on investment for human resources practices, helping organizations evaluate the effectiveness of their recruitment and retention strategies. These and other technological advances, however, require ongoing workforce training and supervision, and they present significant security and privacy concerns (e.g., threats of data breaches, risks to global supply chains) that need to be addressed.

Globally, demographic changes affect every aspect of the economy. Countries are progressing through demographic and epidemiological transitions, which present challenges associated with the aging of the population and the dual burden of communicable and noncommunicable diseases. The aging of the population has a profound effect on the types of services needed by patients, as well as the supply of health professionals. In many Western countries, for example, large segments of the nurse workforce are approaching retirement age, meaning that maintenance of appropriate workforce levels is threatened.

Organization and Management Issues

Globally, the field of healthcare operates under high levels of stress, and we can expect such conditions to continue. Contributing to this stress are the aging of the population, increased chronicity of disease, growing patient complexity, higher levels of consumer demand, and pressures to adopt expensive new technologies and achieve demanding quality goals. In many systems, quality improvement is now tied to organizational reimbursement, meaning that improvement efforts have a major impact on the organization's finances and ultimately on worker salaries. Employees, therefore, are increasingly expected to participate in ongoing quality improvement efforts, meaning that they will require relevant training in the various improvement methodologies. In sum, managers may find it increasingly challenging to recruit, motivate, and retain engaged employees in an environment where the employees are expected to do more with less, and where levels of employee compensation reflect the overall financial pressures on the organization.

Given that organizations often lack the ability to sufficiently reward employees through financial means, they will need to seek alternative methods for enhancing job satisfaction and creating a safe and optimistic work environment. At a minimum, managers—and middle managers in particular—will require training in the ways of motivating employees in the workplace. Possible strategies include job enrichment and job enlargement, where employees perform a wider range of tasks, assume greater responsibility, and, in some instances, gain greater decision-making authority. Following evidence-based strategies and the proven characteristics of high-performance work organizations, organizations should look to select employees based in part on their fit with the organization's culture and values, reward employees contingent on performance, decentralize decision making and empower self-monitoring teams where appropriate, reduce status differences among different levels of employees, enhance job security, and create a climate of psychological safety.

The present and future challenges facing the healthcare workforce highlight the need for effective management in a context of changing conditions, growing pressures, and limited resources. Managers must be competent and well trained, with the ability to manage resources of all kinds, especially human resources. The roles and expectations of managers must be clearly defined, and the individuals who assume managerial roles must be carefully selected. Furthermore, managers must receive extensive training in the ways of motivating employees, both extrinsically and intrinsically, and creating a safe environment in which professionals feel they can develop and flourish.

Future Implications of Information Technology for Global Health

Innovations in IT are transforming both the field of medicine and healthcare systems throughout the world. Although some advanced technologies are quite expensive and out of reach of many people, particularly in developing countries, lower-cost IT innovations hold great potential to improve access to care and quality outcomes for individuals everywhere (Jackson 2016). This section will discuss future implications of IT innovations on health and healthcare systems globally.

Key Drivers

Three overarching drivers are challenging healthcare and IT systems across the world: cost, access, and quality. The cost of healthcare is significant and growing. In the United States, the cost of healthcare as a percentage of the gross domestic product is predicted to increase from 17.5 percent in 2014 to 20.1 percent in 2025 (Centers for Medicare & Medicaid Services 2016). In India, healthcare costs have been identified as a leading cause of poverty (Levinson 2016). Many countries are working both individually and collaboratively to address the costly chronic diseases associated with the aging population (Deloitte 2014). Such chronic diseases are expected to increase drastically in both developing and developed countries (Deloitte 2016). The International Diabetes Federation reports that China and India have the largest numbers of people with diabetes in the world, at more than 96 million and 66 million, respectively (Deloitte 2016). The costs associated with these trends are a key factor driving the development and application of health IT globally. Health IT advances are also driven by the emphasis placed on healthcare access and quality in health reform efforts around the world (Deloitte 2014). The wealth of information generated by electronic health records, payer claims, pharmacy data, and mobile health technologies offers great opportunities for the use of "big data" to help tackle issues of cost, access, and quality in healthcare (EY 2015).

Point-of-Care Health Technologies

Dhawan and colleagues (2015) describe **point-of-care (POC) healthcare technologies** as a "paradigm shift" in global healthcare, with applicability to both wealthy and developing countries. POC technologies can be broadly defined as those technologies that improve the capability for healthcare to be provided *where the patient is* (Dhawan, personal communication, October 2016). Key elements of POC technologies include personal care and precision medicine, connected health applications, and data and analytics.

Personalized Care and Precision Medicine

Experts believe that the long-awaited personalized medicine revolution is now arriving (Van Alstin 2016; Deloitte 2016). In a Center of Digital Transformation white paper, Vitalari (2014) predicts: "By 2030, the [health] industry will move toward a structure that supports personalized medicine, which at its core is predictive and preventative, driving medical practice to be predominantly

point-of-care (POC) healthcare technology Technology that focuses on improving the capability for healthcare to be delivered where the patient is, with an emphasis on remote monitoring, diagnosis, treatment, and communication for personalized care.

precision medicine
An emerging approach for disease prevention and treatment that takes into account individual variability in genes, environment, and lifestyle.

connected health (cHealth)
A technology-enabled approach to integrated care delivery, with an emphasis on remote monitoring, diagnosis, treatment, and communication.

telehealth
The use of technology to deliver health-related services and support remotely.

mobile health (mHealth)
The delivery of health-related services via mobile electronic devices.

focused on wellness." **Precision medicine**, a closely related concept, is an emerging approach for disease prevention and treatment that takes into account individual variability in genes, environment, and lifestyle. Now that the price of personal genome sequencing has fallen, manufacturers have become increasingly focused on personalized medicine approaches. The greater availability of genetic and genomic information is expected to enable development of more effective and targeted therapies in the years ahead (EY 2015).

Connected Health Applications

Connected health (cHealth) is "digital and technology-enabled integrated care delivery that allows for remote communication, diagnosis, treatment, and monitoring" (Deloitte 2016, 18). The broad concept of cHealth encompasses **telehealth**, **mobile health (mHealth)**, electronic health records (EHRs), wearable devices, and social media. Telehealth technologies include home monitoring devices that can help reduce hospital readmissions and support independent living for people with congestive heart failure, diabetes, depression, and other chronic conditions. A 2015 survey of US healthcare consumers showed that telehealth and consultations via phone and email are increasingly recognized as acceptable care alternatives (Deloitte 2016).

Kappal and colleagues (2014) report that India has invested significant research and resources for the provision of medical services and healthcare education in rural areas via telemedicine technologies. Indeed, Asia is noted to be the fastest growing continent for the telemedicine market, with India and China leading the way (Knowledge@Wharton 2012). Mobile technology and devices are improving access to care in rural areas in Africa as well (Deloitte 2014).

Today, more than 20,000 health-related smartphone applications (apps) are available for consumers. These apps and wireless connected medical devices can provide real-time data and enable real-time interventions to support the delivery of care (Deloitte 2016). In India, for instance, the mobile service provider Airtel collaborates with Healthfore and Fortis Healthcare to allow users to access basic medical guidance about nonemergency health problems by phone; such guidance is available 24 hours a day at a cost of less than $1 per consultation (Kappal et al. 2014). India has also begun developing diabetic monitoring systems based on mobile phones. As technology has advanced, wearable bio-sensing devices have become smaller, easier to use, and less expensive, and they now allow for the convenient collection and communication of critical health information such as blood pressure, glucose levels, and heart rate (Szczerba 2014). As adoption rates continue to climb, experts have predicted that telemedicine will be a $38 billion global market by 2025 (Vaidya 2017).

The growing emphasis on population health (as discussed in chapter 13) is driving the need for integrated electronic records across multiple health and social care providers. The National Health Service in England, for instance, set out to have interoperable electronic health records accessible by patients by 2018 and is expected to be paperless by 2020 (Deloitte 2016). In Turkey, infrastructure was completed for the establishment of a health information system covering all health services and all actors across the health system (Akinci et al. 2012). Mexico is implementing EHR systems in both public and private hospitals, and China is rapidly piloting and exploring health IT applications as a key part of its reform efforts (Deloitte 2014). In addition, social media channels are expected to generate significant healthcare data and play an important role in connecting patients with providers in new ways (EY 2015).

Data and Analytics
Data and analytics represent one of the key investment areas for health systems and IT infrastructure. With the changes in the ways health systems are paid and expected to deliver care, healthcare analytics takes on growing importance (Deloitte 2016). Forecasters have predicted that the global healthcare analytics market will expand with a 12.5 percent compound annual growth rate between 2017 and 2023 (BusinessWire 2018). Raghupathi and Raghupathi (2014) point out that big data analytics has the potential to improve care, save lives, and lower costs by discovering and understanding the patterns, trends, and underlying associations within large data sets.

Roles of Key Stakeholders
All relevant stakeholders—including patients, care providers, public and private payers, healthcare managers, and policymakers—must be willing to work together to optimize the use of POC technologies to improve the overall health status of the populations served. As patients become more empowered with information, they should assume greater responsibility for their own health. Both public and private payers should develop innovative programs to educate patients about the potential benefits of POC technologies.

Sustainability
The successful use of IT innovations for global health will depend on the development of sustainable business models and incentive structures that emphasize value. The full implementation of POC technologies requires the investment of significant resources, which can be an obstacle both for developing countries that have existing IT infrastructure gaps and developed countries that struggle with rapidly growing healthcare expenditures. Therefore, decision makers will likely need clear evidence of return on investment before taking action. Dhawan and colleagues (2015) emphasize that the POC technologies "do not exist in isolation and must be integrated into and adopted by new or existing health services delivery models, be supported by sound business cases, and show demonstrated levels of improvement to patient health outcomes."

Future Opportunities and Challenges

Without question, ongoing technological advances have a profound global effect on healthcare. From the simple use of mobile phones as medical imaging devices to the more advanced application of 3D printers to manufacture prostheses, drugs, or even organs, IT will continue to play a vital role in expanding health systems' capabilities in the years ahead. For the latest technological innovations to result in the desired transformational change, however, every nation needs to address such critical issues as the interoperability of data structures, data security, patient privacy, provider compliance, and active patient engagement.

From Medical Tourism to Globalization of Health Services

The practice of medical tourism—that is, the process of traveling to a distant location to obtain medical care—is growing and evolving. Patients Beyond Borders (2017), an organization that collects and reports data about medical tourism, estimates that the medical tourism market size has grown to as much as $72 billion, with 15 million patients worldwide. Estimates of the number of US travelers expected to travel internationally in a given year for the purpose of receiving medical care is estimated at 1.4 million. Other estimates have been even higher. Bartold (2014, 279) has described medical tourism as "a global industry of around $100 billion and growing at the rate of 20–30% per annum."

Medical tourism is typically regarded as an international practice, though it may also occur between different areas of a single country. For instance, many people in the United States travel across state lines to obtain care at centers of excellence such as MD Anderson, the Mayo Clinic, and the Cleveland Clinic. Research suggests that such travel pays off: People in the United States were found to have a 71 percent lower risk of dying and a 65 percent lower risk of complications at hospitals with a rating of five stars than they do at hospitals with a rating of one star (Healthgrades 2016). Medical tourism is most common across three major categories of services: invasive or surgical, diagnostic testing, and lifestyle (Burns, Jayaram, and Bansal 2014).

The Emergence of Medical Tourism

The rise of medical tourism reflects an increasingly global marketplace for healthcare services. Although services account for only about one-fifth of global trade, they have represented the fastest growing component of international trade since the 1980s. The ease of travel and **neoliberal economic policies** for services—such as the privatization of healthcare, state subsidies to private-sector providers, and reduced restrictions on foreign direct investment—have contributed to the development of this market (Burns, Jayaram, and Bansal 2014). These economic policies were strengthened with the introduction of

neoliberal economic policies
Economic policies that favor free-market capitalism with minimal government intervention.

the General Agreement on Trade in Services (GATS), which came into force for member nations of the World Trade Organization (WTO) in 1995 (Burns, Jayaram, and Bansal 2014; WTO 2018). The GATS identifies four modes of service delivery in international trade: (1) cross-border supply of services, aided by technology; (2) consumption of services abroad; (3) establishment of commercial activity in another country; and (4) temporary movement of professionals to deliver services across borders (Burns, Jayaram, and Bansal 2014). Typically, medical tourism is thought of in terms of the first two modes—in other words, consumers are seeking quality care in distant destinations. However, the third and fourth modes are developing as well, with health organizations globalizing their services and going to international consumers.

Medical tourism can increase the flow of foreign currency, support local economies through tourist spending, slow down the "brain drain" of medical professionals moving elsewhere, help with the development and maintenance of medical and surgical subspecialties, and promote the development of sophisticated medical technology and delivery infrastructure (Burns, Jayaram, and Bansal 2014). It can also encourage changes in government policy with regard to foreign direct investment and tariff levels to enable greater modernization.

Although trade policies and ease of travel have been critical to the growth of medical tourism, changes in consumerism have also played a role. Consumers, via the internet and other means, are generally becoming more adept at searching for value in health services. They typically look for a balance of price, quality, and service, requiring health services organizations to compete over how they address this value proposition (Burns, Jayaram, and Bansal 2014). In the face of medical cost inflation in the United States, both private payers (e.g., employers) and public payers (e.g., Medicare) have been requiring enrollees to take on more of the cost burden, whether through higher deductibles or higher copays, and this shift has heightened consumers' sensitivity to the price dimension (Burns, Jayaram, and Bansal 2014). Similar issues with cost inflation and consumer sensitivity are happening worldwide.

Often, surgical and other procedures at international medical tourism destinations are performed by top physicians with improved hospital stay conditions for a fraction of what the cost would be at home. For example, medical care in countries such as Thailand, India, and Singapore—all of which rank among the top medical tourism destinations (Patients Beyond Borders 2017)—can cost as little as 10 to 20 percent of the equivalent care in the United States; these costs may even include airfare and accommodations at five-star hotels. In general, the cost of building and maintaining high-quality patient care centers is substantially lower internationally than in the United States, in large part because of lower labor costs, lack of unions, less expensive technologies, and lower-cost materials used in construction. With regard to labor costs, for example, a new nursing graduate in a medical tourism hospital in India generally earns $3,600 to $4,200 a year, and an experienced nurse specialist in the intensive care unit earns around $15,000; in both cases, these salaries are 10 to 20 percent of the US rate (Burns, Jayaram, and Bansal 2014).

To ensure quality and service, many hospitals seek international accreditation. The Joint Commission, which accredits and certifies healthcare organizations and programs in the United States, has an international branch, the Joint Commission International, that accredits international hospitals. Many international providers also seek to demonstrate quality through partnerships with top medical academic centers. For instance, Harvard University and Mayo Clinic have partnered with University Hospital in Dubai's Healthcare City, and Johns Hopkins Medicine International has partnered with the Apollo Group Hospitals in India (Burns, Jayaram, and Bansal 2014). The partnering institutions typically share best practices and rotate faculty between the facilities.

To be a successful medical tourism destination, a hospital needs to have excellent processes of care, highly trained providers, strong IT capabilities, state-of-the-art medical equipment, and the necessary accreditations. Hospitals should consider augmenting their medical and nursing staffs with professionals who have international training or service exposure. Hospitals may also try to attract patients through enhanced infrastructure and administration capabilities, including high-quality hotel and concierge services (e.g., translators, assistance with travel plans).

Full Globalization of Health Services

As the international provision of health and medical services has expanded, the term *medical tourism* no longer fully represents what is happening. The larger trend is the overall globalization of health services. Medical tourism has typically included services in such areas as cardiology, orthopedic and bariatric surgery, organ transplantation, cosmetic surgery, in vitro fertilization, eye surgery, and dental reconstruction. Today, however, many nations are seeking international assistance in treatments that require extensive follow-up or repeat procedures, such as chemotherapy or radiation, as well as in the development of private senior care, especially for people with chronic mental illnesses such as Alzheimer's disease. These longer-term care needs have led many nations to host the development of Western hospital care.

The globalization of health services is shaped by a variety of push and pull factors. One pull factor involves the willingness of nations to bring in outside interests in an attempt to limit the loss of large numbers of high-paying patients who might travel elsewhere for health services. In China, for instance, people took an estimated 500,000 outbound medical trips in 2016, representing a 500 percent increase from the prior year (Wee 2017). Nations may also welcome international assistance in an attempt to limit the loss of health professionals who might move to other nations that have higher levels of health services and better compensation. In other cases, nations might be motivated by the need to head off increasing morbidity and mortality from particular illnesses.

A major push factor is the desire of leading-edge health services corporations to scale up their operations and seek foreign markets for their services. A number of major US research institutions—including Duke University, Johns Hopkins University, and the University of Pittsburgh Medical Center (UPMC)—have pursued new markets and sought an international branding of their name. For example, UPMC has established partnerships with multiple teaching hospitals around China (Burns, Jayaram, and Bansal 2014), and Colorado-based DaVita Kidney Care (2018) now has kidney dialysis centers in eleven nations. Organizations around the world are pursuing similar strategies. Parkway Hospitals Singapore, for instance, now has hospitals in a number of Asian and Middle Eastern nations.

The leading organizations do not consider these international partnerships as unique, one-time events. Instead, they recognize that far-reaching international opportunities exist and that healthcare, a traditionally domestic-based service industry, has indeed begun to globalize. As a result, an organization such as MD Anderson is competing for providers, research money, patients, and status not just with similar institutions in the United States; it is competing with oncology centers around the world.

Establishing hospitals in other nations requires all of the capabilities described in our discussion of medical tourism, plus more. For example, the hospital needs to have a strategy team that can accurately assess which foreign markets it is best suited to enter. Once a market or two have been identified, the hospital needs to consider the mode of entry—for instance, whether it will be through clinical services, research/teaching, or a partnership or greenfield venture. Partnerships with local hospitals or medical centers are common and sometimes required by government. However, due diligence needs to be given to the benefits and risks of potential partners. For example, a local hospital partner in China might help an organization navigate the bureaucratic maze of government regulations, better understand the nuances of Chinese business conversations, and guide the hospital administration through the multitude of inspections. On the other hand, the partner might present a variety of risks and potential problems related to a clash of cultures or languages, unrealized expectations, or the surrender of control or corporate sovereignty. Probably the biggest obstacle to overcome involves the capability of local human resources to staff and manage an international hospital facility. Budget plans will need to account for expatriate assignments and initial and ongoing training for locals.

Valuing Women's Health from a Holistic Perspective

The health needs of women have changed dramatically over the past few decades, in line with epidemiological transition. Historically, women's health has been spoken of in terms of prenatal care, childbirth, undernourishment, and infectious diseases. Recently, however, increasing attention has shifted to additional conditions that affect the health of women globally, including obesity, diabetes, cardiovascular disease, stroke, cancer, mental illness, and injury (Langer et al. 2015). The rise in incidence of these mainly chronic conditions, with most directly attributable to changes in lifestyle, is occurring in countries of all levels of income; however, the changes are especially rapid in low- and middle-income countries (LMICs) (Bustreo et al. 2012).

Women between the ages of 15 and 49 experienced about 300,000 deaths during childbirth in 2015—a figure that reflects a 44 percent reduction in maternal mortality rate since 1990 (Alkema et al. 2016; Knaul et al. 2016). In contrast, an estimated 508,000 women per year die from breast cancer (WHO 2018a), and 270,000 die from cervical cancer (WHO 2018b). Still others die from diabetes and other chronic diseases. In other words, deaths from chronic and noncommunicable diseases now far outstrip the number of deaths of women attributable to childbirth (Knaul et al. 2016). Deaths from cervical cancer and many other conditions are particularly prevalent among women in LMICs (Bustreo et al. 2012).

Women face an undue burden in many respects. Women's health is too often focused on a woman's reproductive capacity and reproduction-related ailments, instead of on her overall health (Alsan et al. 2016). A broader framework for women's health is therefore both an ethical obligation and a public health imperative (Knaul et al. 2016). For women, stigma often surrounds chronic diseases, such as cancers, that affect their reproductive capacity. Feelings of shame associated with reproductive cancers and fears of becoming an outcast to society—or even to one's own family—can negatively affect utilization of health screening services, thereby threatening the well-being of a patient. In Latin America, more than 50 percent of cancers in women are found in later stages of the disease (American Cancer Society 2017; Flores-Luna et al. 2008; Justo et al. 2013). These and other women's health issues take on added importance and greater complexity when one considers women's contributions to caregiving and other social, economic, and environmental aspects of overall population health (Langer et al. 2015).

What are the causal factors that explain the challenges to women's health in LMICs? One of the key issues is access. Globally, poor health outcomes for women—especially in areas where social and economic inequalities are prevalent—are largely tied to availability of services, lack of healthcare coverage, travel distance to health clinics, and the quality of care received upon reaching the clinic. A variety of strategies related to human resources, organization of care, financing, resource generation, delivery science, and stewardship have potential to address these concerns about access, leading to improved health outcomes (Althabe et al. 2008; Peters et al. 2008). The use of community health workers to bring care closer to home, for instance, has proved effective in numerous settings (Gilmore and McAuliffe 2013). Other improvements and innovations—such as enhanced transportation services and initiatives to reduce waiting times—have shown similar promise. Through systems innovations, Rwanda experienced a reduction in maternal mortality of 6 percent annually between 1990 and 2015; Cambodia, using similar concepts, saw a reduction of 7.4 percent per year over the same period (Alkema et al. 2016; Bucagu et al. 2012).

Still, larger questions must be asked about why the current framework on women's health exists and how a shift can be made to improve access, quality, and outcomes for women. The traditional value proposition is that Value = Quality / Cost. This equation is a major concept in modern healthcare management, and it suggests that the value of healthcare can be increased by improving quality, by reducing costs, or both. The value of cancer prevention and treatment, for example, is significantly reduced if services are delayed, because later-stage cancers are associated with worse health outcomes and lower quality of life, along with higher costs. The traditional value proposition is useful from a resource allocation perspective; however, it fails to fully account for societal values related to health. In particular, the value of women's health in society must be better understood and integrated into the equation.

Typically, when a woman's health is negatively affected, so is the health of the family. In turn, the productivity and income of the family are reduced, affecting the community's economy and, ultimately, the country's gross domestic product. The problem eventually comes full circle, as funding shortfalls compromise provision of government-supported medical services, causing health to deteriorate further. A public discourse—not just among health system managers but across society as a whole—is therefore needed to better appreciate the value of health across population groups, particularly among women whose holistic care has too often been neglected. Women's health should be approached not simply as an issue for the individual or the family, but rather as a national and global issue. A reconceptualization of value, now with a wider purview, is essential for addressing the current challenges facing women's health.

Hospital Administration in Poorer Nations

More than half of the seven billion people on the planet live on less than $2 per day, and most are in resource-poor environments where health services are either in disarray or nonexistent. In many cases, weak administrative and management systems have led to demand displacement, causing district and other hospitals to serve as primary care units for many, with duplication of work and inefficient use of resources. Problems caused by a lack of funding are compounded by poor policy planning, lack of basic equipment and adequate drugs, and staffs that are demoralized, overwhelmed, and inadequately trained. In these settings, even people who can afford to pay are not guaranteed high-quality services.

In some less developed nations, more than 50 percent of the population have never had access to care from a health professional or been to a clinic or hospital. Also, within a country, a tremendous dichotomy often exists between hospital capabilities in urban areas and in rural areas. In Haiti, for example, only 25 percent of childbirths in rural areas occur in health facilities, and many of those facilities lack key resources (Partners in Health 2014). Countrywide, only 37 percent of Haiti's childbirths occur under the care of a skilled attendant (UN Population Fund 2015). As a result, Haiti has the highest maternal mortality rate in the Western Hemisphere. Given the general lack of health services and the disarray of facilities in many areas, sound management of the services that do exist is especially important in poorer nations.

Moving Forward

Many believe that economic growth is necessary for health improvement in poorer nations. However, research indicates that many poorer nations—especially nations with strong governance and political commitment—are able to build resilience into health systems in the face of political unrest, economic crises, and natural disasters. Such efforts can, in turn, foster institutional and experiential memory and enhance the ability to innovate and adapt to resource limitations.

Cuba—which has 11 million people and a per capita income of $7,602, in US dollars (World Bank 2018a)—provides an example of a poorer nation that has demonstrated institutional stability and political commitment for a strong health system. Despite limited finances and little to no external support from civil society, the nation has world-class research and teaching hospitals in Havana and Santiago and at least one research/teaching hospital and medical school in every province. Cuba's infrastructure of hospitals is complemented by a population health and primary care model centered around "consultorios," which are physician and nurse teams assigned to a local population of families. On average, a consultorio is responsible for about 600 people. The community health outreach provided by consultorios, accompanied by a strong clinic and hospital system, has enabled Cuba to attain life expectancies and infant and mortality rates that are the envy of the developing world and comparable to those of the wealthiest of nations.

structural adjustment policy
A program in which a developing country receives a loan that is tied to its adoption of certain market-oriented adjustments or reforms.

Since the 1980s, poverty, debt, and **structural adjustment policies** have led many developing countries to decrease public expenditure on healthcare and health facilities. In countries where neoliberal economic ideology prevails, health is considered a private commodity that should be left to the market rather than the state. In many cases, market provision in poorer nations has led to a two-tier system, with expensive private hospitals that are unaffordable for the poor and underfunded public hospitals that the poor can access. Many people have hoped that civil society, in the form of nongovernmental organizations (NGOs), will step in to help fill the service gap between the two tiers.

Indeed, many developing nations have seen a proliferation of NGOs that provide health services, especially since the introduction of structural adjustment policies. In some cases, this development has been extreme. Haiti, for instance, has been called an "NGO republic" because a large majority of its hospital beds are owned and managed by external entities. A heavy reliance on NGO-based services often leads to fragmentation of health services and places excessive burdens on health ministries and public hospitals that need to direct and coordinate the aid. In some instances, NGOs that become frustrated by an inefficient and ineffective public sector decide to channel their efforts into parallel programs that further undermine the existing public health system.

In 2009, the WHO began a health systems strengthening (HSS) initiative, highlighting the need for better coordination of health system resources for sustained improvement in fragile nations such as Haiti. The HSS initiative has stressed the importance of primary care and helped make large global health organizations—such as the Global Fund to Fight AIDS, Tuberculosis and Malaria—increasingly willing to support and fund health system development. Primary care and community-based initiatives had previously been acknowledged in the Alma-Ata Declaration of 1978 as keys to the goal of "health for all" (WHO 2018d).

The HSS initiative and other developments—including an NGO Code of Conduct—have contributed to an increase in public–private partnerships whereby local government policies and activities are reinforced by the efforts of NGOs. Generally, the hope is that private ventures will become more empathetic and better coordinated with public needs and system goals and that public ventures will continue to learn from the advanced care management techniques and procedures that NGOs often provide.

Resource-poor environments generally have few professionally trained hospital managers available, and the administration role is often done on a rotating basis by clinical professionals. Thus, knowledge of management systems at a hospital may be limited or even totally lacking. In such instances, basic management education should be provided at the beginning of an administrator's tour of duty, and continuing education and tool kit resources should be made available in the following months. Ideally, administrators should learn project management skills early on, so that they have the ability to frame a problem, consider the resources needed and possible interventions, and then monitor and evaluate the effectiveness of an intervention. Familiarity with basic project management processes will add a scientific management orientation to the various functional components that the administrator will oversee.

The knowledge and experience needed to manage the functional areas of a hospital in a low-resource setting may be relatively basic in comparison to the knowledge required for those areas in a modern Western hospital. However, the area of knowledge to be learned and practiced in low-resource settings may be much wider in scope. Indeed, hospital administrators in poorer nations may need to oversee most all management activities in a hospital. Fortunately, a number of resources are available to help. Management Sciences for Health (MSH), for instance, offers a "Managers Who Lead Toolkit" to provide guidance for new administrators in such areas as clinical services and quality management, financial management, organizational sustainability, organizational strategy and planning, information management, human resources management, community health services, drug and supply management, and leadership development (MSH 2018). Additional resources are available from the International Hospital Federation (2015), Partners in Health (Mura and Holman 2011), and other organizations.

Hospital managers in poorer nations also need to understand the vital support role of a community health worker system, which provides education and preventive care at homes and in villages away from the hospital. A robust CHW system can benefit both poorer and wealthier populations. By decentralizing care and preventive health, such a system can reduce the likelihood that hospitals will become overwhelmed with patient care demands. A variety of tool kits—including one from the US Agency for International Development / Maternal and Child Health Integrated Program (2013)—are available to help with the management of CHWs.

Another major challenge for hospital administrators in low-resource environments involves finding, retaining, and managing a sufficient number of qualified health professionals. Indeed, the dearth of doctors and nurses in poorer nations might be the biggest impediment to the provision of good health services. The WHO maintains that a minimum of 2.3 doctors, nurses, and midwives should be available per 1,000 people in a population. Based on this standard, the nations of Liberia, Sierra Leone, Guinea, and Guinea-Bissau were ill equipped—by 9,020 doctors and 37,059 nurses/midwives (Kamal-Yanni 2015)—to provide care during the Ebola crisis of 2014–2015.

A major reason that qualified health professionals often leave poorer nations for more developed nations—or go from rural to urban areas, or from public to private hospitals—is that they are attracted by higher salaries. To compensate for the higher salaries elsewhere, hospital administrators in poorer and rural areas should seek, to the extent possible, to attract and retain doctors and nurses through good working and living conditions, valuable community experiences, supplemental salary opportunities, and continued training opportunities (WHO 2010).

A Global Perspective on Poverty

The WHO (2017) states: "Poverty is associated with the undermining of a range of key human attributes, including health. The poor are exposed to greater personal and environmental health risks, are less well nourished, have less information and are less able to access health care; they thus have a higher risk of illness and disability. Conversely, illness can reduce household savings, lower learning ability, reduce productivity, and lead to a diminished quality of life, thereby perpetuating or even increasing poverty."

For many years, the World Bank has used a global **poverty line** to measure the number of people living in poverty. For many years, people living on the equivalent of $1 a day were considered to be living in poverty. Over time, the poverty line has risen, first to $1.25 a day and, in 2015, to $1.90 (Roser and Ortiz-Ospina 2017). This poverty measurement is based on the monetary value of a person's consumption, and it is based in international dollars—the amount needed to buy goods and services equivalent to what a US dollar would buy in the United States (World Bank 2018b). For countries where reliable measures of consumption are not available, measurements of poverty may be based on income (Roser and Ortiz-Ospina 2017).

poverty line
A measurement of the monetary value of people's consumption, used to determine the number of people living in poverty.

The World Bank (2017) estimates that, in 2013, 767 million people were living in poverty, based on the $1.90 per day standard. Regions with the highest levels of poverty, ranked from most severe to less severe, include sub-Saharan Africa, South Asia, Pacific East Asia, Latin America and the Caribbean, North Africa and the Middle East, and Europe and Central Asia (Meade 2013).

Poverty is often defined in absolute terms of low income, but, in reality, it encompasses a number of factors. The WHO Commission on Social Determinants of Health (2008, 31) states that "Poverty is not only lack of income" and that efforts to address poverty should include "those at the bottom of the distribution of global and national wealth, those marginalized and excluded within countries, and countries themselves disadvantaged by historical exploitation and persistent inequity." The commission describes a **social gradient in health**—a link between socioeconomic position and health—that is apparent globally, across low-, middle-, and high-income countries. Most experts agree that poverty should be approached not just in terms of pure economic data but also in terms of political and cultural factors, people's quality of life, and people's access to education and opportunities (Meade 2013).

social gradient in health
The link, evident throughout the world, between socioeconomic status and health.

In 2013, the World Bank adopted two ambitious goals: (1) to "end global extreme poverty" and (2) to "promote shared prosperity in every country in a sustainable way." The World Bank Group (2016, 1) explains: "This implies reducing the poverty headcount ratio from 10.7 percent globally in 2013 to 3.0 percent by 2030 and fostering the growth in the income or the consumption expenditure of the poorest 40 percent of the population (the bottom 40) in each country." These two goals are closely related to the UN's Sustainable Development Goals—specifically, number 1 ("No Poverty") and number 10 ("Reduced Inequalities")—already adopted by the global community (World Bank Group 2016; UN 2018).

Despite decades of progress in reducing poverty, significant inequalities remain. Such inequalities not only raise issues of fairness and justice; they also carry a high financial cost, affect economic growth, and create social and political barriers (World Bank Group 2016). The World Bank Group (2016, 2) states: "Generally speaking, poverty can be reduced through higher average growth, a narrowing in inequality, or a combination of the two." Hence, the goal of ending extreme poverty by 2030 "might not be achieved without accelerated economic growth or reductions in within-country inequalities, especially among those countries with large concentrations of the poor" (World Bank Group 2016, 2).

In economies for which detailed information about income distribution is available, within-country inequalities continue to be apparent. In fact, in such nations as Argentina, China, India, South Africa, South Korea, Taiwan, and the United States, the share of national income held by the top 1 percent has been increasing, not decreasing. In South Africa, the top income share roughly doubled between 1990 and 2010 (World Bank Group 2016).

Poverty is often a controversial subject. People hold different ideas about what it means to be poor and about how the problems associated with poverty should be resolved (Meade 2013). Substantial improvements have been made on some levels—notably, the World Bank (2017) points out, "Even as the world's population has grown, the number of poor has gradually fallen." In 1990, nearly 4 out of every 10 people globally were living below the poverty line of $1.90 per day; that number had fallen to just over 1 in 10 by 2013 (World Bank 2017). Nonetheless, poverty remains a serious and complex problem with multiple layers that affect many millions of people around the world (Meade 2013).

Summary

In this chapter, we have identified a number of global problems, challenges, and opportunities that healthcare managers will need to address if they hope to support healthy populations in the present day and the years ahead. Sections of this chapter have dealt specifically with the future of the pharmaceutical industry, the global spread of communicable disease, the threats posed by violence and crime in healthcare settings, and the shift toward increasingly consumer-directed care. The chapter has also discussed a variety of issues related to workforce management and advances in health-related technology. Finally, the chapter has examined medical tourism and the increasingly global nature of health services, with a particular focus on areas with high levels of poverty and inequality.

Global health cannot be perceived as a tangent field that one only experiences when traveling abroad. Rather, today's health landscape involves a global exchange of people, information, technology, and—unfortunately—illness and disease, and it requires healthcare managers who can learn, develop, and apply the appropriate competencies to achieve positive outcomes and promote the health and well-being of society.

Discussion Questions

1. What are some key current trends in the global health workforce? Identify some future challenges, and provide strategies for addressing those challenges.
2. What are some strategies for improving women's health in low-income countries?
3. What are some implications of poverty for global health?
4. Why do healthcare managers who are responsible for the health of specific regional service areas need to be aware of and prepared for global health events?
5. Identify at least five core competencies that managers in healthcare organizations need to develop. Why do you think these competencies will improve global population health?

Vignette: Oncology Care in China

Cancer is responsible for an estimated 374.1 deaths per 100,000 person years, making it the country's leading cause of death (Yao et al. 2016). In 2015, China had about 4.3 million new cancer cases and more than 2.8 million cancer deaths (Chen et al. 2016). Roughly 12,000 new cancer diagnoses are made every day.

The Chinese government initiated health reform in 2009. It invested a tremendous amount of money into health infrastructure development and training, and it began basic universal insurance coverage. Government funding for the health budget increased by about 16.5 percent per year from 2009 to 2015, and much of the money went toward the development of Western allopathic care practices to go alongside traditional Chinese medicine. The increased spending has been helpful, but it has not been enough to contain the country's cancer epidemic. Experts believe that China

(continued)

struggles to provide the physical capacity and health provider capacity to manage cancer care at the level required.

Like many nations, China is trying to catch up with leading cancer treatments and increase facility capacity. The nation is also trying to attract oncologists internationally and also keep its own oncologists from traveling to other countries. As part of its effort to attract international oncology expertise, the Chinese government has been extremely welcoming to American medical centers—such as the MD Anderson Cancer Center—wishing to venture into China. In early 2015, at an event attended by Chinese President Xi Jinping, Premier Li Keqiang, and Vice Premier Liu Yandong, MD Anderson received China's top science and technology award for its partnership programs with Chinese institutions focused on training, education, and patient care (MD Anderson 2015). Collaborations have been particularly productive in the areas of cancer screening, liver and lung cancer treatment, and cooperation in clinical trials and other research. Chinese "sister institutions" working with MD Anderson include the Chinese Academy of Medical Sciences Cancer Institute and Hospital in Beijing, Tianjin Medical University Cancer Institute and Hospital, Fudan University Shanghai Cancer Center, and the Sir YK Pao Centre for Cancer at the Chinese University of Hong Kong (MD Anderson 2015).

In addition, IBM (2016) announced that it is making its Watson computer system available to 21 Chinese hospitals, with the aim of helping Chinese physicians to "personalize cancer care." A partnership between IBM and Hangzhou CognitiveCare will center around a cognitive computing platform for oncology care that was developed in conjunction with Memorial Sloan Kettering physicians. A central goal of the partnership is to help Chinese oncologists stay up to date about best practices in cancer treatment.

References

Akinci, F., S. Mollahaliloglu, H. Gursoz, and F. Ogucu. 2012. "Assessment of the Turkish Health Care System Reforms: A Stakeholder Analysis." *Health Policy* 107 (1): 21–30.

Alkema, L., D. Chou, D. Hogan, S. Zhang, A.-B. Moller, A. Gemmill, D. M. Fat, T. Boerma, M. Temmerman, C. Mathers, and L. Say. 2016. "Global, Regional, and National Levels and Trends in Maternal Mortality Between 1990 and 2015, with Scenario-Based Projections to 2030: A Systematic Analysis by the UN Maternal Mortality Estimation Inter-Agency Group." *Lancet* 387 (10017): 462–74.

Alsan, M., A. Bhadelia, P. Foo, C. Haberland, and F. Knaul. 2016. "The Economics of Women's Health in Low- and Middle-Income Countries: A Life Cycle

Approach." In *World Scientific Handbook of Global Health Economics and Public Policy: The Economics of Health and Health Systems*, vol. 2, edited by R. M. Scheffler, 397–432. Hackensack, NJ: World Scientific Publishing.

Althabe, F., E. Bergel, M. L. Cafferata, L. Gibbons, A. Ciapponi, A. Alemán, L. Colantonio, and A. R. Palacios. 2008. "Strategies for Improving the Quality of Health Care in Maternal and Child Health in Low- and Middle-Income Countries: An Overview of Systematic Reviews." *Paediatric and Perinatal Epidemiology* 22 (Suppl. 1): 42–60.

American Cancer Society. 2017. *The Cancer Atlas*. Accessed May 22. http://canceratlas. cancer.org/the-burden/cancer-in-latin-america-and-caribbean/.

Barnsteiner, J. 2011. "Teaching the Culture of Safety." *Online Journal of Issues in Nursing*. Published September 30. http://ojin.nursingworld.org/MainMenu Categories/ANAMarketplace/ANAPeriodicals/OJIN/TableofContents/Vol-16-2011/No3-Sept-2011/Teaching-and-Safety.html.

Bartold, P. M. 2014. "Medical Tourism—An Established Problem." *Australian Dental Journal* 59 (3): 279.

Bucagu, M., J. M. Kagubare, P. Basinga, F. Ngabo, B. K. Timmons, and A. C. Lee. 2012. "Impact of Health Systems Strengthening on Coverage of Maternal Health Services in Rwanda, 2000–2010: A Systematic Review." *Reproductive Health Matters* 20 (39): 50–61.

Buchbinder, S. 2014a. "Teaching About Violence in Healthcare Settings." *Jones & Bartlett Learning Health Blog*. Published February 3. http://blogs.jblearning. com/health/2014/02/03/2376/.

———. 2014b. "Truth in Advertising: Human Trafficking in Southeast Asia." *Islamic Monthly*. Published September 9. http://theislamicmonthly.com/ truth-in-advertising-human-trafficking-in-southeast.

Buchbinder, S. B., and N. H. Shanks. 2017. *Introduction to Health Care Management*, 3rd ed. Burlington, MA: Jones & Bartlett Learning.

Burns, L. R., P. Jayaram, and R. Bansal. 2014. "Medical Tourism: Opportunities and Challenges." In *India's Healthcare Industry: Innovation in Delivery, Financing, and Manufacturing*, edited by L. R. Burns, 219–289. Delhi, India: Cambridge University Press.

BusinessWire. 2018. "Healthcare Analytics Market 2015–2018—Global Forecasts to 2023." Published April 26. www.businesswire.com/news/home/20180426006687/ en/Healthcare-Analytics-Market-2015-2018---Global-Forecasts.

Bustreo, F., F. M. Knaul, A. Bhadelia, J. Beard, and I. Araujo de Carvalho. 2012. "Women's Health Beyond Reproduction: Meeting the Challenges." *Bulletin of the World Health Organization*. Published July. www.who.int/bulletin/ volumes/90/7/12-103549/en/.

Callahan, D. 2012. *The Roots of Bioethics: Health, Progress, Technology, Death*. New York: Oxford University Press.

Centers for Disease Control and Prevention (CDC). 2006. "Bioterrorism Overview." Published February 28. https://emergency.cdc.gov/bioterrorism/pdf/bioterrorism_ overview.pdf.

Centers for Medicare & Medicaid Services (CMS). 2016. "National Health Expenditure Projections, 2015–2025." Accessed July 12, 2018. www.cms.gov/Research-Statistics-Data-and-Systems/Statistics-Trends-and-Reports/NationalHealth ExpendData/Downloads/Proj2015.pdf.

Chen, W., R. Zheng, P. D. Baade, S. Zhang, H. Zeng, F. Bray, and A. Jemal. 2016. "Cancer Statistics in China, 2015." *CA: A Cancer Journal for Clinicians.* Published January 25. https://onlinelibrary.wiley.com/doi/full/10.3322/caac.21338.

Christensen Institute. 2018. "Disruptive Innovation." Accessed July 12. www.christensen institute.org /key-concepts/disruptive-innovation-2/.

Cowles, D. 2011. "Who Killed Consumer-Directed Health Care?" *Employee Benefit News.* Published September 1. www.benefitnews.com/news/who-killed-consumer-directed-health-care.

DaVita Kidney Care. 2018. "About DaVita Inc." Accessed July 25. www.davita.com/about.

Deloitte. 2016. *2016 Global Health Care Outlook: Battling Costs While Improving Care.* Accessed July 12, 2018. www2.deloitte.com/content/dam/Deloitte/global/Documents/Life-Sciences-Health-Care/gx-lshc-2016-health-care-outlook.pdf.

———. 2014. *2014 Global Health Care Outlook: Shared Challenges, Shared Opportunities.* Accessed July 12, 2018. www2.deloitte.com/content/dam/Deloitte/global/Documents/Life-Sciences-Health-Care/dttl-lshc-2014-global-health-care-sector-report.pdf.

Dhawan, A. P., W. J. Heetderks, M. Pavel, S. Acharya, M. Akay, A. Mairal, B. Wheeler, C. C. Dacso, T. Sunder, N. Lovell, M. Gerber, M. Shah, S. G. Senthilvel, M. D. Wang, and B. Bhargava. 2015. "Current and Future Challenges in Point-of-Care Technologies: A Paradigm Shift in Affordable Global Healthcare with Personalized and Preventive Medicine." *IEEE Journal of Translational Engineering in Health and Medicine.* Published March 5. https://ieeexplore.ieee.org/stamp/stamp.jsp?arnumber=7057715.

Duhart, D. T. 2001. *Violence in the Workplace, 1993–99.* Bureau of Justice Statistics, US Department of Justice. Published December. www.bjs.gov/content/pub/pdf/vw99.pdf.

Ehrhardt, M. 2015. "Is Pharma Ready for the Future?" *Strategy + Business.* Published November 30. www.strategy-business.com/article/00363.

Emergency Nurses Association (ENA). 2010. *ENA Workplace Violence Toolkit.* Accessed July 18, 2018. www.ena.org/docs/default-source/resource-library/practice-resources/toolkits/workplaceviolencetoolkit.pdf.

EY. 2015. *Megatrends 2015: Making Sense of a World in Motion.* Accessed September 10, 2016. www.ey.com/Publication/vwLUAssets/ey-megatrends-report-2015/%24FILE/ey-megatrends-report-2015.pdf.

Flores-Luna, L., E. Salazar-Martinez, R. M. Duarte-Torres, G. Torres-Mejía, P. Alonso-Ruiz, and E. Lazcano-Ponce. 2008. "Prognostic Factors Related to Breast Cancer Survival." *Salud Publica de Mexico* 50 (2): 119–25.

Fraher, E. P., and M. Morrison. 2015. "Workforce Planning in a Rapidly Changing Healthcare System." In *Human Resources in Healthcare: Managing for Success*, 4th ed., edited by B. J. Fried and M. D. Fottler, 427–54. Chicago: Health Administration Press.

Gilmore, B., and E. McAuliffe. 2013. "Effectiveness of Community Health Workers Delivering Preventive Interventions for Maternal and Child Health in Low- and Middle-Income Countries: A Systematic Review." *BMC Public Health* 13: 847.

Hauser, A., and M. Castillo. 2013. "A Heavy Toll for the Victims of Human Trafficking." CNN. Published August 26. www.cnn.com/2013/08/25/us/miami-sex-trafficking/index.html.

Healthgrades. 2016. *Healthgrades 2017 Report to the Nation*. Accessed July 24, 2018. www.healthgrades.com/quality/healthgrades-2017-report-to-the-nation.

Holmes, G. M., M. Morrison, D. E. Pathman, and E. Fraher. 2013. "The Contribution of 'Plasticity' to Modeling How a Community's Need for Health Care Services Can Be Met by Different Configurations of Physicians." *Academic Medicine* 88 (12): 1877–82.

IBM. 2016. "21 Hospitals Across China to Adopt Watson for Oncology to Help Physicians Personalize Cancer Care." Published August 11. www-03.ibm.com/press/us/en/pressrelease/50346.wss.

International Hospital Federation (IHF). 2015. *Leadership Competencies for Healthcare Services Managers*. Accessed July 12, 2018. www.ihf-fih.org/resources/pdf/Leadership_Competencies_for_Healthcare_Services_Managers.pdf.

Jackson, J. 2016. "What Can Technology Do for Global Health?" World Economic Forum. Published February 4. www.weforum.org/agenda/2016/02/how-can-we-leverage-technology-to-bridge-the-global-healthcare-divide/.

Justo, N., N. Wilking, B. Jönsson, S. Luciani, and E. Cazap. 2013. "A Review of Breast Cancer Care and Outcomes in Latin America." *Oncologist* 18 (3): 248–56.

Kamal-Yanni, M. 2015. "Never Again: Building Resilient Health Systems and Learning from the Ebola Crisis." Oxfam. Published April 16. https://policy-practice.oxfam.org.uk/publications/never-again-building-resilient-health-systems-and-learning-from-the-ebola-crisis-550092.

Kappal, R., A. Mehndiratta, P. Anandaraj, and A. Tsanas. 2014. "Current Impact, Future Prospects and Implications of Mobile Healthcare in India." *Central Asian Journal of Global Health* 3 (1): 116.

Knaul, F. M., A. Langer, R. Atun, D. Rodin, J. Frenk, and R. Bonita. 2016. "Rethinking Maternal Health." *Lancet* 4 (4): e227–e228.

Knowlegde@Wharton. 2012. "Can Telemedicine Alleviate India's Health Care Problems?" Wharton School of the University of Pennsylvania. Published March 8. http://knowledge.wharton.upenn.edu/article/can-telemedicine-alleviate-indias-health-care-problems/.

Langer, A., A. Meleis, F. M. Knaul, R. Atun, M. Aran, H. Arreola-Ornelas, Z. A. Bhutta, A. Binagwaho, R. Bonita, J. M. Caglia, M. Claeson, J. Davies, F. A. Donnay, J. M. Gausman, C. Glickman, A. D. Kearns, T. Kendall, R. Lozano, N. Seboni,

G. Sen, S. Sindhu, M. Temin, and J. Frenk. 2015. "Women and Health: The Key for Sustainable Development." *Lancet* 386 (9999): 1165–210.

Levinson, J. 2016. "63 Million Indians Are Pushed into Poverty by Health Expenses Each Year—and Drugs Are the Chief Cause." Center for Disease Dynamics, Economics & Policy. Published June 4. www.cddep.org/blog/posts/63_million_indians_are_pushed_poverty_health_expenses_each_year-and_drugs_are_chief_cause/.

Management Sciences for Health (MSH). 2018. "Managers Who Lead Toolkit—Resources to Support Managers Who Lead." Accessed July 12. www.msh.org/resources/managers-who-lead-toolkit%E2%80%94resources-to-support-managers-who-lead.

MD Anderson. 2015. "MD Anderson Receives Top Chinese Science and Technology Award." Published January 16. www.mdanderson.org/newsroom/2015/01/md-anderson-receives-top-chinese-science-and-technology-award.html.

Meade, A. 2013. "What Is Global Poverty?" Borgen Project. Published August 21. https://borgenproject.org/what-is-poverty/.

Mura, J. B., and S. Holman. 2011. *Program Management Guide*. Partner in Health. Accessed July 12, 2018. www.pih.org/practitioner-resource/pih-program-management-guide.

National Institute for Occupational Safety and Health (NIOSH). 2014. "Violence Occupational Hazards in Hospitals." Updated June 6. www.cdc.gov/niosh/docs/2002-101/default.html.

New York Department of Labor. 2009. *Workplace Violence Prevention Program Guidelines*. Published July 18, 2018. www.labor.ny.gov/workerprotection/safety health/PDFs/PESH/WPV%20Violence%20Prevention%20Guidelines.pdf.

Occupational Safety and Health Administration (OSHA). 2016. *Guidelines for Preventing Workplace Violence for Healthcare and Social Service Workers*. Accessed July 18, 2018. www.osha.gov/Publications/osha3148.pdf.

Partners in Health. 2014. "Saving Mothers and Babies in Haiti." Published April 14. www.pih.org/article/saving-mothers-and-babies-in-haiti.

Patients Beyond Borders. 2017. "Medical Tourism Statistics & Facts." Updated December 14. www.patientsbeyondborders.com/medical-tourism-statistics-facts.

Peters, D. H., A. Garg, G. Bloom, D. G. Walker, W. R. Brieger, and M. H. Rahman. 2008. "Poverty and Access to Health Care in Developing Countries." *Annals of the New York Academy of Sciences* 1136: 161–71.

Phillips, J. P. 2016. "Workplace Violence Against Health Care Workers in the United States." *New England Journal of Medicine* 374: 1661–69.

Raghupathi, W., and V. Raghupathi. 2014. "Big Data Analytics in Healthcare: Promise and Potential." *Health Information Science and Systems* 2: 3.

Rauch, J. 2015. "Disruptive Entrepreneurship Is Transforming US Health Care." Published March. www.brookings.edu/wp-content/uploads/2016/06/rauch.pdf.

Roser, M., and E. Ortiz-Ospina. 2017. "Global Extreme Poverty." Our World in Data. Revised March 27. https://ourworldindata.org/extreme-poverty/.

Seattle Times staff. 2016. "CVS Takes Over Target Pharmacies in Washington, Extending Its Reach." Seattle Times. Published June 17. www.seattletimes.com/business/retail/cvs-takes-over-target-pharmacies-extending-its-reach/.

Shelley, L. 2010. Human Trafficking: A Global Perspective. New York: Cambridge University Press.

Szczerba, R. J. 2014. "Tech Trends Shaping the Future of Medicine, Part 1." Forbes. Published November 23. www.forbes.com/sites/robertszczerba/2014/11/23/tech-trends-shaping-the-future-of-medicine-part-1/#271ab7d580d4.

United Nations (UN). 2018. "Sustainable Development Goals." Accessed July 27. www.un.org/sustainabledevelopment/sustainable-development-goals/.

United Nations (UN) Development Programme. 2018. "Millennium Development Goals." Accessed July 16. www.undp.org/content/undp/en/home/sdgoverview/mdg_goals.html.

United Nations (UN) Office on Drugs and Crime. 2004. United Nations Convention Against Transnational Organized Crime and the Protocols Thereto. Accessed July 18, 2018. www.unodc.org/documents/treaties/UNTOC/Publications/TOC%20Convention/TOCebook-e.pdf.

United Nations (UN) Population Fund. 2015. "Slashing Haiti's Maternal and Infant Death Rates, One Delivery at a Time." Published February 26. www.unfpa.org/news/slashing-haiti%E2%80%99s-maternal-and-infant-death-rates-one-delivery-time.

US Agency for International Development / Maternal and Child Health Integrated Program. 2013. Developing and Strengthening Community Health Worker Programs at Scale: A Reference Guide for Program Managers and Policy Makers. Accessed July 12, 2018. www.mchip.net/sites/default/files/mchipfiles/CHW_ReferenceGuide_sm.pdf.

US Department of Justice. 2018. "Stalking." Updated April 11. www.justice.gov/ovw/stalking#stalking.

Vaidya, A. 2017. "Global Telemedicine Market to Hit $113B+ by 2025: 4 Trends to Note." Becker's Hospital Review. www.beckershospitalreview.com/healthcare-information-technology/global-telemedicine-market-to-hit-113b-by-2025-4-trends-to-note.html.

Van Alstin, C. M. 2016. "Looking Forward: HIT in 2016 and Beyond." Health Management Technology. Published January 19. www.healthmgttech.com/hit-in-2016-and-beyond.

Vitalari, N. P. 2014. "A Prospective Analysis of the Future of the US Healthcare Industry." Center for Digital Transformation White Paper Series. University of California-Irvine, Paul Merge School of Business. Accessed September 19, 2016. http://merage.uci.edu/ResearchAndCenters/CDT/Resources/Documents/N%20Vitalari%20A%20Prospective%20Analysis%20of%20the%20Healthcare%20Industry.pdf.

Wee, S.-L. 2017. "China's Ill, and Wealthy, Look Abroad for Medical Treatment." *New York Times.* Published May 29. www.nytimes.com/2017/05/29/business/china-medical-tourism-hospital.html.

World Bank. 2018a. "GDP per Capita (Current US$): Cuba." Accessed July 26. https://data.worldbank.org/indicator/NY.GDP.PCAP.CD?locations=CU.

———. 2018b. "What Is an 'International Dollar'?" Accessed July 27. https://datahelpdesk.worldbank.org/knowledgebase/articles/114944-what-is-an-international-dollar.

———. 2017. "Understanding Poverty." Accessed September 5, 2017. www.worldbank.org/en/understanding-poverty.

World Bank Group. 2016. *Poverty and Shared Prosperity 2016: Taking on Inequality.* Accessed July 13, 2018. www.worldbank.org/en/publication/poverty-and-shared-prosperity.

World Health Organization (WHO). 2018a. "Breast Cancer: Prevention and Control." Accessed July 25. www.who.int/cancer/detection/breastcancer/en/index1.html.

———. 2018b. "Cervical Cancer." Accessed July 25. www.who.int/cancer/prevention/diagnosis-screening/cervical-cancer/en/.

———. 2018c. "Immunization." Accessed July 17. www.who.int/topics/immunization/en/.

———. 2018d. "WHO Called to Return to the Declaration of Alma-Ata." Accessed July 26. www.who.int/social_determinants/tools/multimedia/alma_ata/en/.

———. 2017. "Poverty." Accessed September 5. www.who.int/topics/poverty/en/.

———. 2010. *Increasing Access to Health Workers in Remote and Rural Areas Through Improved Retention.* Geneva, Switzerland: WHO.

———. 2006a. *Task Shifting: Rational Redistribution of Tasks Among Health Workforce Teams—Global Recommendations and Guidelines.* Geneva, Switzerland: WHO.

———. 2006b. *The World Health Report 2006: Working Together for Health.* Geneva, Switzerland: WHO.

World Health Organization (WHO) Commission on Social Determinants of Health. 2008. *Closing the Gap in a Generation: Health Equity Through Action on the Social Determinants of Health.* Accessed July 9, 2018. www.who.int/social_determinants/thecommission/finalreport/en/.

World Trade Organization (WTO). 2018. "The General Agreement on Trade in Services (GATS): Objectives, Coverage and Disciplines." Accessed July 24. www.wto.org/english/tratop_e/serv_e/gatsqa_e.htm.

Yao, N., J. Wang, Y. Cai, J. Yuan, H. Wang, J. Gong, R. Anderson, and X. Sun. 2016. "Patterns of Cancer Screening, Incidence and Treatment Disparities in China: Protocol for a Population-Based Study." *BMJ Open.* Published August 4. https://bmjopen.bmj.com/content/6/8/e012028.

EPILOGUE

Throughout this book, two central, interrelated themes have been the growing interest in global health issues and the rapidly accelerating globalization of advanced health management practices and education. Both of these trends have been heavily influenced by a commitment, evident throughout the world, to expand healthcare access, improve quality, and control costs; to reform healthcare financing and insurance systems; and to spread new ideas in the practice arena with regard to evidence-based management and performance improvement (e.g., continuous quality improvement, Lean, Six Sigma). The number and variety of academic health management education programs are expanding at a rapid pace, and this text strives to support that growth.

The major goal of this text—the first book of its type ever published—is to inform and advance the disciplines of health management practice and education within and across cultures and societies. The book places a special emphasis on the influence of sociocultural factors on the outcomes of healthcare management practice, and it aims to help faculty from academic health management programs, both domestic and foreign, to effectively incorporate global best practices and evidence-based management instructional methods (e.g., managerial competency development and assessment). To ensure global, diverse perspectives, scholars and practitioners from throughout the world were invited to help prepare the book's chapters, and we are grateful for their contributions and expertise. The book has set out to support and strengthen the core competencies adopted by the International Hospital Federation and the Global Healthcare Management Faculty Forum of the Association of University Programs in Health Administration.

This text was specifically designed to help health management students and/or practitioners to develop a sound background in three interrelated areas of contemporary health management in diverse societies, and these areas correspond with the first three sections into which the book's chapters are organized. The first section—"Essential Health Services Management Concepts and Practices"—provided an overview of the structures and functions of contemporary healthcare organizations, models of healthcare financing and payment, institution-level financial management, human resources concerns, and health management informatics. In the second section—"Leadership, Organizational Design, and Change"—the book's focus shifted to what effective leadership is and how it relates to various factors both within and outside the organization. The section addressed not only basic principles of leadership but also strategic management and marketing, performance/quality improvement, managerial ethics, and the governance of healthcare organizations of various types and in different settings. The third main section of the book—"Managing the Organization–Environment Interface"—expanded the analysis further to include the wide range of issues that arise as an organization attempts to adapt to environmental exigencies. The section addressed health policy design and analysis, changing population demographics, and population health management. A fourth section concluded the book with a look at future trends. The underlying assertion of this text is that managers of healthcare organizations across the globe must continually recognize, clearly understand, and effectively respond to major external threats and challenges.

From a global perspective, healthcare management, policy, and education in the modern era are undergoing a major transformation across all types of systems. This shift is evident in

- the widespread healthcare reform efforts aiming to improve access, costs, and quality;
- the new types of payment systems geared toward understanding and improving health at the population level;
- the significant advances in education and practice in the health professions;
- the continued digital transformation of both clinical and nonclinical functions;
- the focus on how organizations can adopt performance improvement methods to "produce more for less," often aligned with value-based reimbursement;
- the proliferation of health management education and development programs more oriented to the needs of providers; and
- the use of internet-based and blended distance-learning platforms to assist global health management development.

Our goal was to produce the first-ever "academic primer" of essential concepts and methods to support the healthcare leaders who will navigate this global transformation in the years ahead. We hope you have found this text to be both interesting and informative, and we wish you success in incorporating the book's concepts, ideas, and practices into your own healthcare management journey.

Bon voyage!

Michael Counte, PhD
Bernardo Ramirez, MD
Daniel J. West Jr., PhD, FACHE, FACMPE
William Aaronson, PhD

APPENDIX
Body of Knowledge: Global Health Management and Policy

Topic	Description	Subtopics
Healthcare services and systems	**Undergraduate** students should be able to: 1. Describe a basic framework to characterize health services and systems in different countries. 2. Understand how healthcare financing and financial management methods vary across types of healthcare delivery systems. 3. Explain the challenges that developing countries face in meeting the healthcare needs of their populations. 4. Describe how project management could be affected by a country's societal norms and governmental policies. **Graduate** students should **also** be able to: 5. Compare and contrast health services and systems in different countries. 6. Differentiate healthcare challenges in developed versus developing countries. 7. Analyze how the healthcare system in one country can affect the healthcare system in another country. 8. Distinguish between techniques applied for single-country management and those applied for management of international (multiple-country) organizations. 9. Adapt project management techniques to apply in a specific country and to apply in international contexts.	• Hospitals • Clinics • Nongovernmental organizations • Community organizations • Public health • Workforce • Management in low-resource settings
Global burden of disease	**Undergraduate** students should be able to: 1. Describe the prevalence and incidence of major diseases in various countries of the world. 2. Explain how diseases spread globally. **Graduate** students should **also** be able to: 3. Characterize trends in the prevalence and incidence of major health conditions across the globe. 4. Analyze the impact of the spread of contagious disease across the globe on the healthcare delivery systems of respective countries.	• Health determinants • Health disparities • Infectious diseases • Chronic diseases • Longevity and long-term care management
Cultural influences	**Undergraduate** students should be able to: 1. Describe how cultural norms and traditions affect individuals' health behaviors. 2. Describe how cultural norms and traditions affect the way healthcare is organized, financed, and delivered. 3. Demonstrate personal cultural sensitivity. **Graduate** students should **also** be able to: 4. Analyze the impact of cultural norms and traditions on the health behavior of individuals. 5. Evaluate how cultural norms and traditions affect the way healthcare is organized, financed, and delivered. 6. Assess how healthcare organizations manage patients with varying cultural backgrounds. 7. Assess how healthcare organizations manage a workforce of employees from varying cultural backgrounds. 8. Describe challenges to institutional collaboration for organizations based in environments of diverse cultural expectations.	• Cultural competency • Diversity and inclusion • Emotional intelligence • Contextual intelligence

(continued)

485

Topic	Description	Subtopics
Medical tourism	**Undergraduate** students should be able to: 1. Define *medical tourism*. 2. List challenges faced by countries and international facilities seeking to be medical tourism destinations. **Graduate** students should **also** be able to: 3. Analyze the pros and cons of becoming a medical tourism destination.	• Continuity of care • Local equity • Populations and health professional migration
Communications and marketing	**Undergraduate** students should be able to: 1. Describe the challenges of caring for patients or populations who speak different languages. 2. Describe management techniques for resolving language differences between patients and providers. 3. Explain principles for marketing and developing materials for multiple-language target audiences. **Graduate** students should **also** be able to: 4. Develop a marketing plan that communicates effectively with stakeholders of diverse languages and cultures. 5. Apply communications tools to effectively reach audiences with diverse cultures and languages.	• Managerial epidemiology • Social marketing • Social media
Data and measurement	**Undergraduate** students should be able to: 1. Identify tools, techniques, and metrics for measuring community health status in various countries. 2. List challenges to accurate data collection within and across countries. 3. Describe how measures of quality might differ from one country to another. **Graduate** students should **also** be able to: 4. Apply valid data and metrics to compare community health status in various countries. 5. Explain the challenges to accurate data collection within and across countries. 6. Evaluate the impact of a healthcare program on one or more nations using appropriate data and metrics. 7. Relate expectations of quality to healthcare system and cultural differences across countries.	• Measures of health status, access, utilization, safety, and quality • Sources of reliable data • Development of appropriate scorecards for decision making • Healthcare informatics • Clinical decision support systems • Electronic health and medical records • Evidence-based management
Policy and regulatory environments	**Undergraduates** should be able to: 1. Explain how government policies affect the healthcare delivery system. 2. Identify variations in policies and regulations imposed by national governments that result in differences in healthcare delivery across various countries.	• Population health • Social security • Public–private partnerships • Nonprofit and for-profit healthcare • Social empowerment

(continued)

Topic	Description	Subtopics
Policy and regulatory environments *(continued)*	**Graduate** students should **also** be able to: 3. Analyze laws and government regulations to assess their impact on the healthcare delivery system and health status of the population. 4. Describe how to negotiate collaboration and change in another country. 5. Differentiate the roles of government ministries, private corporations, and international stakeholders as they relate to the health and healthcare delivery system of a country.	
Global leadership	**Undergraduates** should be able to: 1. Explain why global health is relevant to health and healthcare in the United States. 2. Contribute to global health initiatives at a local level. 3. Describe how management practices that are standard in the United States might vary in implementation in other countries. **Graduate** students should **also** be able to: 4. Demonstrate the applicability of ethical principles in a context of international management. 5. Construct an effective approach to bringing organizations and individuals together to collaborate on activities or policies related to health status or healthcare systems on a global or multinational level. 6. Adjust management operations to match the societal and governmental norms of a particular country.	• Entrepreneurship • Innovation • Mindfulness • Governance
International best practices	**Undergraduates** should be able to: 1. Identify proven healthcare management models and practices from international healthcare settings. **Graduate** students should **also** be able to: 2. Apply proven healthcare management models and practices from international settings to healthcare settings in other countries, including the United States.	• Value-based management • Finance/accounting • Cross-cultural management • Health supply chain • Human resources management • Quality improvement • Accreditation

GLOSSARY

active life expectancy (ALE): The portion of total life expectancy during which an individual is not affected by disability; also called *disability-free life expectancy.*

activities of daily living (ADLs): Routine and fundamental life activities, such as eating, bathing, and dressing.

aged society: A society in which people aged 65 years or older make up 14 to 21 percent of the population.

aggravated assault: Assault involving weapons or serious injury.

aging in place: The practice of remaining in one's own home and community during old age.

aging society: A society in which people aged 65 years or older make up 7 to 14 percent of the total population.

allocative or redistributive policies: Policies that determine the way public goods or resources are shared.

andragogy: The principles and practices of adult education.

assisted living facility: A facility in which staff help residents with activities of daily living and work to ensure residents' health and well-being.

balanced scorecard: A strategic planning tool that places key metrics on a dashboard to aid with the measurement and assessment of performance.

benchmarking: The process of measuring the performance of an organization against a standard (benchmark).

best in class: The highest current performance level in a field, often used as a benchmark to be equaled or exceeded.

best-of-breed (BoB) approach: An approach to electronic health record (EHR) architecture that involves building or buying the best available option for each component of the EHR while adhering to standards that allow interoperability.

best practice: A method or activity that has been shown to generate superior results.

big data: Huge collections of information that can be mined from various sources.

bioethics: The field of ethical study related to biological or medical practices.

bioterrorism: The deliberate release of viruses, bacteria, or other germs to cause illness or death in people, animals, or plants.

breakeven point: The point at which total revenues equal total expenses.

capability: The abilities reflected in the breadth of a role, usually expressed in strategic, tactical, operational, and transactional terminologies.

capacity: The amount and variety of work that a workforce can accomplish.

capital access: An organization's ability to obtain investment capital through various sources, such as debt and equity.

capital budgeting: The strategic planning process used to evaluate and execute an organization's long-term investments.

capital market depth: The overall level of investment capital collectively made available by investors to organizations for the purpose of strategic investments.

capital project analysis: A formal process that involves the assessment of all the costs and benefits of a potential investment that is large enough to significantly expand the scale or scope of the organization.

capital rationing: The process by which potential projects compete for a limited pool of investment capital.

capital structure: The policy for how a firm finances its overall operations and growth, using debt or equity.

capitation: The payment of a fixed amount for a predefined set of services for a predefined population for a specific period.

cash concentration system: A system for combining funds from separate accounts into a single account for more efficient management.

cash management: The set of procedures associated with monitoring, controlling, and allocating a firm's cash.

chronic health condition: A condition that lasts three months or longer and affects an individual's health or independence.

clinical support system: An information technology system that uses patient information to help guide clinical decision making.

closed colony: A state in which everyone in a community is vaccinated, and no new people come in or out.

cloud computing: Computing through remote servers that provide resources on demand via the internet.

co-design: An approach that seeks the active involvement of all stakeholders (e.g., employees, partners, customers, citizens, end users) in the design process.

commercial paper: Debt issued by firms and sold to investors.

community health needs assessment (CHNA): A comprehensive process for examining the health problems of a population, identifying inequalities, and determining priorities to guide the use of resources.

community health worker (CHW): A worker who provides education and preventive care at homes and in villages away from the hospital.

competence: The knowledge, skills, and attitudes that people possess; what people know and do.

computerized provider order entry (CPOE): An application that allows providers to enter patient orders via a computer system.

connected health (cHealth): A technology-enabled approach to integrated care delivery, with an emphasis on remote monitoring, diagnosis, treatment, and communication.

consequentialism: An ethical theory in which an action is determined to be ethical or unethical based on its consequences.

contingency theory: A leadership theory that focuses on the influence of situational variables (relating to leaders, followers, and the situation) on leadership behavior.

contingent loss: A financial loss that occurs if an adverse health event occurs.

continuing care retirement community (CCRC): A model for long-term care in which a comprehensive range of nursing and housing options are available within a single community and services can be modified as individuals age and their needs change.

continuous manufacturing: A manufacturing process by which pharmaceuticals can be produced in a continuous, efficient process in a single facility, minimizing delays associated with previous methods.

continuum of care: The comprehensive array of health services across all settings, specialties, and levels of intensity.

critical reflection: The practice of identifying and assessing the underlying assumptions and values that influence one's performance.

cultural imperialism: The practice of imposing a society's own culture and morality on people of another society.

cultural proficiency: The ability to relate to and work effectively with members of diverse cultures.

data governance: Efforts to protect data integrity and foster accurate data exchange.

data integrity: The completeness, accuracy, consistency, and timeliness of data.

deontology: An approach to ethics based on moral reasoning, rules, and obligation.

derivative: A financial asset (such as a stock option or a forward/future contract) whose market value is derived from the value of an underlying asset (such as a stock or commodity).

design thinking: A problem-solving discipline that takes a human-centric approach to service innovation and improvement, with the customer/user experience at its core.

determinant: A factor that determines or contributes to an outcome.

diagnosis-related group (DRG): A category of patients whose diagnoses share certain common properties.

digital fabrication: A technology for making small batches of medicines that previously had been considered too costly and impractical to produce.

direct care worker: An individual in the health workforce who provides care and personal assistance to individuals who are frail, sick, or injured or who have physical or mental disabilities.

direct channel: A distribution model in which services are provided directly to consumers by the producer.

directional strategies: The mission, vision, and values that provide the basis for an organization's goals and objectives and guide the organization's strategies.

disability: A physical, sensory, cognitive, or intellectual impairment, or type of chronic disease, that limits a person's ability to function in a given social context.

discounted payback period: A metric that indicates the length of time needed for a project to break even, taking into consideration the buying power of future cash inflows when adjusted for the time value of money.

disruptive innovation: A new development that transforms an existing market or field by introducing new, inexpensive, and straightforward ways of doing things.

DMAIC cycle: A Six Sigma improvement cycle that consists of five phases: define, measure, analyze, improve, and control.

e-health: The use of electronic methods to deliver health-related information and services; often written as *eHealth*.

electronic health record (EHR): A digital version of a patient's records from healthcare providers.

electronic medical record (EMR): A digital record containing the standard medical and clinical data gathered for a patient in a particular provider's office.

emotional intelligence (EI): The capacity for recognizing, understanding, and managing emotions in oneself and in one's relationships.

epidemiology: The scientific discipline dealing with the distribution and determinants of disease and other health-related events in a population.

exclusive distribution: A distribution model in which a product is only available through one outlet or very few outlets.

expected medical cost: A measure calculated by multiplying the health status risk for an individual by the medical care risk.

facility design: The design of the space in which a business's activities take place. The planning and layout of that space have a significant impact on the flow of work, materials, and information through the system.

factoring receivables: An arrangement whereby a lender, at a discount, buys receivables that are owed to another company and then collects the receivables.

fee-for-service (FFS): A payment model in which providers are paid on a per-occurrence basis.

filial piety: A cultural norm, prevalent in much of Asia, emphasizing that younger family members are expected to take care of their elders.

fiscal space: The flexibility of a government in determining where to spend revenue.

flow: A key Lean principle referring to the movement of products or services through the value stream without waits or delays.

forward contract: A type of contract that can "lock in" an exchange rate for a future date to protect against exchange rate fluctuations.

global budget: The payment of a fixed amount to provide for the healthcare needs of a population for a fixed period of time (typically one year).

global health policy: The complex web of rules, both formal and informal, that police vested interests in the attainment of the highest level of health possible for all people.

globalization: Interconnectedness and interdependency across people and cultures, stemming from increased transportation, distribution, communication, and economic activity across international boundaries.

groupthink: A condition in which the group weakens its decision making by inappropriately reaching consensus without considering alternative approaches or assumptions.

health-adjusted life expectancy (HALE): A measure of life expectancy adjusted for the severity of an individual's disability.

healthcare system: The arrangement of people, institutions, and resources that deliver healthcare services to meet the needs of a target population. The system's framework aligns resources to support the key performance domains of access, utilization, efficiency, quality, sustainability, and learning.

health demography: The statistical study of vital events such as fertility, morbidity, mortality, and disability.

health economics: A field of economics that addresses health services consumption and efficiency, as well as the financial arrangements that influence the delivery of healthcare services.

health informatics (HI): The application of information and computer science to all levels and settings of healthcare, including health-related research.

health information and communication technologies (HICT): The professional area dealing with the technological aspects of health information and systems.

health information governance (IG): The professional area dealing with health information as a strategic asset requiring high-level oversight.

health information management (HIM): The professional area dealing with the acquisition, analysis, and protection of health information.

health psychology: A field of psychology that examines behavioral factors, such as attitude, perception, motivation, and preference, as they relate to health.

health registry: A collection of disease-, condition-, or procedure-specific information about individuals.

health status risk: The probability that a member of a target population will need or seek care; also called *population health risk.*

health system financing: The process of collecting, allocating, and distributing revenues to cover health services for a designated population.

health technology assessment (HTA): The systematic evaluation of health technology and its properties, effects, and impacts; a multidisciplinary process for evaluating social, economic, organizational, and ethical issues related to health technology.

healthy life years (HLYs): The estimated number of years an individual will live without disability-related limitations on daily activities.

hedging: The purchasing of a financial investment for the purpose of reducing the risk of adverse price movements in another asset.

herd immunity: A state in which most of a community is vaccinated against a disease, making the disease unlikely to spread throughout the group.

hierarchy of needs: A model, introduced by Abraham Maslow, stating that people are motivated by several levels of needs, with physiological needs at the most basic level and self-actualization at the top level.

high-deductible health plan (HDHP): A variant of private insurance and out-of-pocket systems that covers "catastrophic" services, is often paired with a health savings account, and has high deductibles or copayments.

home and community-based services: Health-related services and assistance that are provided in the home and community in which an individual is already living.

human ecology: The study of human adaptation and lifestyles in varying geo-spatial settings.

human trafficking: The trade of human beings for such purposes as forced labor or sexual exploitation.

hyper-aged society: A society in which people aged 65 years or older make up more than 21 percent of the population.

inputs: The tangible and intangible resources needed to carry out a process or provide a service (e.g., people, expertise, materials, energy, facilities, funds).

instrumental activities of daily living (IADLs): Life activities—such as cleaning, shopping, and managing finances—that enable people to live independently.

intensive distribution: A distribution model in which a product is available in as many outlets as possible.

internal rate of return (IRR): A metric representing the percentage rate that a project earns over the course of its life.

internet of things: The vast network of everyday objects and devices connected via the internet.

interoperability: The ability of systems and devices to exchange and interpret data.

jidoka: The ability, in Lean production, to stop a production process immediately when a problem arises so that defects will not be passed on from one step to the next.

job analysis: The process of evaluating the activities of a job, the requirements of the position, and ways the work can best be performed within the organization.

job design: The process of defining the specific tasks, methods, and responsibilities of a given job or position.

joint venture: A business enterprise developed and co-owned by two or more parties, which otherwise retain their own distinct identities.

just culture: An organization approach that emphasizes truth, integrity, and responsibility rather than blame.

just-in-time (JIT) production: The delivery of the supplies, equipment, and information needed for a production process at the time they are needed and in the right quantity.

kaizen event: A short-term improvement event, or rapid process improvement workshop, aimed at improving a specific process; a key tool of Lean.

kanban: A Lean production tool that uses signs or signals to automatically control the movement of inventory.

Keynesian economics: A school of economics, named after John Maynard Keynes, that maintains that active government involvement to influence demand (primarily) can lead to optimal economic performance.

key success factors (KSFs): A series of factors considered critical for an organization's ability to meet client and customer needs and wants and to achieve sustainability (not for profit) or competitive advantage (for profit).

laissez-faire economics: A school of economics that maintains that government involvement in the economy creates market frictions and interference that detract from optimal economic performance.

leadership: The ability to use influence to motivate individuals in an organization to accomplish a particular goal.

league table: A performance table that compares results of similar organizations.

Lean: A quality improvement methodology, evolved from the Toyota Production System in Japan, that emphasizes the elimination of waste and unnecessary steps.

Lean Six Sigma (LSS): A combined approach in which elements of Lean and Six Sigma are implemented concurrently.

licensing/franchising: A type of agreement in which one organization contracts with another to use its name and business model, normally in exchange for a fee or percentage of profits.

loading factors: The overhead costs incurred while administering to the insured population.

long-term services and supports: Care, services, and assistance provided across various settings to help people address difficulties in performing their activities of daily living.

management by exception: A managerial approach that focuses attention and analysis on items where performance is significantly different from what was planned in the budget.

management by objectives (MBO): A management approach in which clear and measurable objectives are used to guide and assess performance.

managerial ethics: The area of study focused on ethical issues and concerns related to managerial responsibilities.

managerial rounding: A practice in which a manager visits employees at their workstations on a weekly basis to provide feedback, discuss work-related issues, and address employee concerns.

marketing: The aspect of strategy that deals with communication, promotion, and distribution of the ideas, products, or services that are key to the strategy.

marketing integration: The practice of tying together the various elements of an organization's promotional mix.

market research: The process of identifying the information needs for successful market planning, identifying sources of data, collecting the data, and then analyzing and acting on the data.

market segmentation: The process of using the information gathered about a market to divide it into identifiable, actionable subgroups.

market sizing: A step in the market research process that aims to assess the total potential need of a community.

mark-up pricing: A pricing method in which the cost of producing a good or service is computed and grossed up by an amount to allow for additional fixed costs and to add a margin.

meaningful use: Use of certified electronic health record technology in a meaningful manner, consistent with government guidelines.

means-tested: Having eligibility criteria based on income or financial need.

medical care risk: The cost of providing care in the event that an individual seeks an intervention.

medical home: A care approach in which a primary care physician works with other specialists and providers to enable coordinated access to services when and where they are needed.

medical sociology: A field of study dealing with social and environmental factors that influence the health of a population.

medical tourism: The traveling of individuals from one country to another for the purpose of receiving medical treatment.

memory care unit: A unit in a nursing home that focuses specifically on dementia care.

mission statement: A statement of an organization's reason for existing, intended to inspire employees and provide direction and alignment toward a common goal.

mobile health (mHealth): The delivery of health-related services via mobile electronic devices.

monolithic approach: An approach to electronic health record architecture in which all the aspects and components are provided through a single vendor.

moral relativism: The tendency to consider morality relative to one's own society, potentially leading to assumptions that the ethical beliefs of people in another society are appropriate for them without question.

national health insurance: A healthcare delivery model in which providers are independent from the government but receive payment from a government-run insurance plan into which everyone is required to pay.

neoliberal economic policies: Economic policies that favor free-market capitalism with minimal government intervention.

net present value (NPV): A metric that represents the overall dollar value of a project to the organization, considering all cash flows over the life of the project.

operations management: The managerial function of creating and delivering an organization's products or services.

organizational culture: A pattern of beliefs, values, standards, and assumptions that is shared by members of an organization and contributes to a sense of belonging.

outputs: The goods, services, or outcomes produced by a system.

parity pricing: A pricing strategy that involves setting prices as close as possible to those of competitors.

path–goal theory: A leadership theory that focuses on the use of contingent rewards to influence followers.

patient journey map: A visual representation of a patient's journey through a set of clinical services.

payback period: A metric that indicates the length of time needed for a project to break even by bringing in sufficient funding to pay back the initial investment.

pay for performance (P4P): A payment model in which a fixed payment approach is paired with performance and quality incentives; sometimes called *value-based contracting* or *purchasing*.

penetration pricing: A pricing strategy that involves setting a low price with the goal of quickly gaining market share.

performance dashboard: A display of key indicators across various areas to show progress toward goals and to support effective governance.

personal health record (PHR): A web or computer application that patients use to maintain and manage their health information in a private, secure, and confidential environment.

plan-do-check-act (PDCA): A quality-improvement approach in which changes are developed, implemented, tested, and refined in repeated cycles; sometimes written as *plan-do-study-act (PDSA)*.

plasticity: A workforce planning approach that loosens the traditional confines of professional disciplines and enables communities to use existing healthcare workers more efficiently.

point-of-care (POC) healthcare technology: Technology that focuses on improving the capability for healthcare to be delivered where the patient is, with an emphasis on remote monitoring, diagnosis, treatment, and communication for personalized care.

policy: A rule, whether formal or informal, written or unwritten.

policy analysis: The act of examining rules, the problems the rules are meant to address, the goals of the rules, and the criteria used to evaluate the efficacy of the rules.

policymaking: The process of creating the rules of policy.

pooling: The accumulation of health revenues on behalf of a defined population for eventual transfer to providers; pooling mitigates risks by grouping individuals together to share current or future medical expenses.

population aging: A global demographic shift whereby older adults are making up an increasing proportion of the overall population.

population health management (PHM): The use of management strategies to improve the health and well-being of a defined population, to improve quality, to reduce costs, and to improve workforce productivity.

population health science: An interdisciplinary specialty area that integrates elements of human genetics, epidemiology, biostatistics, behavioral science, public health, policy science, medical geography, and health informatics.

poverty line: A measurement of the monetary value of people's consumption, used to determine the number of people living in poverty.

prearchitectural medical functional program: A planning document that serves as a road map for the design of a facility; it identifies functional program areas and defines such aspects as users, operational scenarios, design criteria, and square footage needed.

precision medicine: An emerging approach for disease prevention and treatment that takes into account individual variability in genes, environment, and lifestyle.

preventive medicine: The area of medicine dealing with preventive strategies and interventions for the promotion of community and population health.

principlism: An ethical approach based on four basic principles of bioethics: (1) beneficence, (2) nonmaleficence, (3) autonomy, and (4) justice.

process design: The discipline focused on the set of processes, actions, and steps to produce a product or service that delivers particular results for the customer.

process mapping: A tool for examining the activities involved in the delivery of a service and the ways those activities are managed.

process redesign: The task of modifying an existing process to achieve incremental improvement.

product portfolio: The full line of products offered by an organization.

professionalism: The ability to maintain high professional standards and ethics and to draw on the technical and practical skills appropriate for professional scenarios.

prospective payment system (PPS): A payment model in which providers are paid a predetermined, fixed amount to provide services to a population.

public–private partnership: A strategic arrangement in which a private organization partners with a government or government-controlled entity to share financial risk.

pull: A key Lean principle requiring that the production process be triggered only by customer demand.

regionalization: A broad organizational concept with a variety of applications; its key aims include efficient use of limited and expensive health resources, the provision of accessible health services to a defined population, and the development of standards for health services provision.

regulatory policies: Policies that are designed to affect the behavior or actions of others through rules that dictate what can and cannot be done.

request for information (RFI): A process for gathering information across a broad range of vendors.

request for proposal (RFP): A document in which a potential purchaser invites a vendor to present a proposal tailored to specific project requirements.

request for quote (RFQ): A process wherein a potential purchaser invites a vendor to submit a bid (typically, the upfront cost plus any ongoing expenses), allowing for a comparison of bids across vendors.

resilience: The ability to withstand or rebound from adversity, to overcome difficult circumstances, and to add new capabilities and opportunities.

retained earnings: Earnings not paid out to an organization's owners but rather retained by the organization to be reinvested in business operations.

revenue cycle: The time frame between the delivery of care and the receipt of payment.

risk aversion: A tendency to reduce uncertainty; in healthcare, this uncertainty is primarily associated with adverse medical events and the associated financial costs.

search engine marketing (SEM): A form of advertising in which an organization pays for prominent placement on internet search engine pages.

search engine optimization (SEO): The practice of carefully using words on an organization's website to ensure that the site will appear high on the list of search results for a particular product or category.

selective distribution: A distribution model in which a product is available only through select outlets.

sensei: A master teacher in the Lean improvement methodology.

servant leadership: Leadership that is sensitive and responsive to followers' needs.

service blueprint: An operational planning tool that provides guidance on how a service will be provided, taking into account physical environment, staff actions, support systems, and infrastructure.

service design: An emerging field concerned with the design of services and ways to improve and innovate services through the application of established design processes and skills.

simple assault: Assault that does not involve weapons or serious injury.

situational leadership: An approach based on the idea that the most effective leadership style depends on the situation and the person being influenced.

Six Sigma: A quality improvement methodology, developed at the Motorola corporation in the 1980s, that emphasizes the elimination of variation and error.

skilled nursing facility: A facility that provides medical, nursing, or rehabilitation services on a residential basis.

skill mix: The combination of skills available in an organization.

skimming: A pricing strategy that involves setting a high price, often because of intellectual property protections, lack of competitors, or a desire to establish a sense of "prestige" around an organization or product.

SMART governance: Governance that is stakeholder (S) engaged, is mission (M) driven, is accountable (A) to beneficiaries and resource providers, mobilizes resources (R) to support the mission, and demonstrates transparency (T) in all plans and decision making aimed at accomplishing the mission.

SMART objectives: Objectives that are specific, measurable, attainable, realistic, and time framed.

social and managerial epidemiology: A field of study that examines the patterns and trends of morbidity and mortality associated with social factors and health services.

social determinants of health (SDOH): Factors found in living and working conditions that influence the health of a population; such factors are distinct from individual characteristics and behaviors.

social gradient in health: The link, evident throughout the world, between socioeconomic status and health.

social insurance: A healthcare delivery model in which a benefits package is funded through employment-related taxes; the healthcare infrastructure in such systems can be owned by either the government or private industry.

staff mix: The number, qualifications, and experience of people on staff.

stalking: Following, spying, or making unwanted contact with a specific person in a manner that is likely to cause fear or emotional distress.

strategic management process: The ongoing process by which an organization assesses the environment in which it operates, appraises its current direction and market position, determines the most appropriate strategic direction moving forward, and develops and implements goals, objectives, and action plans to accomplish the strategy.

strategy: The art of devising and implementing plans toward the achievement of short-term or long-term goals and objectives.

structural adjustment policy: A program in which a developing country receives a loan that is tied to its adoption of certain market-oriented adjustments or reforms.

supply chain management: The management of interface relationships in the value system.

sustainability: The capacity for a healthcare organization to function efficiently and in a manner that supports effective service both presently and in the future.

SWOT analysis: An analysis of strengths, weaknesses, opportunities, and threats.

targeting: The process of prioritizing market segments and deciding which to pursue first.

target return pricing: A pricing method in which the organization computes costs and projected volumes and then prices the service or good such that a targeted margin or return on investment is achieved.

task shifting: The redistribution of tasks among workforce teams.

telehealth: The use of technology to deliver health-related services and support remotely.

terms of reference (TOR): Documents used to define the scope of responsibilities for leaders, boards, and organizations.

total quality management (TQM): A management approach that seeks to establish continuous, organized quality-improvement activities and to involve everyone in the organization in an integrated effort to improve performance at every level; also known as *continuous quality improvement (CQI)* or *continuous process improvement (CPI)*.

transfer pricing: Establishing the price at which one unit of an organization transfers a good to another unit of the organization.

transformational leadership: Leadership that focuses on efforts to produce positive change in individuals and systems.

transparency: The degree to which a country's reporting standards lead to full disclosure.

triple aim: An approach for optimizing healthcare services by working to (1) improve the health of populations, (2) improve the patient care experience, and (3) reduce the per capita costs of healthcare; advanced by the Institute for Healthcare Improvement.

triple bottom line: A theory that emphasizes an organization's need to monitor and evaluate results in three areas: profit, people, and planet (sustainability).

underwriting methodology: The process of pooling individuals together and calculating the expected medical costs; it requires prediction of both health status risk and medical care risk for the population.

universal coverage: A healthcare delivery model that is financed through general tax revenue and covers all citizens; also called the Beveridge model.

utilitarian ethics: A theory based on the idea that the most ethical action is the one that produces the maximum good for the greatest number.

utility: The representation of the satisfaction experienced by consumers of goods and services; the higher the satisfaction, the greater the associated utility.

value: In competitive terms, the amount that clients (buyers) are willing to pay for what an organization provides them; in not-for-profit terms, the nonmonetary benefit received by clients, constituents, or users.

value-based healthcare: An approach to healthcare that aims to minimize spending while improving quality and patient safety.

value-based payment (VBP): An approach in which prospective payments to providers are adjusted based on performance on a set of quality indicators; value-based systems aim to reward quality of care rather than quantity of care.

value chain: The sequence of internal and external organizational activities that together create a product or service to meet clients' needs and wants.

value pricing: The practice of setting the price for a good or service based on buyers' perceived value.

values statement: A statement that functions as a sort of moral compass and describes how an organization intends to carry out its work.

value system: The set of internal and external value chain relationships that work together to create products or services.

variance analysis: A form of analysis in which the manager compares actual revenue and resource use with standards that were developed as part of the budget process.

vision: A statement that defines what an organization seeks to become and depicts an ideal future in which the organization has fulfilled its mission and strategic goals.

web portal: A basic website on which all the materials needed for a work function are stored.

white paper: A comprehensive yet concise report that summarizes a position on a complex and often controversial or difficult issue; it aims to increase stakeholders' understanding of the issue to support the development of policy.

working capital management: The area of management concerned with the short-term assets and liabilities used in the day-to-day operations of a firm.

INDEX

Note: Italicized page locators refer to figures or tables in exhibits.

workforce capacity and, 95; health workforce in countries with, 456; in Japan, 404; shift toward value-based healthcare and, 423; in Sweden, 407; in Turkey, 411; in United States, 413. *See also* Long-term care services and supports

Aging societies: definition of, 397

AHIMA. *See* American Health Information Management Association

AHRQ. *See* Agency for Healthcare Research and Quality

AIHA. *See* American International Health Alliance

AIIMS. *See* All India Institute of Medical Sciences

Airtel, 462

ALE. *See* Active life expectancy

All India Institute of Medical Sciences (AIIMS): directional statement of, *220*

Allocative or redistributive policies, 378, 384

Allscripts, 135

Alma-Ata Declaration of 1978, 9–10, 471

Almshouses, 413

Alzheimer's disease, 399, 400, 413, 427, 429, 466

Alzheimer's Disease International, 400

AMA. *See* American Marketing Association

Ambient assistive technology, 416

American College of Healthcare Executives (ACHE): code of ethics, 194, 301; competency assessment tool, 188

American College of Pediatricians, 386

American Health Information Management Association (AHIMA), 126

American Hospital Association: Center for Healthcare Governance, 369n9

American International Health Alliance (AIHA), 191;

community-based primary care proposals, 437

American Marketing Association (AMA), 225

Andragogy: definition of, 192

Annual budget cycle, 62–63, *63*

Ansoff, Igor, 226

Ansoff matrix, 244; market strategy and, 226–27, *227*

Apollo Group Hospitals (India): partnership with Johns Hopkins Medicine International, 466

Appreciative inquiry, 349, 369n15

Aramark Charitable Fund, 180

Aravind Eye Care Systems (India): design thinking approach and, 265

Area Agencies on Aging (AAAs), 415

Argentina: income inequality in, 474

Aristotle, 315, 316

Artificial hip: identifying problems with, 438

Ascension Health, 73; directional statement of, *222*

ASEAN. *See* Association of Southeast Asian Nations

Asia: bond markets in, 74; equity market depth in, 76; fast-track aging in, 427; growth of older population in, 397; long-term services in, 399; telemedicine technology use in, 462. *See also* China; India

Aspirin, 239

Assault: simple and aggravated, 453

Assisted living facilities: definition of, 414

Association of Southeast Asian Nations (ASEAN), 380

Association of University Programs in Health Administration (AUPHA), 6; Global Healthcare Management Faculty Forum, xx, 188, *189*, 193, 483; HIMSTA curriculum guidelines, 126–27

Athena Health, 135

Attribute-based encryption (ABE), 148

facing, 13; organizational responsibilities of, 301; professional arena for, 377; professionalization of, 12; revenue cycle and, 58; successful, characteristics of, 110; workplace violence issues and, 453. *See also* Leaders; Leadership

Healthcare organizations: directional statements of, 217–23; most important functions of, 5–6; operational quality improvement models in, *287*; strategic planning for, 198. *See also* Financial management of healthcare organizations

Healthcare services: demand for, 214; life cycle of, 234

Healthcare settings: reasons for failures in, 173

Healthcare systems: definition of, 6; main functions of, 6; sociocultural perspectives in researching (case study), 100–103

Healthcare units: management of physical resources in, 14–15, *15*; planning process for construction of, 16–17

Healthcare workforce: autonomy of, 96; migration of, 95; mobility of, 95; nonprofessional, 458; planning methods for, 458; positive engagement of, 191; shortages in, 457, 459; task shifting and, 458, 459

Health City Cayman Islands, 73

Health committee, 325

Health demography, 424, 433

Health determinants: integrative approach to, 430

Health economics: definition of, 424, 425

Healthfore, 462

Health Foundation (UK), 269

Health Gap, The (Marmot), 181

Health inequities: social determinants of health and, 432

Health informatics (HI): definition of, 125; IMIA competency-based model of, 126

Health informatics research: optimizing population health through, 433–35

Health information and communication technologies (HICT): definition of, 126

Health information exchange: EHR standards, data exchange, and, 133–34

Health information governance (IG): definition of, 126

Health information management (HIM): definition of, 126

Health Information Management Systems Technology and Analysis (HIMSTA): modules within curriculum, 126–27, 130

Health information professions: academic programs in, 126

Health information technology (HIT), 123, 152, 448; advances in, 426; effective application of, 141; long-term care and, 403

Health Information Technology for Economic and Clinical Health (HITECH) Act, 132

Health insurance: mechanics of, *44*, 44–46

Health Insurance Portability and Accountability Act (HIPAA), 146; PCI DSS rules linked with standards of, 148; standards and implementation specifications, *144–45*

Health Level Seven (HL7) International, 133, 134

Health literacy, 448

Health management education: in Slovakia, 181

Health Management School (Bratislava), 181, 191

Health neocolonialism, 313

development, 185–88, *186, 187*; motivation and, 169–70; nurse, 197–98; organizational culture and, 173; organizational strategy, effective communication, and, 214; performance and effectiveness of, 183–84; physician, 197; professionalism and, 171, 193–94; research, science, and, 179–82; self-understanding and, 183; servant, 185; strategic planning and, 198; styles and types of, 181, 185; transformational, 185; triple aim and, 191; values and spirituality in, 195–96; work design and, 196–97
"Leadership Challenge" (Kouzes and Posner), 182
Leadership competence: developing, 171–72
Leadership Competencies for Healthcare Services Managers (IHF Global Consortium), 106–7
Leadership development: components of, 172
League tables, 276, 290
Lean, 275, 286, 483; definition of, 279; in health organizations and systems, *287*; jidoka in, 280, 283; just-in-time production and, 280, 283–84; kaizen improvement events, 280, 283; kanban system in, 284; primary goal in, 283; principles of, 280; Six Sigma compared with, *285*; waste reduction and, 280, 283
Lean Six Sigma (LSS), 284
Learning: basic model of, 185, *186*; as core performance domain, 6, 7, 8; lifelong, 183, 188
Least developed countries (LDCs), xx
"Leftover medicine," 308–9
Legacy cost-plus system, 60
Lending interest rates: across countries with varying levels of economic development, 75, *75*
Licensing/franchising agreement: definition of, 72

LICs. *See* Low-income countries
Life expectancy: extension of, 427
Lifelong learning, 183, 188
Lines of credit, 82
Lithuania: healthy life years in, 399
LMICs. *See* Lower middle-income countries
Loading factors, 39, 46
Local community leaders: good governing bodies and, 324
Locally based providers: cooperation with, 314
Locke, John, 314, 316
Longevity: increasing, 397. *See also* Aging population
Long-term care services and supports: aging population and, 397–98; in China, 409–11; chronic health conditions and, 398–99; definition of, 397; demographic and cultural forces affecting demand and supply of, 397–400; informal caregiving, 401; in Japan, 404, 406; mandatory insurance programs and, 403; mixed systems for, 404; public spending on, *398*; supply issues affecting, 399–400; in Sweden, 407–8; technology and, 402–3; in Turkey, 412–13; in United States, 414–15; universal coverage systems for, 403; workforce challenges in, 401–2, 416
Losses: in fee-for-service model, *47*; in prospective payment system, 48, *48*
Lower middle-income countries (LMICs), xx, 177, 468
Low-income countries (LICs), xx, 177
Low performers, 113, 114, *115*, 117
LSS. *See* Lean Six Sigma
LUX MED, 73

MacArthur Foundation, 176
MACRA. *See* Medicare Access and CHIP Reauthorization Act
Maintenance: equipment, 21–22; of facilities, 20–21; of public areas, 21

ABOUT THE EDITORS

Michael Counte, PhD, is a professor of health management and the director of the International Center for Advances in Health Systems Management in the Department of Health Management and Policy at the Saint Louis University College for Public Health and Social Justice. He has been on the department's faculty since 1994. Previously, from 1975 to 1994, he served as the assistant chairman of the Department of Health Systems Management and as the associate director of the Center for Health Management Studies within Rush-Presbyterian-St. Luke's Medical Center in Chicago. Dr. Counte was also a cofounder of the Rush Center for Research on Health and Aging.

Since completing his graduate work in organizational behavior and health services research at the University of Illinois at Urbana-Champaign, Dr. Counte has been extensively involved in the design of multidisciplinary programs that address public health, medical practice, and health services management. His primary research interests include the multidimensional assessment of hospital performance; the diffusion and impact of large-scale organizational change (especially the implementation of comprehensive management information systems and quality management initiatives); and the effects of healthcare policy changes, such as value-based payment initiatives and managed care programs, on affected populations, particularly older adults. Presently, Dr. Counte is continuing his domestic and global efforts to support the diffusion of performance improvement–oriented, competency-based academic health management education programs and targeted health management development programs for clinicians in management roles.

Dr. Counte has served as a research and healthcare management development consultant to numerous organizations and agencies in the United States, including the National Institute of Nursing Research, the National Institute on Aging, the National Institute on Drug Abuse, the Agency for Healthcare Policy and Research, the US Agency for International Development (USAID), the Department of Veterans Affairs, the Centers for Disease Control and Prevention, and the National Cancer Institute. He has also contributed to major healthcare management practice and educational improvement initiatives in Europe, China, and Taiwan. Dr. Counte has coauthored several professional texts and more than 60 refereed research articles and chapters.

Bernardo Ramirez, MD, is the director of global health initiatives for the Department of Health Management and Informatics at the University of Central Florida (UCF) in Orlando. An associate professor at UCF, he teaches courses on the US health system, international health systems, issues and trends in the health professions, quality improvement, leadership and organizational behavior, and strategic planning in the graduate and undergraduate online and residential programs. Dr. Ramirez is actively engaged in the promotion of global healthcare management education, efforts to address health disparities, and diversity and cultural competency. He has extensive experience in distance education, learning outcomes measurement, and global learning techniques. He has designed and provided instruction through massive online open courses (MOOCs), virtual study abroad programs, and other innovative and engaging learning methodologies. He also conducts research and serves as an adviser for graduate and doctoral students at UCF and other universities in the United States and around the world.

Dr. Ramirez received his MD and MBA degrees from the National Autonomous University of Mexico (UNAM). After beginning his medical career as a general surgeon, he took on a number of positions as a health services administrator in public and private organizations, ranging from clinical and administrative practice at the hospital departmental level to health system reform, planning, and policy at the national level. He has provided technical assistance, research, and training under the auspices of USAID, the Pan American Health Organization, the International Hospital Federation (IHF), the World Bank, the Inter-American Development Bank, and the W. K. Kellogg Foundation, serving for 40 years in more than 60 countries across five continents.

Dr. Ramirez has served as director of the master's program in hospital and health services management at the business school at UNAM, as the general director of health standards for the Ministry of Health of Mexico, and as the president of the Mexican Hospital Association. For 15 years, he was the vice president and director of international programs at the Association of University Programs in Health Administration (AUPHA), and during the last six years he served on AUPHA's board of directors. He is currently a member of the Candidacy Committee and the Global Advisory Council of the Commission on Accreditation of Healthcare Management Education (CAHME), and he serves as the lead facilitator of the IHF Project to Develop Collaboration with Academia of the Special Interest Group in Health Management. Dr. Ramirez is the author of numerous publications, the creator of a variety of training materials, and a presenter in many national and international forums. He has served as a Rotarian and as a board member for the Celebration Foundation and the Florida Hospital Foundation's SHARES International.

Daniel J. West Jr., PhD, FACHE, FACMPE, is chairman and professor in the Department of Health Administration and Human Resources at the University of Scranton in Pennsylvania. He teaches in the Graduate School, specializing in global health management, international accreditation, and healthcare leadership. Dr. West is an adjunct faculty member in the Department of Medicine at the Geisinger Commonwealth Medical College in Scranton, and he also holds professorships at two universities in Slovakia—Trnava University and St. Elizabeth University. In 2007, he received an honorary doctorate of public health from St. Elizabeth University for his international leadership. Dr. West is the president and CEO of HTC Consulting Group, Inc.

Dr. West is a dedicated and hardworking teacher, consultant, and scholar with more than 45 years of healthcare management, advisory, and leadership experience. He received his master's and doctoral degrees from the Pennsylvania State University and has achieved success and recognition through international healthcare projects in such areas as Central Europe, Haiti, Slovakia, Mexico, Brazil, and Georgia. He is recognized as an International Fellow at the University of Scranton and is codirector and cofounder of the Center for Global Health and Rehabilitation. Each year, Dr. West conducts study-abroad tours for graduate health administration students to countries in Central and Eastern Europe and Central and South America. He is board certified in healthcare management by the American College of Healthcare Executives (ACHE).

Dr. West has been CEO for a hospital, a medical practice, and several other healthcare businesses. He maintains fellowship with ACHE, the American College of Medical Practice Executives, the American College of Health Care Administrators, and the Healthcare Financial Management Association. He serves on the board of directors for the Eastern Pennsylvania Healthcare Executive Network (a chapter of ACHE) and the ACHE Regents Advisory Council, and he was recently appointed to the board of trustees of Moses Taylor Hospital, an affiliate of Commonwealth Health. He was chairman of CAHME's board of directors for two years and currently serves on CAHME's Executive Committee, Membership Committee, Strategic Issues Committee, and Governance Committee.

Dr. West has authored more than 300 articles about various aspects of health services administration and leadership. He serves on a number of editorial committees and has delivered more than 575 presentations at regional, national, and international conferences. Current research efforts focus on international accreditation, global health management education partnerships, and public–private partnerships.

William Aaronson, PhD, is associate professor and founding chair of the Department of Health Services Administration and Policy in the College of

Public Health at Temple University in Philadelphia. He previously served as associate dean for graduate programs and assistant dean for research and doctoral programs at Temple's Fox School of Business. Known for his strategic outlook, innovative approaches to curriculum management, and collaborative leadership style, Dr. Aaronson has successfully led the restructuring of doctoral and master's programs at Temple. In his current role, he is applying his experience and skills to the strategic management of his department, with a focus on curriculum revision and the development of new programs.

Dr. Aaronson is a recognized leader in healthcare management education who has served as program director and department chair for CAHME-accredited programs. He has worked in long-term care management, been a consultant to hospitals and long-term care organizations, and served on boards of directors for long-term and primary care organizations. He has also provided consulting services to academic units engaged in curriculum development. Dr. Aaronson has extensively researched the relationship between health policy and healthcare organizational efficiency, quality, and strategy. His work has appeared in top-tier research journals such as *Health Economics*, *Medical Care Research and Review*, *Medical Care*, *Health Services Research*, the *Gerontologist*, the *Journal of Health Politics, Policy and Law*; and the *Journal of Healthcare Management*.

Dr. Aaronson has considerable international experience, having delivered executive training programs for health system leaders and conducted collaborative research with local faculty in numerous countries. He has particular expertise in the health systems, history, culture, languages, and educational systems of Central Europe and the former Soviet Union. He was the recipient of a J. William Fulbright Senior Teaching Scholarship at the University of Matej Bel, Slovakia. An AUPHA International Faculty Fellow, Dr. Aaronson led a five-year, $1.4 million project—funded by USAID and managed by the American International Health Alliance—in which a coalition of Philadelphia-based healthcare providers partnered with the City Health Administration of Kiev, Ukraine, to develop a system of community-based primary healthcare clinics and the infrastructure to support it.

Dr. Aaronson is active in numerous professional and academic organizations. He is currently the chair of AUPHA's Global Healthcare Management Faculty Forum, and he has served on accreditation teams for CAHME, the Pennsylvania Department of Education, the New England Association of Schools and Colleges, and the United Arab Emirates Ministry of Education.

ABOUT THE CONTRIBUTORS

Irene Agyepong, MBChB, DrPH, FGCPS, is a public health physician in the Research and Development Directorate of the Ghana Health Service and a Foundation Fellow of the Ghana College of Physicians and Surgeons (Public Health Faculty). She leads the health policy, management, and leadership sub-specialty track in the public health membership and fellowship training programs of the college. She is an honorary professor in the Division of Health Systems and Policy at the School of Public Health and Family Medicine, University of Cape Town.

Fevzi Akinci, PhD, is dean of the John G. Rangos Sr. School of Health Services at Duquesne University in Pittsburgh, Pennsylvania. Dr. Akinci's current research interests include the burden of disease and chronic care management research, access and utilization studies, and comparative international studies.

Eduardo Álvarez-Falcón, MPhil, is CEO and founding partner of Proxture Ltd. (www.proxture.com), a software-based start-up company that was established in the United States and currently has headquarters in London. He has more than 15 years of experience in senior leadership positions and strategy consultancy, addressing large-scale and complex change management projects (health reforms) and the development of balanced scorecards in various sectors. He has experience working with a variety of teams; public and private organizations; and international clients, partners, stakeholders, and political environments. He has been active in live and distance strategy consulting, training, and education efforts in Latin America, the United States, Canada, Nigeria, Germany, the United Kingdom, and Romania. He concluded his MPhil and MSc studies at Imperial College London Business School, in health policy and health management respectively, in relation to the balanced scorecard implementation at the English National Health Service. He also holds an MBA, a diploma in total quality management, and a degree in medicine from ITAM and La Salle universities in Mexico.

Ellen Averett, PhD, MHSA, is a professor in the Department of Health Policy and Management and the director of the master of health services administration (MHSA) degree program at the University of Kansas School of Medicine. She earned her PhD in clinical psychology from Duke University and her MHSA from the University of Kansas. She is past president of the Kansas Public Health Association and serves on the American Public Health Association's Science Board.

Robert Babela is a professor of public health who teaches at the St. Elizabeth University in Slovakia. He currently serves as the head of the Institute for Healthcare Disciplines and lectures in the field of health administration, healthcare management, and pharmacoeconomics / health technology assessment.

Suzanne Babich, DrPH, is associate dean of global health and professor of health policy and management at the Richard M. Fairbanks School of Public Health at Indiana University in Indianapolis. There, she directs the doctoral program in global health leadership. Dr. Babich works across the school and campus—and around the world—to advance teaching, research, and service in public and global health. She has a special interest in interdisciplinary education and applications of technology for innovative approaches to programming. A champion of public universities, she believes that excellence in local public health requires a global perspective.

Afsan Bhadelia, PhD, is a visiting scientist within the Global Health Systems Cluster in the Department of Global Health and Population at Harvard's T. H. Chan School of Public Health, where she conducts health systems analysis on chronic diseases, particularly cancer. She also manages the *Lancet* Commission on Global Access to Pain Control and Palliative Care and co-coordinates the Commission's Scientific Advisory Committee. She earned her PhD in the health systems program in the Department of International Health at the Johns Hopkins School of Public Health, with a focus on bioethics and health economics. Between 2009 and 2015, she held various research roles at the Harvard Global Equity Initiative, including research director and research associate. She previously coordinated the Global Task Force on Expanded Access to Cancer Care and Control.

David Briggs, PhD, DrPH honoris causa, FCHSM, FHKCHSE, is an adjunct professor in health management at Naresuan University in Thailand and at the University of New England in Australia. He is a Fellow of the Australasian College of Health Service Management, a Foundation Fellow of the Hong Kong College of Health Service Executives, and editor for the *Asia Pacific Journal of Health Management*.

Kevin D. Broom, PhD, is an associate professor of health policy and management in the Graduate School of Public Health at the University of Pittsburgh.

He is also the director of the master of health administration program. He holds a PhD in business administration (finance) from the University of Mississippi and an MBA from Syracuse University. Dr. Broom also has more than 20 years of practice experience as a health administrator and hospital chief financial officer within the US Army Medical Department.

Walter Cintra Ferreira Jr., MD, PhD, is the associate dean of the specialization course in hospital and healthcare systems administration at the Getúlio Vargas Foundation Business School in São Paulo, Brazil. He has served as a director of public and private hospitals and as a public manager in the state and municipal health secretariats of São Paulo. He has teaching experience in postgraduate courses in public health, with an emphasis on healthcare services administration. He received a degree in medicine from the University of São Paulo and an MBA and a PhD in business administration from the Getúlio Vargas Foundation.

Min Cole is a PhD candidate in applied gerontology and a consultant, operator, educator, and researcher specializing in long-term services and supports. She is the founder of Quality of Life Group and Cole Global Care Management, and she has developed, operated, and promoted person-directed care research in Adult Day Health Care and Program of All-Inclusive Care for the Elderly projects in Southern California. She is a member of the California Department of Aging Quality Advisory Committee and an adjunct professor, mentor, recruiter, and researcher at the University of La Verne.

Ariel Cortés, MD, PhD, is an associate professor of health management in the Business Department at the Pontificia Universidad Javeriana in Colombia. He holds a PhD in epidemiology and public health from the Universidad Rey Juan Carlos, a health MBA from the Universitat Pompeu Fabra, an MSc in economics from the Pontificia Universidad Javeriana, an MD from the Universidad Nacional de Colombia, and a degree in public administration from the Escuela Superior de Administracion Publica. Dr. Cortés also has more than 20 years of practice experience as a health administrator and hospital chief financial officer in various organizations in Colombia.

Michael M. Costello, JD, is a member of the full-time faculty in the Department of Health Administration and Human Resources at the University of Scranton in Pennsylvania. He has more than 30 years' experience as an executive in a large regional healthcare system that included two acute care hospitals and a 65-physician group practice. His academic interests are in the areas of health law, healthcare ethics, long-term care administration, health economics, and the delivery of health services.

Serif Esendemir, PhD, received his BA and MS degrees from the Middle East Technical University in Ankara, Turkey, and his doctorate from the applied gerontology PhD program at the University of North Texas. The first applied gerontologist of Turkey, Dr. Esendemir is an assistant professor at Yildiz Technical University in the Faculty of Arts and Sciences in the Department of Humanities and Social Sciences. He is also a member of the Administrative Council of the Darulaceze Presidency, under the Ministry of Family and Social Policies.

Gary L. Filerman, PhD, the president of the Atlas Health Foundation, has been engaged in global health administration and system development for 50 years. His work with the Association of University Programs in Health Administration, the World Health Organization, the United States Agency for International Development (USAID), the International Finance Corporation, Joint Commission International, and the World Bank has taken him to more than 40 countries. His degrees from the University of Minnesota include an MA in Latin American government.

Myron Fottler, PhD, is professor emeritus of healthcare management and former director of health services management programs at the University of Central Florida (UCF). He earned his PhD in business from Columbia University and has published more than 25 books and 150 journal articles during his career at the State University of New York at Buffalo, the University of Alabama, the University of Alabama at Birmingham (UAB), and UCF. He has also been active in the Academy of Management Healthcare Management Division, the Association of University Programs in Health Administration, and the Southern Management Association. Over the course of his career, he has mentored 60 doctoral students at UAB and UCF. He was one of the founding editors of the annual book series *Advances in Health Care Management*, which publishes cutting-edge empirical and theoretical papers. Since his retirement, he has served on several nonprofit boards of directors on the east coast of Central Florida.

Bruce J. Fried, PhD, is associate professor in the Department of Health Policy and Management at the University of North Carolina at Chapel Hill. His research and teaching span the areas of human resources management, quality improvement, managerial epidemiology, the healthcare workforce, international and comparative health systems, and globalization and health. He has coauthored several books, including *Fundamentals of Human Resources in Healthcare* (Health Administration Press, 2018), *Human Resources in Healthcare: Managing for Success* (2015), and *World Health Systems: Challenges and Perspectives* (2012). Dr. Fried received his master's degree from the University of Chicago and his PhD in health administration from the University of North Carolina at Chapel Hill.

Leonard H. Friedman, PhD, FACHE, is a professor of health policy and management and director of the executive master of health administration degree at the George Washington University. He earned his PhD from the University of Southern California School of Public Administration, where his dissertation examined technology acquisition in hospitals in Southern California. Dr. Friedman has been the chair of the healthcare management division of the Academy of Management and the Association of University Programs in Health Administration. He is a Fellow of the American College of Healthcare Executives (ACHE) and is the past president of the National Capital Healthcare Executives Chapter of ACHE.

Mark Gaynor, PhD, is a professor of health management and policy at the College for Public Health and Social Justice at Saint Louis University. Mark's PhD in computer science is from Harvard University. His research interests include distributed sensor networks for medical applications, innovation with distributed architecture, healthcare information technology (HIT), design of network-based healthcare services, interoperability of HIT systems, and emergency medical services. His first book was *Network Services Investment Guide: Maximizing ROI in Uncertain Times* (Wiley, 2003). His current teaching areas include health operations management, health information systems, security and privacy of healthcare information, and Green Belt Six Sigma for healthcare.

Blair Gifford, PhD, is a professor of global health management in the MBA/health programs in the Business School at the University of Colorado at Denver. He also is the founder of the Center for Global Health at the University of Colorado and served as the center's first director. He is currently involved in global health research projects in China, Haiti, and Kenya. Dr. Gifford was recognized as a New Century Fellow by the US Department of State (Fulbright) in 2008. He has a BA degree in economics from the University of California at Santa Cruz and MA and PhD degrees in sociology from the University of Chicago. He has had visiting professor positions at Tsinghua University (Beijing), Yale University, and Northwestern University.

Eva Grey, MD, PhD, is a professor at St. Elizabeth University of Health and Social Work in Bratislava, Slovakia. She has conducted research in bioethics, social work ethics, and palliative care and has participated at conferences in Warsaw, Florence, Vienna, Hamburg, Paris, and Chicago. She was a national delegate at the Fourth World Conference on Women in Beijing.

Shivani Gupta, PhD, is an assistant professor in the College of Nursing and Health Professions at the University of Southern Mississippi (USM). She holds an MBA from USM and a PhD in administration–health services, with a concentration in strategic management, from the University of Alabama at Birmingham. Her research has dealt primarily with strategies employed by healthcare organizations in response to the changes in their environment. She has focused specifically on issues related to the healthcare workforce and organizational structure, and their association with organizational performance; the use of large secondary data sets to address staffing challenges; and improving patients' transitions between acute and post-acute care or community settings.

Steven W. Howard, PhD, is an assistant professor in the Department of Health Management and Policy at Saint Louis University. He has an MBA from the University of Oregon and a PhD in public health, with a concentration in health management and policy, from Oregon State University. His organizational-level work has included economic and outcomes research on unique care models at children's hospitals. At the state level, his work has included analysis of the development of the Coordinated Care Organization health reform model being implemented by the state of Oregon. Dr. Howard's current federal-level research program involves study of the relationships between the market penetration of the Medicare Advantage program and changes in the chronic disease burden at the population level.

Antonio Hurtado, MD, is a medical doctor who earned a graduate healthcare executive management certificate from the School of Public Health in Mexico and Harvard University. He is currently the medical and quality management director for IGSA Medical Services, a health management and construction company with several hospitals operating in Mexico. He has more than 40 years of national and international experience as a consultant, faculty member, and field expert in the planning, design, construction, and operation of public and private hospitals.

Godfrey Isouard, PhD, is director of health management programs in the Faculty of Medicine and Health at the University of New England, Australia. Dr. Isouard is also national vice president of the Australasian College of Health Service Management and former president of the Society for Health Administration Programs in Education.

Bo Jordin, MD, has worked as a specialist in family medicine at Karolinska Institute in Stockholm, Sweden; as a senior medical officer in Stockholm County; as director of primary care for the National Board of Health and Welfare; and as a board member of the European Health Telematics Association. He holds a master of public health degree from the University of Stockholm.

Felicia Knaul, PhD, is a professor at the Miller School of Medicine and director of the Institute for Advanced Study of the Americas at the University of

Miami. She is also senior economist at the Mexican Health Foundation. Knaul received her BA in international development from the University of Toronto and her MA and PhD in economics from Harvard University.

Gilbert Kokwaro, PhD, is director and professor of health systems research at Strathmore University in Kenya. He holds a PhD in pharmacokinetics from the University of Wales. His current research interest is health systems strengthening in developing countries.

Vladimir Krcmery, MD, PhD, ScD, FRCP, received his PhD in infectious diseases at Comenius and his ScD at Bratislava. He has been a lecturer in Brno, Munich, Boston, Nairobi, Bangkok, Phnom Penh, and Taipei. He has served at Trnava University School of Public Health as department chair and dean and at St. Elizabeth University as president and chair of the global health and tropical diseases program. He is a Fellow of the Royal College of Physicians, Edinburgh, and of the American College of Physicians. He holds honorary degrees from the universities of Scranton, Warsaw, Varna, Krasnodar, Cambridge, and Budweis.

Zhanming Liang, PhD, FCHSM, is senior lecturer at La Trobe University, Australia, and the president of the Society for Health Administration Programs in Education. She has spent the past decade researching and teaching in the areas of management competency, healthcare quality, and program planning and evaluation. Prior to becoming an academic, she worked in such roles as medical practitioner, planning and evaluation consultant, and senior manager.

Xinliang Liu, PhD, is an assistant professor in the Department of Health Management and Informatics at the University of Central Florida. His research focuses on health services utilization, costs, quality of care, and performance evaluation of healthcare organizations. His teaching interests include healthcare research methods, healthcare operations management, and healthcare quality management. Dr. Liu received an MD-equivalent degree from China and a PhD degree in health services research from Virginia Commonwealth University.

Ana Maria Malik, MD, PhD, full professor at Escola de Administração de Empresas de São Paulo (São Paulo Business School), Fundação Getúlio Vargas (Getúlio Vargas Foundation), in Brazil. She is a former director of public and private hospitals in Brazil and health coordinator of the São Paulo metropolitan region.

Mariepi Manolis Cylwik is a University of Cambridge graduate and a senior clinician in the United Kingdom, where she has 15 years' experience working in the National Health Service. She is completing an MPhil in service design at the Royal College of Art, London, and has unique experience in the design, delivery, and management of health service projects, both within the United Kingdom and abroad. Her chief interest lies in healthcare innovation strategy—more specifically, the design of health systems and service platforms that redefine the future of the healthcare experience. She is a visiting lecturer and tutor at the Imperial Medical School.

Egil Marstein, PhD, is an adjunct associate professor who has spent most of his academic career teaching master's and doctoral students in public health management and comparative public health systems. His research and publications focus on health policy reforms and global health governance, with special attention to the influence of actor agents of transnational health initiatives, such as intergovernmental institutions, nongovernmental organization, and philanthropic and charitable organizations, as well as public–private partnerships. Marstein is a guest lecturer at universities in both the United States and Europe.

Maysoun Dimachkie Masri, ScD, is a health system financing analyst advising the Division of Health System Financing at the Department of Health in Abu Dhabi, United Arab Emirates, about new healthcare financing initiatives and projects. She holds a doctorate of science in health systems management from Tulane University, in addition to an MBA in healthcare management. She also has an MPH in health services administration from the American University of Beirut, Lebanon. Previously, Dr. Masri was an assistant professor teaching healthcare finance and economics at the Department of Health Management and Informatics at the University of Central Florida. Prior to entering academia, Dr. Masri worked as a consultant in the insurance industry and as a director of a not-for-profit hospital.

Mary Helen McSweeney-Feld, PhD, is an associate professor in the healthcare management program in the College of Health Professions at Towson University, in Towson, Maryland. She is a licensed nursing home administrator and Fellow of the American College of Healthcare Administrators. Dr. McSweeney-Feld has been involved in local and national grant and demonstration programs focusing on such areas as long-term care direct care workers, Alzheimer's disease and dementia, and emergency preparedness for long-term care communities. She is the lead editor of *Dimensions of Long-Term Care Management: An Introduction*, second edition (Health Administration Press, 2017), and has written extensively about long-term care administration issues for a variety of publications. She is a member of the Programming Committee of the Maryland Chapter of ACHE.

Carol Molinari, PhD, is a professor in the health systems management program at the University of Baltimore, where she teaches undergraduate and graduate courses. Her areas of research include diversity management, cultural competence, and governance for acute and long-term healthcare facilities. She has authored several chapters and coedited a textbook related to long-term care management in the United States and other countries. Dr. Molinari has a PhD in health policy and management from the Johns Hopkins School of Hygiene and Public Health, an MBA from the University of Baltimore, and an MPH from the University of North Carolina at Chapel Hill.

Alice Noblin, PhD, RHIA, CCS, is an associate professor and director of the health informatics and information management undergraduate program at the University of Central Florida. Her research interests include electronic health records, patient engagement in health information technology, and health literacy. She received her PhD in public affairs from UCF.

Egbe Osifo-Dawodu, MD, is a partner at the Anadach Group, a global healthcare strategic firm that focuses on bringing innovative advice and services to clients and partners in the public and private sectors. Dr. Osifo-Dawodu has more than 30 years' experience in healthcare policy, care provision, and financing in Africa, Asia, Europe, Latin America, and the United States. She holds an MBA from Cranfield School of Management, an MSc from Oxford University, and an MBBS from the University of Ibadan. She is also a member of the United Kingdom's Royal College of Physicians.

Xiaomei Pei, PhD, is a professor of sociology at Tsinghua University in China who specializes in studies of health and aging in contexts of social change. She received her doctoral degree from the University of North Texas and has been executive director of the Tsinghua University Gerontology Center for the past decade.

Anatoliy Pilyavskyy, PhD, is the chair of the Department of Mathematics and Quantitative Methods at the Lviv University of Trade and Economics, Ukraine. He has more than 43 years of research and teaching experience and has authored three books and more than 100 scientific and educational articles in Ukrainian, Russian, and English. In 1996, Dr. Pilyavskyy received a USAID funded International Research and Exchanges Board scholarship at Temple University to study healthcare organization and finance. His areas of research include mathematical methods in economics and the efficiency and effectiveness of medical institutions in Ukraine. He is a member of the International Association of Health Economics.

Benjamin K. Poku, DrPH, has 20 years of experience in healthcare. He is currently teaching healthcare-related courses in Abu Dhabi, United Arab Emirates. His passion is global health management and policy.

Cherie L. Ramirez, PhD, is a lecturer in biochemistry and the inaugural Center for Excellence in Teaching Science, Technology, Engineering, and Mathematics Faculty Fellow in the Chemistry and Physics Department at the College of Arts and Sciences of Simmons College. She earned her PhD in genetics at Harvard University and completed her postdoctoral training at Harvard's T. H. Chan School of Public Health. Dr. Ramirez has held appointments at the Harvard Global Health Institute and the Global Health Education and Learning Incubator at Harvard, where she led faculty, graduate, and postdoctorate professional development activities related to global health teaching. Her current research interests include improving access to medicines and promoting healthy workplaces. She has worked in Mexico, South Africa, and Turkey and has presented papers on the topic of public–private healthcare partnerships at several international conferences.

James A. Rice, PhD, FACHE, has more than 35 years of experience in the US health sector and has also worked in more than 30 countries to strengthen their health financing, management, and governance systems. At Gallagher Integrated, he is responsible for helping clients enhance the effectiveness of their governance strategies and structures, as well as enabling physician leaders to engage in modern leadership and governance processes. Dr. Rice was a senior officer actively involved in building the Allina Health system in Minnesota. He also managed a large health system reform program in Russia in the mid-1990s and recently led a $200 million USAID project to strengthen the leadership and governance of health systems in Asia, Africa, and Latin America. He holds faculty positions at the business school of Strathmore University in Nairobi, Kenya; the Judge Business School at Cambridge University in England; and the School of Public Health of the University of Minnesota.

Martin Rusnák, MD, PhD, is full professor of public health at the University of Trnava, Slovakia. He is a physician with professional interests in public health, health services quality, healthcare systems research, informatics and statistics, project management, and healthcare information systems. His scientific interests focus on the effectiveness of healthcare systems, treatment outcomes for severe traumatic brain injuries, and the health of minorities and population groups facing complicated economic and social conditions. As a full professor of public health, he teaches public health policy, epidemiology, and statistics of healthcare.

Viera Rusnáková, MD, PhD, MBA, is full professor of public health at the University of Trnava, Slovakia. She first completed specialization study in medical informatics and neurology and then dedicated her professional career to healthcare and public health informatics, as well as quality of healthcare and public health. She obtained a PhD from the Slovak Academy of Sciences and an MBA from the University of Leeds in the United Kingdom. She teaches informatics, biostatistics, and management for students of public health.

Godfrey Gwaze Sikipa, MD, is the founder and CEO of Compre Health Services, a private health consulting and service delivery company registered in Zimbabwe and based in the city of Harare. He is also chairman of the Hospital Management Board of the Parirenyatwa Group of Hospitals, the largest hospital group in Zimbabwe. Dr. Sikipa worked in Zimbabwe's Ministry of Health for 17 years, starting as a junior hospital clinician and rising through the ranks to the position of permanent secretary of the ministry. Internationally, he has worked for the Joint United Nations Programme on HIV/AIDS and several health consulting companies, including Family Health International, RTI International, and Management Sciences for Health. He has provided technical assistance for projects in a number of countries, including Kenya, South Africa, Uganda, Namibia, Nigeria, Zambia, and Zimbabwe. He is a current member of the Technical Evaluation Reference Group of the Governing Board of the Geneva-based Global Fund to fight AIDS, Tuberculosis, and Malaria.

Steven J. Szydlowski, DHA, holds a full-time faculty position in the Department of Health Administration and Human Resources at the University of Scranton in Pennsylvania. He also is director of the graduate health administration program. Dr. Szydlowski received a doctoral degree in health administration and leadership from the Medical University of South Carolina. He also earned two master's degrees. Dr. Szydlowski's work has been published in peer-reviewed journals, and he has presented at more than 100 national and international conferences. He also serves as a journal editor. Dr. Szydlowski has affiliated faculty appointments at St. Elizabeth University and Trnava University in Slovakia and at Tbilisi State Medical University and the University of Georgia, in the Republic of Georgia.

Jason S. Turner, PhD, is an associate professor of health service management at the University of Cincinnati College of Medicine. He holds a PhD in health services organization and policy (finance cognate), as well as an MA in applied economics, from the University of Michigan. Prior to entering academia, Dr. Turner spent time in the health sector as a hospital and insurance executive.

Steven G. Ullmann, PhD, is professor and chair of the Department of Health Sector Management and Policy and director of the Center for Health Management and Policy at the University of Miami. He holds a bachelor's degree in economics from the University of California, Berkeley, and has master's and PhD degrees in economics from the University of Michigan, Ann Arbor.

Thomas T. H. Wan, PhD, is a professor of public affairs, health management and informatics, and medical education at the University of Central Florida. He is also an associate dean for research for the College of Health and Public Affairs. Dr. Wan has taught at Cornell, Maryland, and Virginia Commonwealth University. He received an MA in sociology/criminology and a PhD in sociology/demography from the University of Georgia. He completed his postdoctoral fellowship and earned his MHS degree from the Johns Hopkins University School of Public Health. His engagement in health services management research and consultation has helped the development of formal MHA graduate programs in Kazakhstan, the Czech Republic, and Taiwan.

David Wyant, PhD, is an assistant professor of management in the Jack C. Massey College of Business at Belmont University in Nashville, Tennessee. He holds a PhD in health services research policy and administration (finance) from the University of Minnesota and an MBA (finance) and MA in economics (international trade) from the Ohio State University. Dr. Wyant began his career in healthcare in 1977 as staff economist for the Ohio Nursing Home Commission of the Ohio Legislature. Since that time, he has held positions with healthcare providers, in healthcare policy, and as a university faculty member in healthcare management. He also worked for three years in banking.

Francisco Yepes, MD, DrPH, is professor of public health and health administration in the Institute of Public Health at the Pontificia Universidad Javeriana in Bogotá, Colombia. He holds a DrPH and an MSc in health administration from Harvard University and an MPH from Antioquia University. Dr. Yepes also has served as secretary general of the Ministry of Health, vice president of the Social Security Institute, and as an international consultant in health services.

Feliciano (Pele) Yu Jr., MD, MSHI, MSPH, is a pediatrician with expertise in health informatics and health services research. He is the chief medical information officer at Arkansas Children's Hospital and professor of pediatrics and biomedical informatics at the University of Arkansas for Medical Sciences College of Medicine. Dr. Yu's primary focus lies in the intersection of health informatics, outcomes research, and quality of care.